Targeted Cancer Immune Therapy

Joseph Lustgarten • Yan Cui • Shulin Li
Editors

Targeted Cancer Immune Therapy

Springer

Editors
Joseph Lustgarten
Mayo Clinic Scottsdale Arizona
Cancer Center Scottsdale
13400 East Shea Boulevard
Scottsdale, AZ 85259
USA
lustgarten.joseph@mayo.edu

Yan Cui
Gene Therapy Program
Louisiana State University
Health Sciences Center
533 Bolivar Street, CSRB 601F
New Orleans, LA 70112
USA
ycui@lsuhsc.edu

Shulin Li
Department of Comparative Biomedical Sciences
Louisiana State University
Skip Bertman Drive
Baton Rouge, LA 70803
sli@vetmed.lsu.edu

ISBN 978-1-4419-0169-9 e-ISBN 978-1-4419-0170-5
DOI 10.1007/978-1-4419-0170-5
Springer Dordrecht Heidelberg London New York

Library of Congress Control Number: 2009926174

Printed on acid-free paper

Springer is part of Springer Science+Business Media (www.springer.com)

Preface

Stimulation of the immune system's ability to control and destroy tumors continues to be the goal of cancer immune therapy; but the scope has rapidly expanded; approaches are constantly updated; new molecules are continually introduced; and immune mechanisms are becoming better understood. This book has no intention of covering every aspect of immune therapy but rather focuses on the novelty of cancer immune therapy in an attempt to give readers an opportunity to absorb the new aspects of immune therapy from a single source. In this regard, three areas were selected: cytokine immune therapy, cell-based immune therapy, and targeted immune therapy. In each of these three sections, only the novel aspects of immune therapy were described instead of attempting to cover any historical achievement. In the first section, Cytokine Immune Therapy, the IL12 family, IL18, IL21, IL24, IL28, and IL29 were emphasized in regard to the antitumor function and application in treating tumors. Most of these selected cytokines were discovered in last 10 years. In the second section, Cell-based Immune Therapy, the focus was engineering potent immune regulatory or effector cells such as dendritic cells, T cells, and stem cells. Cell engineering design is primarily based on the increased understanding of the interaction of tumor antigen-presenting cells, antigen- specific effector cells, and the tumor microenvironment. Rapidly evolving stem cell research presents us with additional promising measures to incorporate engineered stem cells in order to augment the immune function of T cells and DCs for long-term therapeutic efficacy. In the third section, Targeted Immune Therapy, the focus was rearticulating the antibody therapy for boosting immune response, which includes immunocytokines, "T-body," and tumor targeted CpG ODN. Immunocytokines represent a new class of biopharmaceuticals composed of two well known immune components–antibodies and cytokines – with the unique ability to target cytokines to the tumor microenvironment and thereby activate antitumor responses. The "T-body" approach uses the antitumor antibodies and the efficient tissue rejection of T- cells for adoptive cancer therapy. Tumor-targeted CpG ODN targets Toll-like receptors within the tumor using hybrid molecules of antibody conjugated CpG-ODN for the induction of antitumor responses. Some or all of these innovative approaches may ultimately become effective future immune therapies for treating malignancy.

Scottsdale, AZ Joseph Lustgarten
New Orleans, LA Yan Cui
Baton Houge, LA Shulin LI

Contents

Contributors

Sita Aggarwal William Hansel Cancer Prevention Laboratory, Pennington Biomedical Research Center, Louisiana State University System, Baton Rouge, LA, USA

Wesley M. Burnside Gene Therapy Program, Louisiana State University Health Sciences Center, New Orleans, LA, USA

Lisa H. Butterfield Department of Medicine, University of Pittsburgh Cancer Institute, Pittsburgh, PA, USA
Department of Surgery and Immunology, University of Pittsburgh, Pittsburgh, PA, USA

Chintana Chirathaworn Faculty of Medicine, Center of Excellence in Clinical Virology, Chulalongkorn University, Bangkok, Thailand

Yan Cui Gene Therapy Program, Stanley S. Scott Cancer Center, Louisiana State University Health Sciences Center, New Orleans, LA, USA

Jeffry Cutrera Department of Comparative Biomedical Sciences, School of Veterinary Medicine, Louisiana State University, Baton Rouge, LA, USA

Eduardo Davila Department of Pediatrics and the Stanley S. Scott Cancer Center, Louisiana State University Health Sciences Center, New Orleans, LA, USA

Ian D. Davis Ludwig-Austin Joint Medical Oncology Unit, Austin Health, Melbourne, Australia

Denada Dibra Department of Comparative Biomedical Sciences, Louisiana State University, Baton Rouge, LA, USA

Haidong Dong Departments of Urology and Immunology, College of Medicine, Mayo Clinic, Rochester, MN, USA

Maria Adelaida Duque Cancer Center Scottsdale, Mayo Clinic Arizona, Scottsdale, AZ, USA

Zelig Eshhar Department of Immunology, The Weizmann Institute of Science, Rehovot, Israel

Dinorah Friedmann-Morvinski Laboratory of Genetics, The Salk Institute for Biological Studies, La Jolla, CA, USA
Department of Immunology, The Weizmann Institute of Science, Rehovot, Israel

Stephen D. Gillies Provenance Biopharmaceuticals Corp., Waltham, MA, USA

William Hansel William Hansel Cancer Prevention Laboratory, Pennington Biomedical Research Center, Louisiana State University System, Baton Rouge, LA, USA

Dominique Hoelzinger Cancer Center Scottsdale, Mayo Clinic Arizona, Scottsdale, AZ, USA

Naomi Hunder ZymoGenetics, Seattle, WA, USA

Chien-Fu Hung Department of Pathology, Johns Hopkins School of Medicine, Baltimore, MD, USA
Department of Oncology, Johns Hopkins School of Medicine, Baltimore, MD, USA

Jessica B. Katz Lankenau Institute for Medical Research and Division of Hematology/Oncology, Department of Medicine, Lankenau Hospital, Philadelphia, PA, USA

Shulin Li Department of Comparative Biomedical Sciences, Louisiana State University, Baton Rouge, LA, USA

Joseph Lustgarten Cancer Center Scottsdale, Mayo Clinic Arizona, Scottsdale, AZ, USA

Noweeda Mirza Cancer Center Scottsdale, Mayo Clinic Arizona, Scottsdale, AZ, USA

Archana Monie Department of Pathology, Johns Hopkins School of Medicine, Baltimore, MD, USA

Alexander J. Muller Lankenau Institute for Medical Research, Department of Microbiology and Immunology, Jefferson Medical School and Kimmel Cancer Center, Thomas Jefferson University, Philadelphia, PA, USA

William J. Murphy Department of Microbiology and Immunology 320, School of Medicine University of Nevada, Reno, NV, USA

Muneo Numasaki Department of Nutrition Physiology, Pharmaceutical Sciences, Josai University, Saitama, Japan

Yong Poovorawan Faculty of Medicine, Center of Excellence in Clinical Virology, Chulalongkorn University, Bangkok, Thailand

George C. Prendergast Lankenau Institute for Medical Research and Department of Pathology, Anatomy & Cell Biology, Jefferson Medical School and Kimmel Cancer Center, Thomas Jefferson University, Philadelphia, PA, USA

Jian Qiao Departments of Urology and Immunology, College of Medicine, Mayo Clinic, Rochester, MN, USA

Faisal Razzaqi Department of Pediatrics, Louisiana State University Health Sciences Center, New Orleans, LA, USA

Carl E. Ruby Earle A. Chiles Research Institute, Portland Providence Medical Center, Portland, OR, USA

Pallavur V. Sivakumar ZymoGenetics, Seattle, WA, USA

Kresten Skak Novo Nordisk A/S, Bagsværd, Denmark

Shannon Smith Cancer Center Scottsdale, Mayo Clinic Arizona, Scottsdale, AZ, USA

Mark J. Smyth Peter MacCallum Cancer Centre, East Melbourne, Australia

Rajasree Solipuram William Hansel Cancer Prevention Laboratory, Pennington Biomedical Research Center, Louisiana State University System, Baton Rouge, LA, USA

Lazar Vujanovic Department of Medicine, University of Pittsburgh Cancer Institute, Pittsburgh, PA, USA

Andrew D. Weinberg Earle A. Chiles Research Institute, Portland Providence Medical Center, Portland, OR, USA

Danice E.C. Wilkins Department of Microbiology and Immunology 320, School of Medicine University of Nevada, Reno, NV, USA

T.-C. Wu Department of Pathology, Johns Hopkins School of Medicine, Baltimore, MD, USA; Department of Oncology, Johns Hopkins School of Medicine, Baltimore, MD, USA; Department of Molecular Microbiology and Immunology, Johns Hopkins School of Medicine, Baltimore, MD, USA; Department of Obstetrics and Gynecology, Johns Hopkins School of Medicine, Baltimore, MD, USA

Lolie Yu Department of Pediatrics, Louisiana State University Health Sciences Center, New Orleans, LA, USA

Part I
Cytokine Immune Therapy

Role of IL12 Family in Regulation of Antitumor Immune Response

Denada Dibra and Shulin Li

Abstract The efficacy of immune therapy is partially dependent upon the tumor microenvironment. This microenvironment could either promote or demote tumor growth. Cytokines, which are secreted either by tumor, immune, or stromal cells, are key players that govern the outcome of this microenvironment. One such cytokine family is interleukin (IL)12 and the members of this family include IL12, IL27, IL23, and IL35. In this review, the expression and function of these family members and the cognate receptors in tumor microenvironment and other tissues are summarized and discussed. Our review indicates that, although these heterodimeric cytokines share subunits p35, p40, p19, EBI3, and p28 among these family members, each of them have distinct function. The same gene may also play different function when the expression is localized in different tissues.

Introduction

Tumor eradication or progression is dependent on interaction and communication with immune cells. Such crosstalk between tumors and immune cells is partially conducted through cytokines. In reality, the tumor microenvironment is frequently immunosuppressive and contributes to a state of immune tolerance [1]. As such, delivery of potent immune enhancer cytokines such as Interleukin (IL)12 may reverse immune tolerance because IL12 is a potent proinflammatory and immunoregulatory cytokine that plays a central role in tumor eradication via induction of IFNγ and cytotoxic T lymphocytes [2]. IL12 therapy for treating tumors was successful in a variety of murine models [3–5]. Although it is a promising immunotherapeutic agent, excess toxicity in preclinical trials is associated with systemic delivery of IL12 [6]. Decreasing the amount of IL12 administration reduces its therapeutic

S. Li (✉)
Department of Comparative Biomedical Sciences, Louisiana State University, Skip Bertman Drive, Baton Rouge, LA 70803, USA
e-mail: sli@vetmed.lsu.edu

J. Lustgarten et al. (eds.), *Targeted Cancer Immune Therapy*,
DOI 10.1007/978-1-4419-0170-5_1, © Springer Science+Business Media, LLC 2009

efficiency. Only immunogenic cancers are susceptible to this cytokine; therefore, local expression of IL12 or alternative cytokines in the tumor microenvironment is needed in cancer therapy.

The IL12 family is composed of IL12, IL23, IL27, and IL35, and although they are in the same family, these cytokines have different functions. IL12 is the key cytokine that promotes Th1 differentiation, while IL23 promotes Th17 differentiation [2, 7]. IL35 enhances the function of T regulatory cells (Tregs), while IL27 exerts pro and antiinflammatory functions [8]. Interestingly, while these family members perform such diverse functions they share many receptors and subunits. As such, IL12 and IL23 share subunit p40 and receptor IL12Rβ1, IL27, and IL35 share subunit EBI3 and receptor gp130, while IL12 and IL35 share subunit p35 and receptor IL12Rβ2 [9]. Many reviews have heavily described how these cytokines affect autoimmune diseases [10–12] as well as the behavior of immune cells [13, 14]. But the literature lacks reviews that focus on how IL12 family members signal in tumors and how they affect the crosstalk between tumors and immune cells. In summary, this review focuses on the expression and function of IL12 family members and their cognate receptors in tumors and how these cytokines affect Tregs.

Aberrant Expression of IL12 Family Member Receptors and Subunits

The IL12 cytokine family is composed of IL12, IL27, IL23, and IL35. IL27 is a heterodimeric cytokine that consists of EBI3, an IL12p40-related protein, and p28, a newly discovered IL12p35-related polypeptide [15]. IL-27 is produced by dendritic cells, monocytes, and endothelial cells [16, 17]. This cytokine exerts its biological functions through the heterodimeric receptor WSX1/TCCR and gp130 [18]. gp130 is ubiquitously expressed and is a receptor of other cytokines such as IL6, while WSX1 is specific for IL27 [19]. WSX1 is expressed mainly in monocytes, dendritic cells, T and B lymphocytes, NK cells, mast cells, and endothelial cells [18].

Recent discoveries have found that subunits or receptors of the IL12 family members are expressed not only in immune cells but also in tumor cells. Tumors have many ways to outfox the immune system such as retention of certain receptors while eliminating others or modulation of the downstream signaling of a receptor. IL23 subunits p19 and p40 are upregulated in multiple human cancers such as colon, ovarian, head and neck, lung, breast, stomach, and melanoma cancers [20]. IL12 is not upregulated in these tumors, as IL12p35 expression in tumors was similar to adjacent tissues. We have shown that WSX1 is expressed and functional in human breast cancer cells [21], while others later have confirmed its expression in human melanoma cells [22] and leukemia cells [23]. In addition to the IL27 receptor WSX1, the EBI3 subunit of IL27 is expressed in a variety of blood-related tumors [24–26]. We will carefully examine the role that each subunit/receptor plays.

While overexpression of WSX1 in epithelial cells delayed IL27-mediated tumor cell proliferation [22], WSX1 expression in leukemia cells transformed two leukemia cell lines, 32D and BaF3, by eliciting antiapoptotic and mitogenic signals [23]. Overexpression of WSX1 not only induces cytokine (IL3)-independent growth, but also activates Jak2, ERK1/2, and STAT5, which are all markers of acute myeloid leukemia (AML) transformation. However, the activation of these genes via WSX1 is not the determining factor to induce cell transformation. The key factor is the presence of a point-mutation of Jak2 at V167F. [27–29]. WSX1-dependent transformation of the leukemia cells is dependent upon activation of Jak2-V617F. The coexpression of WSX1 and mutated Jak2, but not wildtype Jak2, results in phosporylation of STAT3 and Jak2. Therefore, overexpression of WSX1 does not transform cells per se but instead acts as a scaffold receptor to activate tumor cells with already mutated JAKs. On the contrary to the leukemia cells lines, overexpression of WSX1 in melanomas enhances IL27-mediated antiproliferative activities [22]. Enhanced signaling of IL27/WSX1 signaling is dependent on the presence of STAT1 and upregulation of MHC class I. IL27 signaling also enhances transcription factor IRF1 and IRF8 expression. IL27-mediated delayed tumor growth is partially dependent on IRF1, as downregulation of IRF1 with siRNA partially reversed the aforementioned process [22]. As a synopsis, human and mouse melanoma cells downregulate WSX1 as a mechanism to enhance cell survival.

The Pradhan group also showed that WSX1-dependent transformation of the leukemia cells is independent of gp130 and IL27, as gp130 is not expressed in the tested leukemia cells [30]. In accordance with other publications, they also show the IL27 downstream signaling is inhibited, which demonstrates that IL27 needs a heterodimeric receptor to signal [31]. As the study in the melanoma cells showed the protective role of IL27/WSX1 signaling, the study in leukemia cells did not evaluate the role of IL27 signaling by overexpression of the missing receptor gp130 on these WSX1-transformed leukemia cells. One possibility is that leukemia cells downregulate gp130 while maintaining WSX1 therefore inhibiting IL27 signaling while preserving scaffold receptor WSX1.

Not only IL27 receptor WSX1 is expressed in dissociation to gp130 in cancers, but also its subunit EBI3 is selectively expressed in dissociation to p28 in a series of Epstein-Barr virus (EBV) and human T cell leukemia virus (HTLV) type associated lymphomas [26]. EBV associated lymphomas are associated with several human malignancies such as Burkitt lymphoma, Hodgkin's lymphoma, and nasopharyngeal carcinoma [32]. Although these tumors express antigen-presenting molecules such as HLA-1 and immune costimulatory molecules, such as CD80 and CD86, are susceptible to CTL in vitro, CTL specific against EBV are rarely found in patients' lymph nodes [33]. One question is how these tumors downregulate immune surveillance. IL10 is one of the cytokines associated with the immunosuppressive environment in EBV-positive tumor cells [34]. Another possible factor associated with EBV-derived tumors is the IL27-EBI3 subunit. EBI3 is a downstream factor of NFkB activation, and its expression is associated with other oncogenes responsible for T cell transformation such as LMP1 and Tax [26]. Nearly 90% of tumor cells in each case tested from Hodgkin's lymphoma patients were positive for EBI3, but only 5% were positive for p28 subunits. Similarly, in EBV-associated lymphoproliferative disorders (EBV-LPDs), EBI3 was expressed at high levels, whereas p28 or IL27 were not detected. In addition, EBI3 levels were detected in follicular lymphomas and in diffuse large B cell lymphomas of both germinal centre and nongerminal B cell like types [25]. Also, EBI3 was overexpressed in a subset of adult T cell leukemias that are dependent on IL2. These lymphomas upregulate EBI3 and express significant levels of the WSX1 receptor but lack p28, a necessary subunit to form a bioactive IL27 [26]. Although normal T cells express EBI3 after activation, these levels are 16 times lower than HTLV-positive T cells. Interestingly, the EBI3 expression level in EBV-LPDs was correlated with LMP1, an oncogene that plays a role in EBV-mediated growth transformation. EBI3 induction in HTLV positive T cells is dependent on NFkB activation via Tax protein, which plays an important role in T cell transformation. The inhibition of NFkB signaling reduces EBI3 expression only in the presence of wildtype Tax, but not mutated Tax, which is defective in NFkB activation [26]. These studies suggest that EBI3 is a downstream factor of oncogenes that are associated with lymphoma transformation and might play a role in tumor progression and immune evasion.

Another independent study revealed that EBI3 is expressed in Hodgkin's lymphoma and nasopharyngeal carcinoma [24]. In addition to EBI3, IL12p35 was also expressed, but IL12p40 subunit was not expressed. The copresence of IL12p35 and EBI3 and the absence of IL12p40 could result in the production of immunosuppressive cytokine IL35. It seems logical that immune evasion of these lymphoma cells may be attributed to IL35 function. In accordance with these conclusions, others have indicated that nasopharyngeal carcinoma cells are not capable of inducing IL12p70 [35]. These findings suggest that EBV HTLV-type associated lymphomas selectively modulate IL12 family members by enhancing EBI3 and/or p35 while downregulating p40 and/or p28 to attain a favorable tumor microenvironment.

The dissociated expression of EBI3 and p35 expression is observed not only in a pathogenic scenario but also in normal settings such as the intestinal tract [36]. The intestinal tract is the initial contact site between host and pathogens. In a balanced system, proinflammatory signals are cancelled with antiinflammatory signals. Overexpression of proinflammatory cytokines, such as IL12, in this environment would result in an autoimmune disease. Defining the mechanism on how the intestinal tract differentiates between pathogenic and commensial bacteria is of crucial importance. It would not only provide insight into the control processes in the peripheral tolerance but also indicate several potentially important therapeutic targets. One potential use of these targets would be cancer therapy since immune cells develop tolerance toward tumor cells. Human mucosal epithelial cells produce EBI3, IL12p35, and IL23p19 but not their counterpart subunits, such as p28 and IL12p40, which are necessary to form bioactive and functional IL12, IL27, and IL23. Proinflammatory mediators such as IL1α and TNFα induce EBI3 and p19 but not IL12p35 [36]. p35 is induced after IFNγ responses and its expression was delayed when compared with EBI3 and p19. This model suggests that in a balanced system such as the intestinal tract induction of p35 to make a functional IL35 is pushed to a later time point; therefore, only after a prominent cell-mediated immune response are both subunits of IL35 induced.

IL27 signaling in tumors is inhibited by dissociated and/or aberrant expression of its receptor WSX1 and gp130 [21–23]. As mentioned earlier, one possibility is that certain tumors preferentially lower one or the other receptor as a mechanism to enhance cell survival. Although modulation of IL27 receptors in tumors might be useful therapeutically, clinical translation as a therapy would require further investigation of (I) the pathways that are activated by WSX1 receptor and (II) the critical pathways activated by this receptor that are malfunctioning in tumor-bearing patients. Further mechanisms are needed to establish how this receptor activates downstream pathways in either epithelial or blood-related tumors; nonetheless, its therapeutic potential is promising.

Role of IL23 in Tumor

IL23 is another member of the IL12 family. This cytokine is composed of two subunits: p19 and p40 [9]. Although IL23 shares subunit p40 and receptor IL12Rβ1 with IL12, they drive quite different immune pathways. IL12 drives the classical IFNγ pathway, and IL23 is an essential factors required for the expansion of already committed Th17 cells into pathogenic cells [37]. Although many reviews and research articles have focused on the role of IL23 in autoimmune diseases, only a few articles have focused on the role of IL23 in cancers [38–40].

The role of IL23 in tumor biology is double-faced because the lack of IL23 shows protection against tumor initiation while IL23 used as a therapeutic or vaccine adjuvant reduces tumor growth [20, 41, 42]. To study the role of IL23 expression in epithelial tumorigenesis, the authors tested susceptibility of IL12p35$^{-/-}$, IL12/23p40$^{-/-}$, and IL23p19$^{-/-}$ mice to tumor formation during cancer progression [20]. Mice lacking IL23 subunits p19 and p40 but not p35 were resistant to tumor initiation and papilloma formation. Reduced tumor initiation in IL23 deficient mice was consistent with reduction of inflammatory markers, which are essential for tumor promotion such as IL17, GCSF, MMP9, and CD31. Another interesting factor is that the lack of IL23 in the tumor microenvironment enhanced CD8 infiltration in vivo. Lack of CD8 T cell infiltration was dependent on IL23, as intradermal injection of IL23 reduced CD8 T cell infiltration while IL12 enhanced CD8 infiltration as previously observed [43].

Contrary to the discovery described above, local and systemic administration of IL23 reduces tumor growth. Local overexpression of single chain IL23 in cell lines such as immunogenic CT26 grew in Balb/c mice but then spontaneously regressed in a CD8 T cell-dependent matter [41]. This same phenomena was also observed using a poorly immunogenic melanoma cell line such as B16F10 [42]. IL23-mediated tumor growth inhibition was dependent on CD8 T cell and IFNγ production. In another study by Overwijk, overexpression of IL23 in nonimmunogenic B16 tumors did not show tumor growth inhibition. Nonetheless, this group studied how IL23 could be used as an adjuvant to vaccination of already established nonimmunogenic melanoma tumors [44]. They used a gp100 peptide vaccination after adoptively transferring antigen-specific pmel CD8 T cells toward this peptide. IL23 aided tumor suppression by vaccine-induced T cells and enhanced function of intratumoral T cells. The enhanced T cell effector functions were characterized by high ability of antigen specific CD8 T cells to produce IFNγ without need of in vitro stimulation with the peptide. Although IL23 enhances IFNγ production by tumor-specific T cells, they conclude that IFNγ production by CD8 T cells does not have a major role in enhancing the role of IL23 as an adjuvant; however, adoptive transfer of $IFN\gamma^{-/-}$ pmel T cells still remains responsive to IL23 therapy. Contrary to the statement that IFNγ is dispensable, others have shown that IFNγ is absolutely necessary for IL23 antitumor activity [45]. In IFNγ knockout (KO) mice, IL23 antitumor effects were nonexistent, and in IL12 KO mice, the effects were partially abrogated. In addition, this study shows that IL23 administered systemically reduces tumor growth and is dependent on CD4, CD8, and partially on NK cells. The authors suggest that once a Th1 response is fully established, IL23 does exert its potent antitumor activity. This claim is not in disagreement with Overwijk study since their argument solely depends on $IFN\gamma^{-/-}$ CD8 transfer, but not on the endogenous IFNγ. In summary, IFNγ is primarily involved in IL23-mediated antitumor activities while IFNγ production from CD8 is dispensable in this process. Further conclusive studies are needed to elucidate whether prevalence of Th1 response is necessary to mediate IL23 antitumor response and molecular mechanism associated with it.

IL23-mediated antitumor effects are observed not only in mouse tumor models but also in human pancreatic cancer cell lines such as AsPC [46]. Interestingly, AsPC overexpressing IL23 showed retarded tumor growth in nude mice but not in SCID mice. In addition, depletion with anti-asialo GM1 antibody did not affect tumor growth inhibition in nude mice. In this particular tumor model, IL23 mediates its antitumor effect mainly through γδ T and/or NKT cells.

One of the downfalls of using IL23 systemically is weight loss, which is toxicity dependent on the expression of TNFα [44]. Depletion of TNFα reduces side effects; nonetheless, it is not feasible as it mediates not only weight loss but also antitumor activity. Therefore, local rather than systemic administration of this cytokine would improve its antitumor activities as a direct immune stimulator or as a vaccine adjuvant. Indeed, local expression of IL23 augmented vaccine-induced antitumor activity without weight loss.

Contradictory to the aforementioned role of IL23 as an anticancer therapeutic agent/adjuvant, IL23 expression in the microenvironment enhances tumor growth partially by activating a tumor-promoting inflammation and angiogenesis. It is well known that IL23 promotes pathogenic Th17 lineage. It also promotes tissue restructuring and neovascularization and all tumor-adopted strategies to thrive and grow. To explain the contradictory role of IL23, these authors suggest that high expression of IL23 in the tumor microenvironment induces an overwhelming myeloid infiltration of DC, macrophages, and granulocytes that destroy tumors [40]. Others indicate that a Th1 priming microenvironment in the host is necessary for systemic delivery of IL23 to eradicate tumors as IL23 was noneffective to eradicate tumors in $INF\gamma^{-/-}$ mice [45]. IFNγ also has been shown to downregulate Th17 while promoting Th1 induction [47, 48]. On the one hand, it is also reasonable to assume that exogenous IL23 can serve as a potent adjuvant/therapeutic anticancer agent to enhance an already established but probably weak Th1/IFNγ immune response. On the other hand, endogenous IL23 produced at the local microenvironment together with other inflammation-promoting agents from tumors, such as TGFβ, might reroute the immune response toward more of wound-healing tumor-promoting Th17.

Role of IL27 in Tumor

One of the earlier functions attributed to IL27 is its ability to synergize with IL12 to induce IFNγ and proliferation of naive CD4 T cells [15]. IL27 also induces T-bet expression and IL12Rβ expression, key components to Th1 commitment, through STAT1 [49]. Given its role in initiation of Th1 response and induction of IL12 receptor, several researchers evaluated the role of IL27 in cancer immunotherapy. The function of IL27 was examined in different tumor models such as colon cancer 26 (CT26), neuroblastoma (TBJ), and aggressive melanoma (B16F10) [50–54].

IL27 possesses T cell and NK cell-mediated antitumor activities. In an immunogenic colon cancer system, IL27 mediates antitumor activities mainly though CD8 T cells and epitope-specific CTL. Immunogenic CT26 overexpressing IL27 showed reduced tumor growth in vivo. IL27 expression induced IFNγ and increased CTL against CT26 cells. The mechanism was dependent on CD8 and IFNγ, since antitumor activity was abolished in nude mice or mice depleted of IFNγ and CD8. Interestingly, in T-bet$^{-/-}$ mice, IL27 did not display any antitumor activities [55]. Not only CD8 T cells but also other subsets of T and NK cells account for IL27 antitumor properties. In nude mice, CT26-IL27 tumor growth was retarded when compared with parent CT26. These phenomena were partially reversed upon administration of anti-asialo GM1 depletion antibody [50]. This result suggests that γδ T cells or NKT are the possible effector cells that are mediated by IL27 and contribute to antitumor effect. Others show that in highly aggressive melanoma B16F10, NK cells were mainly involved [53].

IL27 antitumor activity does not depend on either STAT4 or IL12 [56]. Since IL27 exerted antitumor effects in either IL12p40 or STAT4 KO mice, IL12 is not necessary for IL27-mediated antitumor activity. In contrast to IL27, IL23 is partially dependent upon IL12 to exert antitumor activity [45]. The mechanism associated with IL27 as an anticancer agent depends upon CTL induction and enhancement of cytolytic molecules such as granzyme B and perforin [56]. STAT1 was the important transcription factor necessary for induction of T-bet, IL12Rβ2, perforin, granzyme B, and synergistic induction of IFNγ with IL12 [56]. T-bet was important for induction of IL12Rβ2, perforin, granzyme B, and synergistic induction of IFNγ with IL12. IL27 is known to enhance T-bet expression, suggesting an important role of IL27 in regulating the expression of these genes. However, IL27 could enhance allogeneic CTL activity independent of T-bet [56]. Although IL27 increased CTL activity in a T-bet independent matter, this transcription factor is important for IL27-mediated antitumor activities in vivo, as tumors grew much faster in T-bet$^{-/-}$ mice but not in wildtype mice. These phenomena could be explained by a later study, which emphasizes that T-bet and WSX1 expression in CD8 T cells are indispensable for IFNγ production in CD8 T cells in vivo but not in vitro [57].

In the neuroblastoma TBJ cell line, overexpression of IL27 completely eradicated more than 90% of tumors and rendered these mice resistant to tumor challenge [58]. IL27 producing tumors, TBJ27, but not control TBJ tumors reduced adjacent parental tumor cells. IL27 overexpression conferred tumor memory not only on neuroblastoma but also in another independent tumor model such as CT26 [55]. In addition to inducing tumor memory, overexpression of this cytokine in the tumor microenvironment also reduced metastasis of primary tumors. TBJ27 reduced the number of metastatic tumors in the liver, and 40% of the mice were free of their metastatic tumors. The mechanism responsible for IL27-mediated tumor regression was dependent on CD8 T cells but not on NK or CD4 T cells. IL27 also enhanced IFNγ and MHC class I expression in the tumor microenvironment [58]. Such great antitumor effect associated with IL27 production in the tumor could be attributed to IL27 signaling in the host as well as in the tumor itself. Although this study did not determine WSX1 levels on the TBJ cell line, enhanced MHC class I induction in the tumor environment suggests the presence of a functional WSX1.

IL27 antitumor effect has been shown not only in immunogenic models such as CT26 and neuroblastoma but also in B16F10, a mouse melanoma that is a model of poor immunogenicity characterized by low MHC class I expression. B16F10 that overexpress single chain IL27 show reduced tumor growth of primary tumors and pulmonary metastases [59]. Interestingly, IL27-mediated antimetastatic activities were not dependent on the host as T, B, and NK deficient mice still retained tumor growth inhibition. The authors also showed that IL27 enhanced expression of anti-angiogenic markers such IP10 and MIG while it reduced in vivo angiogenesis. What seems to be quite impressive is that IL27 acts independently of IFNγ to induce anti-angiogenesis markers. Even in IFNγ$^{-/-}$ mice, IL27 expressing B16F10 tumors, B16F10-IL27, showed reduced tumor growth and metastasis. Similarly, another group using the same tumor model, B16F10, showed that IL27 exerts anti-tumor activities in the absence of IFNγ [42]. This phenomenon is quite different from IL12 and IL23 as both these cytokines depend on IFNγ to induce antitumor activity [45]. It also seems that IL27, a downstream molecule of IFNγ and IL12, might act synergistically or independently of IL12 to suppress tumor growth.

As we have previously seen, IL27 antitumor effects are not only attributed to signaling in tumors or immune cells but also to vascular endothelial cells that surround the tumor microenvironment [59, 60]. During tumor progression, endothelial cells can have two roles: promoting or inhibiting tumor growth. On the one hand, endothelial cells act as a support matrix in tumors and provide many growth factors to tumors through enhancing angiogenesis. On the other hand, endothelial cells can function as antigen-presenting cells and can upregulate MHC class I and II to aid CTL activity [61]. In addition, they can upregulate certain receptors to recruit innate immune cells [62]. The balance between anti and protumor environments depends on the cytokine profiles and the level of each cytokine expressed in these cells. The IL27 receptor WSX1 was present in endothelial cells, and IL27 signaling directly on endothelial cells has increased antiangiogenic molecules such as IP10 and MIG [59]. IL27 also upregulated MHC class II and MHC class I together with microglobulin and *Tap* genes [60]. It also increases fractaline expression in endothelial cells, a chemokine that attracts and activates CX3CR1 NK positive cells and DC cells [63, 64]. Activation of NK and maturation of DC cells in the local microenvironment leads to an enhanced expression of IL12 and IFNγ, both factors necessary to tip the microenvironment balance toward an antitumor response.

IL27 overexpression exerts antitumor effects not only in mouse carcinoma but also in human oesophageal carcinoma Eca cell line [65]. When injected into nude mice, Eca cells overexpressing IL27 showed a retarded tumor growth and enhanced survival. Similar to previous tumor models, NK cells from mice overexpressing IL27 showed increased IFNγ production and cytolytic activities when compared with splenocytes from control mice. The retarded tumor growth could not be due to direct effect of IL27 signaling into the tumor cells as IL27 did not increase MHC class I or reduced cell proliferation. While IL27 showed an increase in NK cell function, IL27 did not increase NK cell infiltration or NK cell activation marker CD69 [65]. Although IL27 has been shown to increase the antiangiogenic markers MIG and IP10 in other reports [59], this study showed no change in IP10, MIG, or vessel number. One possibility could be that IFNγ induction in nude mice is limited, although other reports show that IL27 can have anticancer properties independent of IFNγ [42, 59]. Once again, this suggests that IL27 employs different antitumor pathways depending on the tumor microenvironment that particular tumors create.

Contradictory to the aforementioned role of IL27 in reducing tumor growth, this cytokine has been shown to have an antiinflammatory role. Other groups have shown that IL27 receptor knockout mice have a prolonged cytokine expression, while DC cells have a prolonged expression of activation markers CD80/86 after LPS stimulation [66]. In addition, IL27 directly downregulates these activation markers in LPS-stimulated DC. The IL27 receptor WSX1 was upregulated in DC cells after LPS stimulation and IL27 also downregulates IL2 production in activated T cells. These authors propose a model that IL27/WSX1 delivers little inhibitory signals at the initial immune response, while at later phases upregulation of IL27/WSX1 promotes more profound inhibitory functions. In vivo this model does not hold true as constant IL27 expression enhanced NK and T cells functions. Immature dendritic cells reside primarily in peripheral tissues where they uptake antigens and process it, while mature DC reside in the lymphoid tissue to interact with antigen-specific T cells. One of the problems associated with tumor microenvironment is lack of DC maturation such as in human breast, ovarian, and prostate cancers [67]. These immature DC rarely leave the tumor environment to mature and travel to the lymphoid organs as tumor-associated factors such as IL-10, TGFβ, and VEGF inhibit DC cell differentiation [68, 69]. Therefore, the role of IL27 to downregulate activation markers would mean that these DC need to be matured in the first place.

Role of IL12 Family in Treg Cells

T regulatory cells are part of the T cell repertoire that keep the immune system in check by inhibiting proliferation and function of T cells and attenuating responses against self and non-self. There are two types of Treg cells: naturally occurring Treg cells that are generated in the thymus and inducible Treg, which are generated in the periphery from naïve T cells via TGFβ [70–72]. Treg cells express Foxp3, a transcription factor that controls both development and function of these cells [73]. Besides Foxp3 Tregs, there are other types of regulatory T cells, such as Tr1 and Th3, which also contribute to suppression in the periphery. Tr1 and Th3 are characterized by secretion of immunosuppressive IL10 and TGFβ, respectively [74, 75]. In a clinical setting, high numbers of Treg is an indication of poor prognosis for cancer patients [76–78]. Many tumors enhance number of Treg as a mechanism to evade tumor recognition. A high accumulation of Treg in the tumor microenvironment, lymph nodes, or blood is not a result of high trafficking into these areas but rather a result of proliferation and de novo induction [79]. TGFβ is a key player in this process, as it increases the proliferation as well as the induction of de novo Treg. Tumors release TGFβ or induce immature DCs to release TGFβ that can enhance the number of Tregs [80]. Tregs not only suppress CD8 T cell proliferation but also inhibit NK cell function [79]. Tregs and TGFβ inhibit NK cell cytolysis, IL12-mediated IFNγ secretion, and NKG2D expression.

The IL12-associated cytokines modulate induction and function of Treg. Induction of $Foxp3^+$ Treg via TGFβ is completely inhibited by IL6 [81, 82]. The combination of IL6 and TGFβ diverts induction of Foxp3 Treg into Th17 cells. Not only IL6, but also IL27 has a prominent role in induction of Treg. Recent reports have shown that IL27 not only suppressed Th17 induction via TGFβ and IL6 but also suppressed the number of inducible Treg in vitro [83, 84]. IL27 suppresses number of TGFβ-induced Treg in a dose and time-dependent manner. This suppression was not dependent on either IL2 or STAT1 as high doses of recombinant IL2 did not rescue IL27-mediated suppression of Treg while IL27 retained Treg suppression in $STAT1^{-/-}$ splenocytes [83].

Although IL27 suppresses induction of Treg, the lack of IL27 does not attenuate naturally occurring Treg as $WSX1^{-/-}$ mice and wt mice have a similar number of Treg [85, 86]. In addition, EBI3 deficiency does not affect the population of Foxp3 CD25+ T cells. Moreover, IL27 itself does not aid Treg in suppression of T cell proliferation. In a classical Treg functional assay, $WSX1^{-/-}$ Treg suppressed T cell proliferation in the same manner as wt cells in the presence or absence of IL27 [81]. Thus, IL27 seems to not play a role in T cell development or function, but rather plays a role during Treg induction.

In addition to Foxp3 inducible Treg, other regulatory T cells such as Tr1 contribute to active suppression in the periphery. Tr1 cells express IL10 and exert their immune suppression mainly through this cytokine [87]. IL27 not only suppresses the induction TGFβ-mediated Treg, but also enhances generation of Tr1-like cells to produce IL10 [88]. The presence of TGFβ produced from Treg converts immature

DC into tolerogenic ones. These modified DC produce IL27 and TGFβ. Production of IL27 and TGFβ by these tolerogenic DC in turn induces T effector cells to produce IL10. Other groups also confirmed that IL27 upregulated IL10 expression in CD4 and CD8 effector cells [89]. Interestingly, IL27 enhances production of IL10 in these cells only once activation of T cells has occurred (Fig. 1).

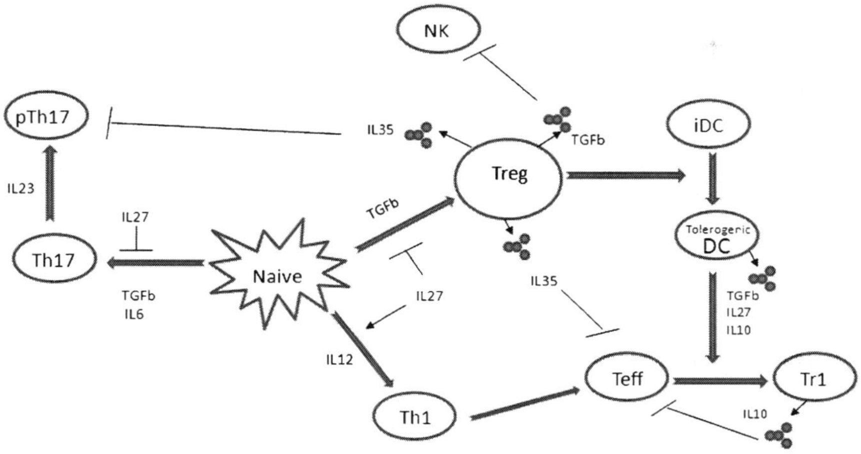

Fig. 1 IL12 family affects different pathways of immune system

Not only does IL27 neutralize the TGFβ effect on Treg but it also neutralizes IL6-induced T cell hyperproliferation [81]. IL6 renders effector T cell refractory to Treg cell-mediated suppression while inducing hyperproliferation of these cells [90]. Therefore, although IL6 and IL27 share the same receptor, these cytokines exert different functions.

The mechanistic cues on how IL27 in some instances promotes a proinflammatory environment by reducing Treg numbers [83, 84] while on others promotes an antiinflammatory by neutralizing IL6-induced T cell proliferation and inducing Tr1 cells still needs to be clarified [81, 88, 89]. Probably timing and state of T cells dictates the role of IL27. IL27 priming of naïve CD4T cells inhibits Treg induction, resulting in a proinflammatory environment. Addition of this cytokine at a later time when the Treg cells have already acquired Foxp3 enhances Treg function indirectly by converting IL6 mediated refractory T cells into T cells susceptible to Treg cytolysis. In addition, production of IL27 in the presence of TGFβ gears effector cells toward production of IL10. Therefore, IL27 has opposing roles during different stages of an immune response.

Many questions need to be answered on the role of IL27 in Treg. First, Villarino et al. show that WSX1 expression is modulated during an immune response. WSX1 is increased not only in activated T cells and memory T cells but also in Treg CD62L^{high}CD25^{high} when compared with naïve CD62L^{high}CD25^{low} [85]. Although others have shown that IL27 does not affect Treg suppression, why is there a higher expression in Treg rather than in naïve T cells? Next, there is no evidence whether IL27 suppresses inducible Treg in vivo or whether IL27 exerts antitumor effects partially by effecting Treg. Although many authors and studies have described IL27 as a future candidate for cancer therapies, caution should be made when interpreting these studies. The timing of expressing IL27 will determine whether IL27 suppresses or enhances Treg. Primarily, most studies use tumors transduced with single chain overexpressing IL27, thus expressing this cytokine at the initial stage of mounting an immune response. Presence of IL27 at the initial stage establishes a Th1 proinflammatory environment. There are no studies showing the prophylactic properties of IL27 administration after tumor establishment. Systemic delivery of IL27 has little to no effect on already established tumors (our unpublished data). In such, the tumors that are clinically detectable have already established an immunosuppressive environment characterized by the presence of Treg. In this perspective, IL27 might promote an immunosuppressive environment; therefore, the use of IL27 as a therapeutic agent alone might not be effective. Administration of IL27 in addition with Treg suppressors such as cyclophosphamide might provide a synergistic effect. The timing and sequence of administration between these two agents should be considered as well. The first phase should consist of cyclophosphamide, followed by IL27 after a lag period. In the presence of lower numbers of Treg, IL27 might stimulate T cells and NK to produce cytotoxic molecules against tumors. The lag period should provide enough stimuli to revert the immune-suppressive tumor environment at least for a short time. In addition, the lag period should be in reverse proportion to tumor size and aggressiveness. In other words, the lag period in aggressive tumors models should be shorter than immunogenic tumors. Also, lower number of Treg would translate into fewer tolerogenic DC; therefore, there is less chance that IL27 might enhance induction of Tr1 cells. In light of new antiinflammatory properties, further in-depth studies are needed to explore the anticancer role of IL27.

Il35

IL35 is the newest member of IL12 family, which expands not only IL12 family but adds complexity in modulating the immune system by this family [8]. IL35 is composed of the IL27 subunit EBI3 and IL12 subunit p35, a complex already known but with no attributable function [91]. EBI3 was shown to be a downstream gene induced by Foxp3. From all the alpha chain cytokines of IL12 family that are expressed, only p35 and EBI3 are expressed by Treg. Treg upregulates this cytokine only during active suppression of T cells while in contact with T effector cells (Teff), suggesting that proximity to Teff is required for induction of this cytokine [92]. IL35 suppresses Teff proliferation and IFNγ production in response to activation in an antigen-specific and nonspecific manner [8]. Downregulation in either subunit might be necessary to reduce IL35 suppressive activity, as either subunit alone does not suppress proliferation of effector T cells.

IL35 expression may not be constricted only to Treg, as APC do induce all subunits of the IL12 family. Although both IL27 and IL35 compete for EBI3, the only known preferential expression difference between these two cytokines is location, as IL27 is mainly constrained to APC while IL35 is constrained to Treg. Moreover, since EBI3 is shared by IL27 and IL35 and $TCCR^{-/-}$ mice display a different phenotype than $EBI3^{-/-}$ mice in T cell-mediated hepatitis [93, 94], then caution should be used when interpreting results from these two different strains. Further studies are needed to establish the mechanism necessary to produce one cytokine over another in APC. In addition, future studies should elucidate whether APC produce IL35 and whether it exerts immunosuppressive role during APC-T cell interactions.

Acknowledgement This study was supported by National Institutes of Health (Bethesda, MD) grant RO1CA120895 and NIH/NIBIB grant R21EB007208

References

1. Neeson, P., and Paterson, Y. (2006) Immunol Investig 35, 359
2. Trinchieri, G. (1995) Annu Rev Immunol 13, 251
3. Brunda, M. J., Luistro, L., Rumennik, L., Wright, R. B., Dvorozniak, M., Aglione, A., Wigginton, J. M., Wiltrout, R. H., Hendrzak, J. A., and Palleroni, A. V. (1996) Cancer Chemother Pharmacol 38 Suppl, S16
4. Brunda, M. J., Luistro, L., Warrier, R. R., Wright, R. B., Hubbard, B. R., Murphy, M., Wolf, S. F., and Gately, M. K. (1993) J Exp Med 178, 1223
5. Rakhmilevich, A. L., Turner, J., Ford, M. J., McCabe, D., Sun, W. H., Sondel, P. M., Grota, K., and Yang, N. S. (1996) Proc Natl Acad Sci USA 93, 6291
6. Car, B. D., Eng, V. M., Lipman, J. M., and Anderson, T. D. (1999) Toxicologic Pathol 27, 58
7. Aggarwal, S., Ghilardi, N., Xie, M. H., de Sauvage, F. J., and Gurney, A. L. (2003) J Biol Chem 278, 1910
8. Niedbala, W., Wei, X. Q., Cai, B., Hueber, A. J., Leung, B. P., McInnes, I. B., and Liew, F. Y. (2007) Eur J Immunol 37, 3021
9. Oppmann, B., Lesley, R., Blom, B., Timans, J. C., Xu, Y., Hunte, B., Vega, F., Yu, N., Wang, J., Singh, K., Zonin, F., Vaisberg, E., Churakova, T., Liu, M., Gorman, D., Wagner, J., Zurawski, S., Liu, Y., Abrams, J. S., Moore, K. W., Rennick, D., de Waal-Malefyt, R., Hannum, C., Bazan, J. F., and Kastelein, R. A. (2000) Immunity 13, 715
10. Alber, G., Al-Robaiy, S., Kleinschek, M., Knauer, J., Krumbholz, P., Richter, J., Schoeneberger, S., Schuetze, N., Schulz, S., Toepfer, K., Voigtlaender, R., Lehmann, J., and Mueller, U. (2006) Ernst Schering Res Found Workshop 107
11. Becker, C., Wirtz, S., and Neurath, M. F. (2005) Inflamm Bowel Dis 11, 755
12. Gaddi, P. J. and Yap, G. S. (2007) Immunol Cell Biol 85, 155
13. Goriely, S., Neurath, M. F., and Goldman, M. (2008) Nat Rev 8, 81
14. Beadling, C., and Slifka, M. K. (2006) Arch Immunol Ther Exp (Warsz) 54, 15
15. Pflanz, S., Timans, J. C., Cheung, J., Rosales, R., Kanzler, H., Gilbert, J., Hibbert, L., Churakova, T., Travis, M., Vaisberg, E., Blumenschein, W. M., Mattson, J. D., Wagner, J. L., To, W., Zurawski, S., McClanahan, T.K., Gorman, D.M., Bazan, J.F., de Waal Malefyt, R., Rennick, D., and Kastelein, R.A. (2002) Immunity 16, 779
16. Villarino, A. V., Huang, E., and Hunter, C. A. (2004) J Immunol 173, 715
17. Wirtz, S., Becker, C., Fantini, M. C., Nieuwenhuis, E. E., Tubbe, I., Galle, P. R., Schild, H. J., Birkenbach, M., Blumberg, R. S., and Neurath, M. F. (2005) J Immunol 174, 2814

18. Pflanz, S., Hibbert, L., Mattson, J., Rosales, R., Vaisberg, E., Bazan, J. F., Phillips, J. H., McClanahan, T. K., de Waal Malefyt, R., and Kastelein, R. A. (2004) J Immunol, 172, 2225
19. Chen, Q., Ghilardi, N., Wang, H., Baker, T., Xie, M. H., Gurney, A., Grewal, I. S., and de Sauvage, F. J. (2000) Nature 407, 916
20. Langowski, J. L., Zhang, X., Wu, L., Mattson, J.D., Chen, T., Smith, K., Basham, B., McClanahan, T., Kastelein, R. A., and Oft, M. (2006) Nature 442, 461
21. Li, S., Zhu, S., and Dibra, D. (2007) United States Patent Application 20070280905
22. Yoshimoto, T., Morishima, N., Mizoguchi, I., Shimizu, M., Nagai, H., Oniki, S., Oka, M., Nishigori, C., and Mizuguchi, J. (2008) J Immunol 180, 6527
23. Pradhan, A., Lambert, Q. T., and Reuther, G. W. (2007) Proc Natl Acad Sci USA 104, 18502
24. Niedobitek, G., Pazolt, D., Teichmann, M., and Devergne, O. (2002) J Pathol 198, 310
25. Larousserie, F., Bardel, E., L'Hermine, A.C., Canioni, D., Brousse, N., Kastelein, R., and Devergne, O. 2006, J Pathol 209, 360
26. Larousserie, F., Bardel, E., Pflanz, S., Arnulf, B., Lome-Maldonado, C., Hermine, O., Bregeaud, L., Perennec, M., Brousse, N., Kastelein, R., and Devergne, O. (2005) Am J Pathol 166, 1217
27. Baxter, E. J., Scott, L. M., Campbell, P. J., East, C., Fourouclas, N., Swanton, S., Vassiliou, G. S., Bench, A. J., Boyd, E. M., Curtin, N., Scott, M. A., Erber, W. N., and Green, A. R. (2005) Lancet 365, 1054
28. James, C., Ugo, V., Le Couedic, J. P., Staerk, J., Delhommeau, F., Lacout, C., Garcon, L., Raslova, H., Berger, R., Bennaceur-Griscelli, A., Villeval, J. L., Constantinescu, S. N., Casadevall, N., and Vainchenker, W. (2005) Nature 434, 1144
29. Jones, A. V., Kreil, S., Zoi, K., Waghorn, K., Curtis, C., Zhang, L., Score, J., Seear, R., Chase, A. J., Grand, F. H., White, H., Zoi, C., Loukopoulos, D., Terpos, E., Vervessou, E. C., Schultheis, B., Emig, M., Ernst, T., Lengfelder, E., Hehlmann, R., Hochhaus, A., Oscier, D., Silver, R.T., Reiter, A., and Cross, N. C. (2005) Blood 106, 2162
30. Pradhan, A., Lambert, Q. T., and Reuther, G. W. (2007) Proc Natl Acad Sci USA 104, 18502
31. Pflanz, S., Hibbert, L., Mattson, J. D., Rosales, R., Vaisberg, E., Bazan, J. F., Phillips, J. H., McClanahan, T. K., de Waal malefyt, R., and Kastelein, R. A. (2004) J Immunol 2225
32. Kutok, J. L. and Wang, F. (2006) Ann Rev Pathol 1, 375
33. Frisan, T., Sjoberg, J., Dolcetti, R., Boiocchi, M., De Re, V., Carbone, A., Brautbar, C., Battat, S., Biberfeld, P., Eckman, M., et al. (1995) Blood 86, 1493
34. Herbst, H., Foss, H. D., Samol, J., Araujo, I., Klotzbach, H., Krause, H., Agathanggelou, A., Niedobitek, G., and Stein, H. (1996) Blood 87, 2918
35. Schwaller, J., Tobler, A., Niklaus, G., Hurwitz, N., Hennig, I., Fey, M. F., and Borisch, B. (1995) Blood 85, 2182
36. Maaser, C., Egan, L. J., Birkenbach, M. P., Eckmann, L., and Kagnoff, M. F. (2004) Immunology 112, 437
37. Langrish, C. L., Chen, Y., Blumenschein, W. M., Mattson, J., Basham, B., Sedgwick, J. D., McClanahan, T., Kastelein, R. A., and Cua, D. J. (2005) J Exp Med 201, 233
38. Layh-Schmitt, G. and Colbert, R. A. (2008) Curr Opin Rheumatol 20, 392
39. McGeachy, M. J. and Cua, D. J. (2008) Immunity 28, 445
40. Langowski, J. L., Kastelein, R. A., and Oft, M. (2007) Trends Immunol 28, 207
41. Wang, Y. Q., Ugai, S., Shimozato, O., Yu, L., Kawamura, K., Yamamoto, H., Yamaguchi, T., Saisho, H., and Tagawa, M. (2003) Int J Cancer 105, 820
42. Oniki, S., Nagai, H., Horikawa, T., Furukawa, J., Belladonna, M.L., Yoshimoto, T., Hara, I., and Nishigori, C. (2006) Cancer Res 66, 6395
43. Mortarini, R., Borri, A., Tragni, G., Bersani, I., Vegetti, C., Bajetta, E., Pilotti, S., Cerundolo, V., and Anichini, A. (2000) Cancer Res 60, 3559
44. Overwijk, W. W., de Visser, K. E., Tirion, F. H., de Jong, L. A., Pols, T. W., van der Velden, Y. U., van den Boorn, J. G., Keller, A. M., Buurman, W. A., Theoret, M. R., Blom, B., Restifo, N. P., Kruisbeek, A. M., Kastelein, R. A., and Haanen, J. B. (2006), J Immunol 176, 5213
45. Kaiga, T., Sato, M., Kaneda, H., Iwakura, Y., Takayama, T., and Tahara, H. (2007) J Immunol 178, 7571

46. Ugai, S., Shimozato, O., Yu, L., Wang, Y. Q., Kawamura, K., Yamamoto, H., Yamaguchi, T., Saisho, H., Sakiyama, S., and Tagawa, M. (2003) Cancer Gene Ther 10, 771
47. Murphy, C. A., Langrish, C. L., Chen, Y., Blumenschein, W., McClanahan, T., Kastelein, R. A., Sedgwick, J. D., and Cua, D. J. (2003) J Exp Med 198, 1951
48. Willenborg, D. O., Fordham, S., Bernard, C. C., Cowden, W. B., and Ramshaw, I. A. (1996) J Immunol 157, 3223
49. Takeda, A., Hamano, S., Yamanaka, A., Hanada, T., Ishibashi, T., Mak, T. W., Yoshimura, A., and Yoshida, H. (2003) J Immunol 170, 4886
50. Chiyo, M., Shimozato, O., Yu, L., Kawamura, K., Iizasa, T., Fujisawa, T., and Tagawa, M. (2005) Int J Cancer 115, 437
51. Hisada, M., Kamiya, S., Fujita, K., Belladonna, M. L., Aoki, T., Koyanagi, Y., Mizuguchi, J., and Yoshimoto, T. (2004) Cancer Res 64, 1152
52. Morishima, N., Owaki, T., Asakawa, M., Kamiya, S., Mizuguchi, J., and Yoshimoto, T. (2005) J Immunol 175, 1686
53. Oniki, S., Nagai, H., Horikawa, T., Furukawa, J., Belladonna, M. L., Yoshimoto, T., Hara, I., and Nishigori, C. (2006) Cancer Res 66, 6395
54. Salcedo, R., Stauffer, J. K., Lincoln, E., Back, T. C., Hixon, J. A., Hahn, C., Shafer-Weaver, K., Malyguine, A., Kastelein, R., and Wigginton, J. M. (2004) J Immunol 173, 7170
55. Hisada, M., Kamiya, S., Fujita, K., Belladonna, M. L., Aoki, T., Koyanagi, Y., Mizuguchi, J., and Yoshimoto, T. (2004) Cancer Res 64, 1152
56. Morishima, N., Owaki, T., Asakawa, M., Kamiya, S., Mizuguchi, J., and Yoshimoto, T. (2005) J Immunol 175, 1686
57. Mayer, K. D., Mohrs, K., Reiley, W., Wittmer, S., Kohlmeier, J. E., Pearl, J. E., Cooper, A. M., Johnson, L. L., Woodland, D. L., and Mohrs, M. (2008) J Immunol 180, 693
58. Salcedo, R., Stauffer, J. K., Lincoln, E., Back, T. C., Hixon, J. A., Hahn, C., Shafer-Weaver, K., Malyguine, A., Kastelein, R. A., and Wigginton, J. (2004) J Immunol 173, 7170
59. Shimizu, M., Shimamura, M., Owaki, T., Asakawa, M., Fujita, K., Kudo, M., Iwakura, Y., Takeda, Y., Luster, A. D., Mizuguchi, J., and Yoshimoto, T. (2006) J Immunol 176, 7317
60. Feng, X. M., Chen, X. L., Liu, N., Chen, Z., Zhou, Y. L., Han, Z. B., Zhang, L., and Han, Z. C. (2007) Hum Immunol 68, 965
61. Epperson, D. E. and Pober, J. S. (1994) J Immunol 153, 5402
62. Cook-Mills, J. M. and Deem, T. L. (2005) J Leukoc Biol 77, 487
63. Guo, J., Zhang, M., Wang, B., Yuan, Z., Guo, Z., Chen, T., Yu, Y., Qin, Z., and Cao, X. (2003) Int J Cancer 103, 212
64. Lavergne, E., Combadiere, B., Bonduelle, O., Iga, M., Gao, J. L., Maho, M., Boissonnas, A., Murphy, P. M., Debre, P., and Combadiere, C. (2003) Cancer Res 63, 7468
65. Liu, L., Wang, S., Shan, B., Shao, L., Sato, A., Kawamura, K., Li, Q., Ma, G., and Tagawa, M. (2008), Scand J Immunol 68, 22
66. Wang, S., Miyazaki, Y., Shinozaki, Y., and Yoshida, H. (2007) J Immunol 6421
67. Zou, W., Machelon, V., Coulomb-L'Hermin, A., Borvak, J., Nome, F., Isaeva, T., Wei, S., Krzysiek, R., Durand-Gasselin, I., Gordon, A., Pustilnik, T., Curiel, D. T., Galanaud, P., Capron, F., Emilie, D., and Curiel, T. J. (2001) Nat Med 7, 1339
68. Gabrilovich, D. I., Chen, H. L., Girgis, K. R., Cunningham, H. T., Meny, G. M., Nadaf, S., Kavanaugh, D., and Carbone, D. P. (1996) Nat Med 2, 1096
69. Fricke, I., and Gabrilovich, D. I. (2006) Immunol Investig 35, 459
70. Fontenot, J. D., Dooley, J. L., Farr, A. G., and Rudensky, A. Y. (2005) J Exp Med 202, 901
71. Chen, W., Jin, W., Hardegen, N., Lei, K. J., Li, L., Marinos, N., McGrady, G., and Wahl, S. M. (2003) J Exp Med 198, 1875
72. Apostolou, I., and von Boehmer, H. (2004) J Exp Med 199, 1401
73. Gavin, M. A., Rasmussen, J. P., Fontenot, J. D., Vasta, V., Manganiello, V. C., Beavo, J. A., and Rudensky, A. Y. (2007) Nature 445, 771
74. Chen, Y., Kuchroo, V. K., Inobe, J., Hafler, D. A., and Weiner, H. L. (1994) Science 265, 1237
75. Groux, H., O'Garra, A., Bigler, M., Rouleau, M., Antonenko, S., de Vries, J. E., and Roncarolo, M. G. (1997) Nature 389, 737

76. Curiel, T. J., Coukos, G., Zou, L., Alvarez, X., Cheng, P., Mottram, P., Evdemon-Hogan, M., Conejo-Garcia, J. R., Zhang, L., Burow, M., Zhu, Y., Wei, S., Kryczek, I., Daniel, B., Gordon, A., Myers, L., Lackner, A., Disis, M. L., Knutson, K. L., Chen, L., and Zou, W. (2004) Nat Med 10, 942
77. Sasada, T., Kimura, M., Yoshida, Y., Kanai, M., and Takabayashi, A. (2003) Cancer 98, 1089
78. Sato, E., Olson, S. H., Ahn, J., Bundy, B., Nishikawa, H., Qian, F., Jungbluth, A. A., Frosina, D., Gnjatic, S., Ambrosone, C., Kepner, J., Odunsi, T., Ritter, G., Lele, S., Chen, Y. T., Ohtani, H., Old, L. J., and Odunsi, K. (2005) Proc Natl Acad Sci USA 102, 18538
79. Ghiringhelli, F., Menard, C., Terme, M., Flament, C., Taieb, J., Chaput, N., Puig, P. E., Novault, S., Escudier, B., Vivier, E., Lecesne, A., Robert, C., Blay, J. Y., Bernard, J., Caillat-Zucman, S., Freitas, A., Tursz, T., Wagner-Ballon, O., Capron, C., Vainchencker, W., Martin, F., and Zitvogel, L. (2005) J Exp Med 202, 1075
80. Ghiringhelli, F., Puig, P. E., Roux, S., Parcellier, A., Schmitt, E., Solary, E., Kroemer, G., Martin, F., Chauffert, B., and Zitvogel, L. (2005) J Exp Med 202, 919
81. Bettelli, E., Carrier, Y., Gao, W., Korn, T., Strom, T. B., Oukka, M., Weiner, H. L., and Kuchroo, V. K. (2006) Nature 441, 235
82. Bettelli, E., Oukka, M., and Kuchroo, V. K. (2007) Nat Immunol 8, 345
83. Neufert, C., Becker, C., Wirtz, S., Fantini, M. C., Weigmann, B., Galle, P. R., and Neurath, M. F. (2007) Eur J Immunol 37, 1
84. Huber, M., Steinwald, V., Guralnik, A., Brustle, A., Kleemann, P., Rosenplanter, C., Decker, T., and Lohoff, M. (2008), Int Immunol 20, 223
85. Villarino, A. V., Larkin, J. I., Saris, C. J. M., Canton, A. J., Lucas, S., Wong, T., de Sauvage, F. J., and Hunter, C. A. (2005) J Immunol 174
86. Batten, M., Li, J., Yi, S., Kljavin, N. M., Danilenko, D. M., Lucas, S., Lee, J., de Sauvage, F. J., and Ghilardi, N. (2006) Nat Immunol 1
87. Battaglia, M., Gregori, S., Bacchetta, R., and Roncarolo, M. G. (2006) Semin Immunol 18, 120
88. Awasthi, A., Carrier, Y., Peron, J. P., Bettelli, E., Kamanaka, M., Flavell, R. A., Kuchroo, V. K., Oukka, M., and Weiner, H. L. (2007) Nat Immunol 8, 1380
89. Fitzgerald, D. C., Zhang, G. X., El-Behi, M., Fonseca-Kelly, Z., Li, H., Yu, S., Saris, C. J., Gran, B., Ciric, B., and Rostami, A. (2007) Nat Immunol 8, 1372
90. Pasare, C. and Medzhitov, R. (2003) Science 299, 1033
91. Devergne, O., Birkenbach, M., and Kieff, E. (1997) Proc Natl Acad Sci USA 94, 12041
92. Collison, L. W., Workman, C. J., Kuo, T. T., Boyd, K., Wang, Y., Vignali, K. M., Cross, R., Sehy, D., Blumberg, R. S., and Vignali, D. A. (2007) Nature 450, 566
93. Siebler, J., Wirtz, S., Frenzel, C., Schuchmann, M., Lohse, A. W., Galle, P. R., and Neurath, M. F. (2008) J Immunol 180, 30
94. Yamanaka, A., Hamano, S., Miyazaki, Y., Ishii, K., Takeda, A., Mak, T. W., Himeno, K., Yoshimura, A., and Yoshida, H. (2004) J Immunol 172, 3590Role of IL12 Family in Regulation of Antitumor Immune Response

IL-18 in Regulation of Antitumor Immune Response and Clinical Application

Chintana Chirathaworn and Yong Poovorawan

Abstract Interleukin-18 (IL-18) is a member of the IL-1 family. Since IL-18 has been identified as an IFN-γ-inducing factor, its role in the immune response related to IFN-γ function has been widely investigated. IFN-γ is one of the Th1 cytokines, which enhances cell-mediated immune response such as macrophage and cytotoxic T cell activation. In addition, NK cell activity is activated by IFN-γ. For those reasons, IL-18 has been studied as a cytokine involved in host defense especially in killing intracellular organisms. Furthermore, NK cell activity and Th1 response are crucial in tumor cell surveillance and elimination so the application of IL-18 for cancer immunotherapy has been widely investigated. Currently, IL-18 has been known to play roles not only in cancer and defense against infection but also in pathologies of various inflammatory diseases. However, this review will gather information on IL-18 functions and applications focusing only on its role in anticancer immune response. Studies using IL-18, alone or in combination with other cytokines or proteins, have provided promising results for cancer immunotherapy. However, various data implicating that IL-18 is involved in cancer progression have also been reported. In addition, the level of IL-18 is associated with poor prognosis in various cancers. Clinical application of IL-18 in cancer immunotherapy may not be as simple as giving IL-18 to any cancer patients and expecting enhancement of antitumor immunity.

Introduction

Interleukin-18 was initially discovered in 1995 as an interferon-gamma-inducing factor (IGIF). It was cloned from the liver of mice inoculated with *Propionibacterium acne* and challenged by lipopolysaccharide (LPS) to induce toxic shock. In humans,

Y. Poovorawan (✉)
Center of Excellence in Clinical Virology, Faculty of Medicine, Chulalongkorn University, Bangkok 10330, Thailand
e-mail: Young.P@Chula.ac.th

J. Lustgarten et al. (eds.), *Targeted Cancer Immune Therapy*,
DOI 10.1007/978-1-4419-0170-5_2, © Springer Science+Business Media, LLC 2009

the *IL-18* gene is located on chromosome 11q22 and encodes a 193 amino acid precursor protein. It is a cytokine of the interleukin-1 cytokine superfamily and displays 12% and 19% amino acid sequence homologies with IL-1α and IL-1β, respectively [1–3].

IL-18 is expressed in biologically inactive form. Its precursor protein contains interleukin-1 beta converting enzyme (ICE-caspase-1) cleavage site. Caspase-1 processing of the IL-18 precursor is similar to that of IL-1β. Both IL-18 and IL-1β precursors are cleaved at the aspartic acid P1 position. The 24-kDa pro-IL-18 is cleaved by ICE-caspase-1 resulting in an 18-kDa functional molecule [4–6].

An extracellular serine esterase, proteinase-3 (PR-3), which is able to cleave pro-IL-18 into its active form, has been identified. This suggests that pro-IL-18 could also be processed extracellularly [7]. When epithelial cells are primed with IFN-γ and then stimulated with PR-3 in the presence of LPS, these cells release IL-18. Caspase-3 (CPP32) cleaves both precursor and mature forms of IL-18 into biologically inactive degraded products [8, 9]. This cleavage may potentially contribute to the down-regulation of IL-18. The release of IL-18 is caspase-1 independent [10].

Endotoxin, exotoxin, and a variety of microbial components induce IL-1, IL-6, and TNF-α production in macrophages. Those components can also stimulate IL-18 production. The predominant cell sources of IL-18 are macrophages and dendritic cells. However, IL-18 can be produced by other cell types such as Kupffer cells, T cells, B cells, osteoblasts, keratinocytes, and astrocytes [11]. IL-18 can also be produced in other epithelia such as intestinal epithelial cells and the stratified epithelium of the esophageal mucosa [12, 13]. Keratinocytes of the stratified epithelium of the skin and airway epithelium are also important sites of IL-18 production [13, 14].

IL-18 Receptor

Interleukin-18 receptor (IL-18R) belongs to the IL-1 receptor/TLR family, which has three conserved extracellular immunoglobulin-like domains and a TIR (Toll-IL-1 receptor) motif in cytoplasmic domain. IL-18R is composed of a constitutive ligand-binding α chain, which binds IL-18 with low affinity (Kd 20–40 nM) and inducible β chain which does not bind IL-18. IL-18Rα and IL-18Rβ chains form high affinity IL-18R. The tricomplex of IL-18, IL-18Rα, and IL-18Rβ forms a high affinity complex (Kd 600 nM) (Fig. 1) [15–17].

The principle cellular targets of IL-18 are NK cells and T cells. IL-18R is expressed on various cell types such as T lymphocytes, B lymphocytes, natural killer cells, and nonlymphoid cells such as macrophages, endothelial cells, fibroblasts, melanocytes, cardiomyocytes, and numerous epithelial cells. IL-18R expression is increased after activation by IL-2, IL-12, and mitogen whereas IL-4 inhibits its expression [9].

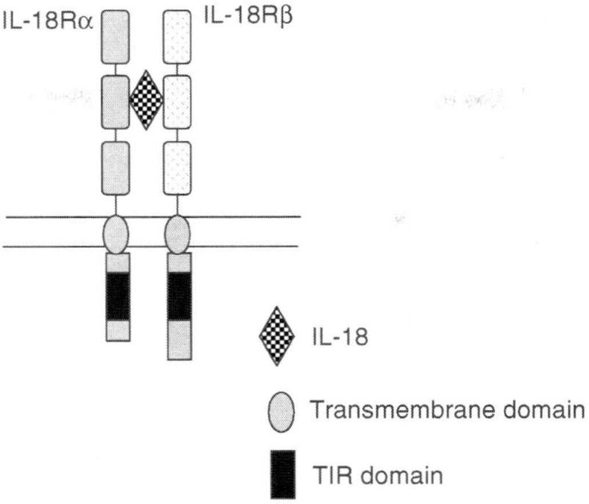

Fig. 1 IL-18 receptor: IL-18R is composed of three extracellular Ig-like domains. The cytoplasmic TIR domain is indicated by the black box. Upon binding of IL-18 to the IL-18Rα chain, the IL-18β chain is recruited to the complex and a high affinity receptor is formed

IL-18 Receptor Signal Transduction

IL18Rα, previously known as IL-1R-related protein (IL-1Rrp), is a member of the IL-1R family and represents the ligand-binding chain of IL-18R. Upon IL-18Rα binding to IL-18, IL-18Rβ, the second chain, is recruited to the signaling complex. IL-18Rβ is structurally related to IL-18Rα; however, it will not bind to IL-18 unless IL-18α is already bound to IL-18. Since the IL-18Rβ structure is also related to the IL-1 signal-transducing chain, the IL-1R accessory protein, IL-18Rβ was originally termed the IL-18R accessory protein-like chain (IL-18RAcP).

IL-18 signals IL-18R through a pathway shared with the IL-1R pathway. IL-18R is a member of the IL-1R family. Receptors in this family contain a Toll/IL-1 receptor (TIR) homology domain in the cytoplasmic tail, which is crucial for signal transduction. The IL-18R extracellular domain is composed of three Ig-like domains. Both IL-18Rα and IL-18Rβ are required for signal transduction.

The IFN-γ promoter region has binding sites for various transcription factors such as AP-1, NF-kB, NFAT, and STAT4 [18–20]. After binding of IL-18 to IL-18Rα, the IL-18Rβ is recruited to the signaling complex. Signal transduction includes recruitment of an adaptor molecule, MyD88 (myeloid differentiation factor 88) and the kinase IRAK (IL-1 receptor-associated kinase). Phosphorylated IRAK then dissociates from the IL-18R complex and interacts with TRAF-6 (TNF receptor-associated factor-6). TRAF-6 phosphorylates NIK (NF-kB-induced kinase), which in turn phosphorylates IKK resulting in NF-kB and AP-1 activation. Binding of IL-18 to IL-18R also stimulates the MAPK pathway involved in IFN-γ production (Fig. 2) [21].

Mice deficient in MyD88 do not produce acute phase protein, and do not respond to IL-1 or IL-18 [22]. Mice deficient in IRAK lack responsiveness to IL-18, and activation of NF-kB and IFN-γ production induced by IL-18 are significantly reduced [23].

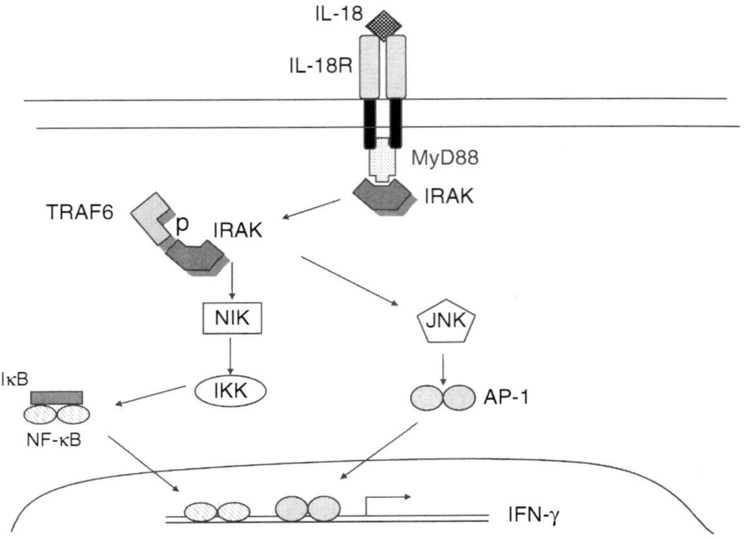

Fig. 2 IL-18R signal transduction. Binding of IL-18 to the IL-18 receptor induces recruitment of MyD88 to the cytoplasmic tail. MyD88 then recruits and activates IRAK to the receptor. Phosphorylated IRAK dissociates from the IL-18R receptor and interacts with TRAF6, which in turn activates IKK and JNK resulting in NF-κB and AP-1 activation. The activated transcription factors activate IFN-γ gene expression

IL-18 directly induces activation of the IFN-γ promoter in primary human CD4$^+$ T cells transfected with the IFN-γ promoter whereas activation of the IFN-γ promoter by IL-12 requires CD3/CD28 costimulation. Both AP-1 and STAT4 are required for IL-12-dependent IFN–γ promoter activation since mutation of the AP-1 or STAT site has been shown to abrogate IL-12-mediated IFN-γ promoter activation. However, IL-18-induced IFN-γ promoter activation is only diminished by mutation of AP-1 thus demonstrating the difference between IL-18 and IL-12 in inducing IFN-γ expression [18].

IL-18 Regulation by IL-18-Binding Protein

The regulation of IL-18 function is different from IL-1 regulation. Regulation of IL-18 function is accomplished by the soluble IL-18 binding protein (IL-18BP). IL-18BP is a naturally occurring soluble protein in the immunoglobulin superfamily. It is constitutively expressed in lymphoid tissues. In human, *IL-18BP* gene is located on chromosome 11q13. IL-18BP abrogates IFN-γ production induced by IL-18, which implicates that this protein functions in inhibition of Th1 response [24].

Binding of IL-18BP to IL-18 prevents IL-18 from binding to IL-18Rα on the target cell membrane resulting in interference with high affinity IL-18R formation (Fig. 3).

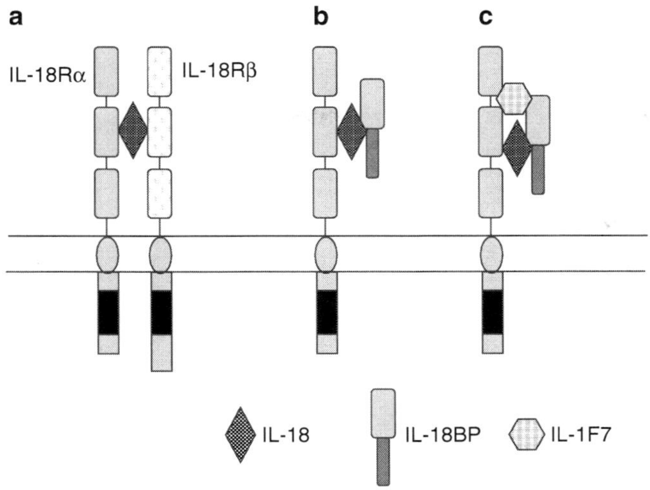

Fig. 3 IL-18 regulation by IL-18BP and IL-1F7. (**a**) Binding of IL-18 to the IL-18 receptor (**b**) Binding of IL-18BP to IL-18 prevents recruitment of the IL-18β chain to form a high affinity receptor. (**c**) Binding of IL1F7 enhances the ability of IL-18BP to inhibit binding of the IL-18β chain to IL-18Rα

IL-18BP has a high affinity (400 pM) for mature IL-18. IL-18BP is not the soluble form of IL-18R. It has only one Ig-like domain. There are four isotypes (IL-18BPa, b, c, and d) of human IL-18BP generated from alternative mRNA splicing. Only IL-18BPa and IL-18BPc have intact Ig-like domains and can neutralize IL-18. The role of the other two isoforms is still unknown [25, 26].

Binding of IL-18 glutamic acid at position 35 and lysine at position 89 to amino acids of opposite charge in IL-18BP are thought to participate in IL-18 and IL-18BP binding. Mutation analysis has demonstrated that these two amino acids are functionally important for biological activity and for neutralization.

A fusion construct of human IL-18BP-linked to Fc of IgG1 (IL-18BP-Fc) was used to demonstrate IL-18 binding and neutralization. IL-18BP-Fc binds human, mouse, and rat IL-18 with high affinity and it blocks IL-18-induced IFN-γ production in KG-1 cells. IL-18BP-Fc blocks IFN-γ production in mice challenged with LPS. Moreover, IL-18BP-Fc prevents liver damage induced by *Pseudomonas aeruginosa* exotoxin suggesting that IL-18BP can function as a natural inhibitor of IL-18 [27].

IFN-γ up-regulates and induces the release of IL-18BP. Besides endothelial cells and monocytes/macrophages, IL-18BP expression has also been shown in epithelial cells, spleen, and intestinal tract. The 20- to 30-fold molar excess of IL-18BP over IL-18 and the high binding affinity of IL-18BP to IL-18 make IL-18BP an important natural occurring inhibitor of IL-18 [28–30].

Another regulator of IL-18 activity is binding of a member of the IL-1 family, IL-1F7. IL-1F7b shares two conserved amino acids (Glu-35 and Lys-124) with IL-18. These amino acids participate in binding to the IL-18Rα chain and IL-18BP.

The IL-1F7b isoform can be cleaved by caspase-1 resulting in a mature protein that can bind IL-18Rα with low affinity. Binding of IL-1F7b results in failure of IL-18Rβ chain recruitment to form a functionally active complex. Binding of IL-1F7b to IL-18BP enhances the ability of IL-18BP to inhibit IL-18-induced IFN-γ production [31, 32].

IL-18 in Regulation of Antitumor Immune Response

Antitumor immunity is mainly affected by natural killer (NK) cells and cytotoxic T cells (CTL). In addition to macrophage-derived cytokines such as IL-12, NK cells can be activated by IFN-γ. IL-12 can act in synergy with TNF-α to stimulate IFN-γ production from NK cells. IFN-γ induces NK cell activation. IL-12 also induces specific $CD4^+$ T cells to secrete IFN-γ and TNF-α.

Activation of T helper cells generates two types of immune response: Th1 and Th2. Th1 immune response is activated by IL-2, IFN-γ, and TNF-β. Th1 cytokines such as IL-2, IFN-γ activated macrophages and cytotoxic T cells generate cell-mediated immune response. Th2 response is enhanced by IL-4, IL-5, IL-6, and IL-10. Th1 and Th2 cells regulate each other by cytokines they secrete.

Since IFN-γ is a cytokine involved in stimulation of various cells in the immune system, especially NK cells and CTL, induction of this cytokine is promising for cancer immunotherapy. Besides IL-12, IL-18 is another cytokine known to induce IFN-γ.

IL-18 in IFNγand Th1 Response Induction

IL-18 can stimulate a small amount of IFN-γ production on its own. IL-18 and IL-12 synergistically induce IFN-γ production. Moreover, it has been clearly demonstrated that IL-18 synergizes with IL-12 in induction of Th1 response. IL-12 stimulation increases T cells positive for IL-18R. Then, these T cells respond to IL-18 by proliferation and enhanced IFN-γ production (Fig. 4). Th1 cells, but not Th2 cells, increase IL-18R expression and IFN-γ production in response to IL-18. IL-18 regulates IFN-γ promoter activity by binding to the AP-1 site in the IFN-γ promoter region while IL-12 induces its production only after the activation of a costimulatory signal by CD28 in T cells. [18, 33, 34].

Ovalbumin and IL-18 fusion DNA efficiently increased OVA-specific IFN-γ production, anti-OVA IgG2a isotypes and inhibited IL-4 production in C57BL/6 mice when compared with injection of ovalbumin DNA only [35]. Injection of anti-CD3sFv/IL-18 DNA efficiently increased the production of both ovalbumin-specific IFN-γ and anti-ovalbumin IgG2a, compared with injection of anti-CD3sFv DNA only. This further suggests that stimulation of TCR in the presence of IL-18 promotes Th1 response [36].

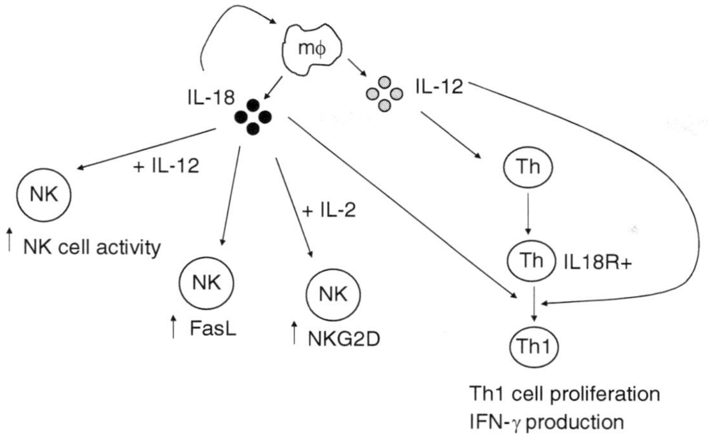

Fig. 4 IL-18 induces Th1 response and NK cell activation. IL-12 induces IL-18 receptor expression. Then, IL-12 and IL-18 synergistically induce IFN-γ production and Th1 cell proliferation. IL-18 induces FasL expression, IL-18 in combination with IL-12 activate NK cells, and IL-18 + IL-2 increase NKG2D expression

IL-18 in NK Cell Activation

NK cells are cells of the innate immune response that are involved in killing cells infected with virus or tumor cells. The effect of IL-18 on NK cell activity has been demonstrated (Fig. 4). Since IL-12 influences NK cell activity, the role of IL-18 on NK cell function has been investigated. NK cells freshly prepared from C57BL/6 spleen cells strikingly proliferated in response to combinations of IL-12 and IL-18 but not to the individual cytokine. The combination of IL-12 and IL-18 also enhances IFN-γ production and NK cell activity. IL-18, like IL-12, fails to enhance NK activity of splenocytes of perforin-deficient mice, which suggests that IL-18 and IL-12 up-regulate perforin-mediated cytotoxic activity of NK cells [37, 38].

It has been shown that IL-18 enhances FasL expression on NK cell lines. Administration of IL-18 to CL8-1 melanoma bearing mice suppressed tumor growth and up-regulated the FasL mRNA expression in splenocytes. The antitumor effect of IL-18 is mediated by NK cells. IL-18 was administered into wild type, Fas deficient and FasL deficient mice to demonstrate the role of FasL in the IL-18 antitumor effect. The antitumor effect of IL-18 was completely abrogated in FasL deficient but not in Fas deficient or wild type mice. This suggests that the antitumor effect of IL-18 is FasL-dependent [39].

The application of IL-18 in cancer therapy has been investigated in various cancer models. The induction of antitumor immunity by IL-18 administration has been shown. Depletion of NK cells abrogates this anticancer activity of IL-18 suggesting that IL-18 induced antitumor immune response is mediated by NK cells [40–42].

Tumor cells can evade being killed by NK cells by various mechanisms. One such mechanism is down-modulation of the activating receptor on NK cells. TGF-β secreted by tumors down-regulate an NK-activating receptor, NKG2D, resulting in poor NK cell activity. Patients with lung cancer or colorectal cancer have elevated levels of TGF-β, and this elevation is inversely correlated with NKG2D expression on NK cells in these patients. TGF-β reduces NKG2D expression on NK cells and lymphokine-activated killer cells and thus decreases their potential to kill tumor cells.

IL-2/IL-18 increases NKG2D expression in TGF-β treated NK cell lines. These two cytokines prevent TGF-β-induced NKG2D down-regulation of NK cells via the JNK pathway. Furthermore, NK cytotoxicity reduced by TGF-β was restored by IL-2/IL-18 treatment. This suggests that IL-18 does not only activate NK cells but is also involved in protecting the NK cell activating receptors from down modulation by TGF-β secreted by tumor cells [43–45].

IL-18 in Cytotoxic T Cell Activation

The effect of IL-18 on cytotoxic T cells has also been reported. Mouse fibroblasts expressing B7-1 and IL-18 were loaded with an ovalbumin (OVA) epitope, and these cells were tested for the induction of OVA-specific CTLs in C57BL/6 mice. Immunization with the IL-18/B7-1-transfected fibroblasts induced strong cytotoxic activities against OVA-expressing EL4 (EG7) tumor cells. The acitvity of OVA-specific cytotoxic $CD8^+$ T cells in mice with the IL-18/B7-1-transfected fibroblasts was significantly higher than the response in mice immunized with IL-18 or B7-1 constructs alone. Moreover, treatment with the IL-18/B7-1-transfected fibroblasts significantly prolonged the survival of EG7 tumor-bearing mice. This suggests that IL-18 enhances the ability to present antigen and thus, induces antigen-specific CTL response [46].

IL-18 as a Precancerous Factor

Although its anticancer effect has been demonstrated, the precancerous effect of IL-18 has also been reported. Park et al. were the first group that reported elevated expression and secretion of IL-18 in cancer patients. Expression and secretion of IL-18 were elevated in squamous cell carcinoma, melanoma, and skin cancer cell lines [47]. In gastric carcinoma patients, IL-18 expression was higher in tumor regions than in nontumor regions [48]. Association of IL-18 levels with tumor progression and metastasis has been reported. The role of IL-18 in cancer immune evasion, increased cancer cell adherence to the microvascular wall and increased angiogenic and tumor growth-stimulating factor production has been shown [49]. According to these observations, the role of IL-18 in cancer progression has been widely studied.

IL-18 in Tumor Growth and Immune Evasion

Cancer cells evade the immune response via various mechanisms such as down regulation of MHC I expression, interference with antigen processing and presentation and increase in FasL expression [50–52]. The effects of IL-18 involvement in tumor immune escape have been reported. IL-18 induces FasL expression in melanoma cells and melanoma cells transfected with antisense IL-18 were more susceptible to NK cell killing than wild type cells [53].

Expression of IL-18R was demonstrated in four gastric cancer cell lines MKN28, MKN45, NUGC3, KATOII. IL-18 enhanced in vitro proliferation of these cell lines and NF-kB activation in a dose-dependent fashion. When IL-18 pretreated gastric cancer cells were incubated with cytokine-activated peripheral blood killer lymphocytes, perforin or interferon-gamma production of killer lymphocytes decreased, resulting in a decreased susceptibility of cancer cells to be killed. IL-18 treated gastric cancer cells showed increased expression of granzyme B and protease inhibitor. IL-18 injection into SCID mice inoculated with gastric cancer cells decreased the animals' survival time. This suggests that gastric cancer cells utilized IL-18 to evade host immune surveillance [54].

IL-18 in Tumor Angiogenesis

Angiogenesis is the process of new vessel formation, which is crucial in inflammatory response, wound healing, and tumor progression [55]. Solid tumors require new blood vessels to supply them with oxygen and nutrients for their growth. Vascular endothelial growth factor (VEGF), platelet-derived growth factor (PDGF), fibroblast growth factor (FGF), TGF-β, and angiogenin are angiogenesis activators [56–58].

Factors or cytokines that help induce angiogenesis or increase angiogenic factors are suspected to be involved in tumor progression. IL-18 induces conditions favorable for tumors not only by facilitating tumor immune evasion but also by involving angiogenesis and metastasis.

The influence of IL-18 on angiogenic factor secretion was demonstrated in rheumatoid arthritis (RA) patients. IL-18 has been suggested to be involved in the pathogenesis of RA. IL-18 up-regulates secretion of angiogenic factors such as stromal cell-derived factor 1alpha (SDF-1alpha)/CXCL12, monocyte chemoattractant protein 1 (MCP-1)/CCL2, and VEGF in synovial tissue fibroblasts of RA patients.

The induction of SDF-1alpha/CXCL12 by IL-18 is dependent on JNK, p38 MAPK, phosphatidylinositol 3-kinase (PI3K), PKCdelta, and NFkappaB. IL-18-induced MCP-1/CCL2 production is mediated by JNK, PI3K, PKCalpha, and NFkappaB. IL-18-induced VEGF production is mediated mainly by JNK-2, PKCalpha, and NFkappaB. This demonstrates that different signaling intermediates are involved in secretion of SDF-1alpha/CXCL12, MCP-1/CCL2, and VEGF in synovial tissue fibroblasts stimulated with IL-18 [59].

A subsequent study on IL-18 and VEGF in RA patients reported that levels of IL-18 and VEGF in sera and synovial fluids of RA patients were significantly higher than those of osteoarthritis (OA) patients. Fibroblast-like synoviocytes (FLS) isolated from synovial tissues of RA patients were stimulated with IL-18. This stimulation increased VEGF secretion and AP-1 biding. AP-1-specific inhibitor inhibited these effects of IL-18. This suggests that IL-18 stimulates binding of AP-1 to the VEGF promoter resulting in VEGF mRNA and protein expression. VEGF induction by IL-18 may thus be involved in enhanced angiogenesis in tumor [60].

In gastric cancer patients, high expression of IL-18 was detected in invasive tissue with high microvessel density, which suggested that IL-18 expression may be associated with new blood vessel formation [48].

Thrombospondin (TSP-1) is known to inhibit angiogenesis in several cancers; however, it has been shown that TSP-1 stimulated angiogenesis in gastric cancer. IL-18 induced TSP-1 mRNA and protein expression in gastric cancer cells. This effect was inhibited by SP600125, a c-Jun N-terminal kinase (JNK) specific inhibitor, which implicates that IL-18 may be involved in angiogenesis by increasing TSP-1 production via the JNK pathway [61].

High levels of IL-18 have been shown associated with poorer prognosis of myeloma patients. The levels were higher in patients at stage III than stages II and I and IL-18 levels decreased after treatment. The levels of IL-18 also correlated with levels of VEGF in these patients [62].

IL-18 in Tumor Metastasis

Cell migration and angiogenesis are the key steps in tumor metastasis. Metastasis is a complex process including degradation of extracellular matrix (ECM) and regulation of various adhesion molecules and chemokine receptors. After ECM degradation, cancer cells migrate to another site by regulation of adhesion molecules. Cancer in patients with metastasis is more aggressive than primary cancer.

The ability of B16F10 cells (murine melanoma cells) to migrate was reduced after transfection with antisense IL-18. Exogenous IL-18 treatment improved migration ability, suggesting that IL-18 enhanced the migration ability of melanoma cells. Reactive oxygen intermediate (ROI) levels and ERK1/2 phosphorylation were increased by IL-18. An antioxidant, *N*-acetyl-L-cystein (NAC), and PD98059, a MAPK inhibitor, blocked these effects induced by IL-18. These results suggest that IL-18 enhances melanoma cell migration through the generation of ROI and activation of the MAPK pathway [63].

The effect of IL-18 on VEGF-induced migration was also investigated in gastric cancer. VEGF induces migration of VEGF receptor-2-expressing SNU-601 cells. An antioxidant and an ERK1/2-specific inhibitor block VEGF-enhanced IL-18 production. In addition, inhibiting IL-18 markedly reduced VEGF-enhanced migration. This suggests that IL-18 is involved in VEGF-enhanced cell migration [64].

The relationship between matrix metalloproteinases (MMPs) and IL-18 has been investigated. MMP-9/-2 and IL-18 are over-expressed in some hematologic malignancies such as acute myeloid leukemia (AML). This over-expression is associated with poor disease prognosis. IL-18 significantly upregulated transmigration of the human myeloid leukemia cell line, HL-60. The migration induced by IL-18 was inhibited by an MMP inhibitor, anti-MMR-9, anti-MMP-2, and anti-IL-18 antibodies. This demonstrates that IL-18 induces gelatinase activity leading to ECM degradation and then transmigration [65].

Lung cancer metastasis induced by IL-18 has been demonstrated. The effect of IL-18 on PLA801D, lung giant cell carcinoma cells, was studied. IL-18 was only detected in the highly metastatic PLA801D subline, which suggests that IL-18 may play a role in metastasis. When the poorly metastatic PLA801C subline was transfected with sense IL-18, cell motility in vitro was significantly increased and the E-cadherin protein was significantly down-regulated. IL-18 antisense decreased cell migration and increased E-cadherin expression in transfected cells. This implicates that IL-18 might play a role in tumor metastasis of lung cancer by down-regulating E-cadherin expression [66, 67].

Interaction between tumor cells and endothelial cells contributes to tumor cell arrest and extravasation during metastasis. Several cytokines such as TNF-α and IL-1β up-regulate vascular cell adhesion molecule-1 (VCAM-1) expression. Conditioned medium from B16M melanoma cells (B16M-CM) induced TNF-α, IL-1β, and IL-18 production from primary hepatic sinusoidal endothelium (HSE). This medium also increased B16M cell adhesion to HSE. In addition, exogenous IL-18 increased the number of melanoma cells adhering to HSE. ICE inhibitors anti-IL18 and IL-18BP inhibit this adhesion. These results demonstrate a role of IL-18 in hepatic metastases of B16M [68, 69].

Accumulating evidences support that IL-18 can enhance tumor progression by various mechanisms such as promoting tumor growth, protecting tumor from being killed by the immune effector cells, and enhancing angiogenesis and metastasis (Fig. 5).

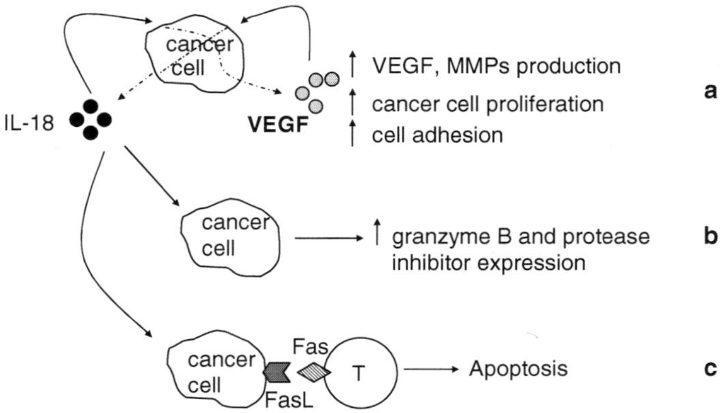

Fig. 5 IL-18 enhances angiogenesis, metastasis and immune evasion. Cancer cells can secrete IL-18 which can induce tumor growth, VEGF and MMP production and increased cell adhesion resulting in tumor progression (**a**). IL-18 induces granzyme B and protease inhibitor expression (**b**) and FasL expression (**c**) to interfere with killing mechanisms and induce apoptosis of effector cells

IL-18 as a Cancer Prognostic Marker

Since high levels of IL-18 have been detected in cancer patients and IL-18 secretion associates with tumor immune evasion, angiogenesis, and metastasis, the levels of IL-18 may be an indicator of unfavorable prognosis in cancer patients. Association of IL-18 levels with cancer progression has been investigated in various types of cancer.

Mean serum IL-18 expression was higher in patients with cutaneous T cell lymphoma and cutaneous natural killer cell lymphoma when compared with controls. Peripheral blood mononuclear cells from patients stimulated with anti-CD3 or IL-18 produced lower levels of IFN-γ than controls [70].

Levels of sICAM-1 have been widely studied as a cancer marker. Since IL-18 enhances ICAM-1, the use of IL-18 serum levels as a marker for metastatic cancer was investigated. IL-18 levels were significantly higher in patients with liver or bone metastases compared with patients without metastases and healthy donors [71]. This suggests that IL-18 levels could be used as a metastasis breast cancer marker.

The IL-18 level was elevated in patients with hemophagocytic lymphohistiocytosis (HLH) when compared with healthy controls. In addition, the level gradually decreased in the course of clinical improvement. IL-18 may be involved in the pathogenesis of HLH patients [72].

Serum IL-18 levels were significantly higher in patients with breast cancer when compared with the controls and the levels in patients whose tumor size was greater than or equal to 5 cm were higher than in patients whose tumor size was less than or equal to 2 cm. Patients who were axillary lymph node negative (ALN) had lower serum IL-18 levels than patients with positive ALN. Moreover, serum IL-18 levels were significantly higher in patients with stage IIB or IIIA when compared with patients with stage I or IIA [73]. IL-18 has been suggested as a marker for breast cancer progression since the IL-18 level was higher in patients with metastasis than in normal volunteers and breast cancer patients without metastasis. Statistically significant differences between the levels of IL-18 in breast cancer patients with or without metastasis and the control group were shown. A significant increase in IL-18 level in metastatic as opposed to nonmetastatic cancer was also observed. This suggests that IL-18 is an important marker for suspected invasive metastasis [71, 74].

Serum IL-18 levels were elevated in ovarian cancer patients and were correlated with overall survival [75]. IL-18 levels increase and correlate with tumor growth in esophageal carcinoma patients. Mean serum IL-18 levels of patients with esophageal carcinoma were significantly higher than of healthy volunteers. Furthermore, the mean levels increased in patients as the disease stage progressed [76].

Renal cell carcinoma patients showed significantly higher IL-18 levels when compared with control subjects. The levels in patients with grade 3 and 4 tumors are higher than in patients with grade 1 and 2 tumors [77].

Serum IL-18 levels were significantly higher in bladder cancer patients when compared with control subjects. Moreover, the level was higher in patients with Ta stage than patients with T1 and T2, T3, T4 stages and in patients with grade 1 tumors than patients with grade 2 and grade 3 tumors [78].

Determining IL-18 levels in combination with other tumor markers increased specificity of detection. IL-18 and FGF-2 were significantly elevated in tumor tissues from patients with ovarian cancer. The combined use of IL-18, FGF-2, and CA125 showed similar sensitivity for ovarian cancer scoring compared with that of CA125 alone; however, the combination significantly improved specificity of detection [79].

Serum IL-18 levels of oesophageal cancer patients were significantly higher than in the control group. The levels were significantly higher in stage IV patients in comparison to patients surgically treated. Statistically significant differences were observed upon comparing IL-18 levels between patients with different stages, tumor depth and lymph node metastasis [80].

IL-18 levels in the gastric cancer patient group were significantly higher than in the gastric ulcer patient group [81].

Investigation of IL-18 as a prognostic factor in hepatocellular carcinoma was also reported. Levels of IL-18 were significantly higher when compared with controls and the levels correlated with advanced tumor stages. Patients with high serum IL-18 levels had a poorer prognosis than patients with lower levels [82].

Besides IL-18, association of IL-18R expression with patient prognosis was reported. IL-18 increases NF-kB activation and the expression of Bcl-xL and xIAP mRNA in hepatocellular carcinoma (HCC) cells and suppresses apoptosis of HCC cells induced by etoposide in vitro. A study in patients with HCC associated with HCV infection demonstrated that the overall survival rate is significantly lower in IL-18 receptor-positive patients than in the IL-18 receptor negative patients. The prevention of apoptosis in HCC cells by IL-18 may be one of the pathogenic mechanisms in HCC [83].

Genetic factors are involved in cancer development and progression. IL-18 is a multifunctional cytokine that induces IFN-γ secretion and plays a role in both antitumor immunity and in cancer progression. Variations in the IL-18 promoter may lead to altered IL-18 production and/or activity resulting in modulation of an individual's susceptibility to cancer.

The relationship between the IL-18 gene promoter −137 G/C and −607 C/A polymorphisms and their haplotypes and the risk of prostate cancer in the Chinese population was demonstrated. There were significant differences in the genotype and allele distribution of −137 G/C polymorphisms of the IL-18 gene between cases and controls. The −137 G/C and C/C genotypes were associated with a significant risk of prostate cancer when compared with −137 G/C genotypes. The −137C/−607A haplotype was associated with a significantly increased risk of prostate cancer when compared with the 137G/−607C haplotype [84].

Polymorphism at −607 A/C in conjunction with the development of colorectal cancer was shown. The proportion of heterozygotes in the patient group was significantly higher than that in healthy controls. This significant increase was detected independently of Duke's tumor stage. The carrier frequency of the mutant A allele was significantly higher in the patient group compared with controls. Heterozygotes for the IL-18 −607 A/C polymorphisms exhibited an increased risk for colorectal cancer development [85].

Currently, there are a few reports on association between IL-18 promoter polymorphisms and risk of cancer development or progression. The results of studies are still controversial. Some reports demonstrate no association between certain IL-18 promoter polymorphisms in cancer development or protection. To investigate genetic susceptibility involving the IL-18 gene is not that simple because IL-18 is a multifunctional cytokine with its expression regulated by various transcription factors and by other cytokines. In addition, anticancer immunity is regulated by various cytokines and different types of cancers and cancer stages may respond differently to certain cytokines or therapy.

IL-18 in Cancer Therapy

Because of its known functions in the enhancement of Th1 response and NK cell activity, IL-18 has been a promising cytokine for cancer therapy. A number of studies that support IL-18 application in tumor elimination have been reported.

The phase I study on toxicity, pharmacokinetics, and biological activities in patients with advanced cancer (such as renal cell cancer, melanoma, and Hodgkin's lymphoma) following recombinant human IL-18 (rhIL-18) administration has been reported. IL-18 was given in doses ranging from 3 to 1,000 μg/kg. Common side effects and laboratory abnormalities included chills, fever, nausea, headache, hypotension, transient, asymptomatic grade 1 to 2 neutropenia, thrombocytopenia, anemia, hypoalbuminemia, hyponatremia, and elevations in liver transaminases. IL-18 plasma levels increased when the given dose was increased. Its administration leads to an increase in serum IFN-γ, GM-CSF, IL-18-binding protein, and soluble Fas ligand. This study suggests that rhIL-18 is safe to be given in biologically active doses to patients with advanced cancer [86].

Antitumor activity of IL-18 has been investigated in various studies by administration of IL-18 alone or in combination with other cytokines or molecules. Furthermore, immunization with DNA vaccine has been widely studied for enhancing humoral and cellular immune responses against cancer and infectious diseases. The IL-18 gene has been used alone or fused with various genes for other cytokines or proteins as DNA vaccines aimed at enhancing the immune response.

The effect of IL-18 in enhancing tumor immunity in hepatic cancer was demonstrated. CT26, murine colon adenocarcinoma cells, were identified in mouse liver before IL-18 naked DNA vaccine was injected directly into the liver. IL-18 treatment augmented the numbers of effector T cells, NK cells, and IFN-γ secreting cells. Tumor growth was reduced with this treatment [87].

Administration of IL-18 into mice before or after challenge with a mouse melanoma cell line, CL8-1, suppressed tumor growth and reduced the number of mice displaying tumor growth. The establishment of CL8-1 was abrogated in all animals. The antitumor effects of IL-18 were abrogated upon elimination of NK cells, which suggests that the antitumor effect is mediated by NK cells [41].

IL-18 administration induced antitumor effects in BALB/c mice challenged intraperitoneally with syngeneic Meth A sarcoma or in tumor bearing mice. Mice pretreated with IL-18 before tumor challenge survived whereas control mice died within 3 weeks of challenge. The antitumor effect was mediated by NK cells. The spleen cells from resistant mice exhibited Meth A cell killing in vitro [40].

The therapeutic potential of IL-18 for patients with glioma has also been reported. Intratumor injection of IL-18 led to brain tumor regression in mice. Intraperitoneally administered IL-18 delayed the growth of subcutaneously inoculated gliomas but not of gliomas in the brain. Tumor regression was not observed in NK cell-depleted mice [42].

In addition, access of IL-18 to the central nervous system has been increased by controlled manipulation aimed at inducing antitumor activity against glioma. IL-18 was loaded onto biodegradable poly(D,L-lactide-*co*-glycolide) (PLGA)sustained-release microspheres for stereotaxic implantation into CNS tumors. Biological activity of IL-18 after release from microspheres was preserved, and the amounts of the active cytokine released were sufficiently relevant to validate therapeutic strategy [88]. Refining this method of cytokine delivery will overcome the difficulty in accessing and subsequently eradicating CNS tumors.

Retroviral constructs expressing IL-18 were introduced into a murine neuroblastoma cell line (N-2a). N-2a cells secreting mature IL-18 (N-2a/IL-18) were nontumorigenic, whereas N-2a cells expressing proIL-18 (N-2a/IL-18p) or parental N-2a cells were tumorigenic. However, N-2a expressing IL-18 could induce tumors in mice lacking $CD4^+$ and $CD8^+$ T cells, which suggests that the antitumor effect is mediated by T cells [89].

The synergistic antitumor effect of IL-18 in combination with cells expressing a costimulatory molecule, B7-1 (CD80), was shown. Murine B16 melanoma cells expressing B7-1 were inoculated alone or in combination with IL-18 into C57BL/6 mice bearing B16 melanoma cells. Administration of B7-1 expressing B16 cells in combination with IL-18 suppressed tumor growth and significantly prolonged survival. Moreover, NK cell activity and INF-γ production were increased by this treatment. NK cell infiltration into tumors was observed. Depletion of NK cells inhibited the antitumor effect. Administration of either B7-1 expressing B16 cells or IL-18 alone has no antitumor effect [90].

The combined effect with another costimulatory molecule, B7-2, has also been studied. Plasmids carrying IL18 and B7-2 genes were injected into melanoma tumor-bearing mice. This administration in combination with X-ray irradiation showed slower B16 tumor growth and a significant increase in cytotoxic T cells, NK cells, TNF-α, and IFN-γ production, when compared with either treatment on its own [91].

Interleukin-12 (IL-12) has been known as a cytokine that induces Th1 polarization. In addition, it can activate NK cell activity. Synergistic effects of IL-12 and IL-18 in antitumor activity have been demonstrated. Tumor-draining lymph node (TDLN) cells were treated with anti-CD3/antiCD28 followed by stimulation with IL-12 and /or IL-18. IL-18 plus IL-12 showed a synergistic effect in augmenting IFN-γ and

GM-CSF secretion. IL-18 alone had only a minimal effect. IL-18 prevented IL-12 stimulated TDLN cells from producing IL-10. Specific NFkB inhibitors significantly suppressed IL-12/IL-18-induced IFN-γ secretion. TDLN cells cultured in medium enriched with a combination of IL-12 and IL-18 infiltrated pulmonary tumor nodes and eradicated established tumor metastases more efficiently than T cells cultured with IL-12 or IL-18 alone [92].

Injection of a vector encoding IL-18 into mice with MCA205 fibrosarcoma completely eradicated tumors and induced protective systemic immunity in all animals. Administration of IL-12 in combination with IL-18 established synergistic antitumor effects. Depletion of NK cells abrogated the antitumor effect [93].

Fusion vaccines of dendritic cells into tumor cells have the advantage of inducing an immune response against various kinds of tumors. In a liver metastasis model, C1300 neuroblastoma cells were used to demonstrate the IL-18 effect on dendritic cell vaccines. Transduction of IL-12 and IL-18 into fusion cells engendered higher IFN-γ, NK cell, and CTL activity than could be observed in the controls [94].

Apoptin is a chicken anemia virus-derived protein that induces apoptosis in tumors but not in normal cells. The genes for apoptin and IL-18 were simultaneously transferred into C57BL/6 mice bearing Lewis lung carcinoma (LLC) to demonstrate the effect of IL-18. The combination of these two genes inhibited the growth of established tumors in mice. Pronounced NK cell and CTL activity was observed in vitro. T cells from lymph nodes of mice vaccinated with either the IL-18 gene alone or with a combination of the *IL-18* gene and the *apoptin* gene secreted high levels of IL-2 and IFN-γ. This implicates that the vaccination inhibited tumor growth by inducing Th1 response. The combination of IL-18 with apoptin may be useful for cancer immunotherapy [95].

Another protein that is fused to IL-18 to enhance its effect is epidermal growth factor (EGF). EGF regulates cell cycle and differentiation. A fusion protein, consisting of the EGFR-binding domain and the mature human IL-18 peptide was constructed and expressed in the insect cell line Sf9 using the baculovirus expression system. This fusion protein induced human PBMC to secrete levels of IFN-γ similar to those induced by native IL-18. This fusion protein can specifically bind the EGF receptor and compete with native EGF.

The antitumor effect of the EGF/IL-18 fusion protein was investigated. This fusion protein induces IFN-γ secretion in KG-1 cells, and promotes PBMC proliferation. It also stimulates $CD4^+$ T cell activation. Furthermore, the EGF-IL-18 fusion protein induces significant tumor regression in SMMC-7721-xenografted Balb/c nude mice when administered together with peritumoral injections of X-ray-irradiated NK-92 cells. The treatment induces tumor cell arrest in the G1 phase and apoptosis [96, 97].

Alpha-Galactosylceramide (alpha-GalCer) activates NK cells through stimulation of cytokine secretion by NKT cells. IL-18 can activate NK cells directly. The antitumor effect of these two NK cell activators was studied in melanoma. NK cell-sensitive mouse B16 melanoma cells injected into a mouse tail vein produced pulmonary metastasis. Administration of either alpha-GalCer or IL-18 subsequent to injection of B16 melanoma cells markedly suppressed the number of pulmonary metastatic foci. Injecting a combination of IL-18 and alpha-GalCer enhanced NK cell cytotoxicity and increased the number of NK cells in the lung. The antitumor effect of this combined administration was abolished by treating mice with anti-asialo GM1 serum to deplete NK cells but not NKT cells. The effect observed upon combined administration is likely due to IL-18 directly stimulating NK cells and alpha-Gal-Cer stimulating NKT cells to produce cytokines such as IL-12, IFN-γ to activate NK cells [98].

MUC1 (mucin 1) is a transmembrane glycoprotein normally expressed on epithelia of the pancreas, breast, prostate, colon, and lung. In adenocarcinomas, MUC1 is overexpressed and aberrantly glycosylated, which makes it an interesting target for immunotherapy. Cancer therapy with a combination of IL-18 with this self-antigen has been reported. DNA plasmids encoding human MUC1 (pMUC1) and mouse interleukin-18 (pmuIL-18) were constructed. Vaccination with this construct protected MUC1 transgenic mice (MUC1.Tg) from subcutaneous tumor challenge and prevented and treated pulmonary metastases in these mice. Moreover, MUC1 in combination with IL-18 reduced the incidence of lung tumor and prolonged survival. Vaccination with plasmid expressing either MUC1 or IL-18 alone was not sufficient to elicit antitumor effects. A combination of MUC1 and IL-18 protected mice from challenge with MUC1-positive tumors, but not MUC1-negative tumors specificity of the antitumor response was also observed. Depletion of $CD8^+$ T cells and IFN-γ demonstrated that antitumor immunity was mediated by $CD8^+$ T cells and IFN-γ. It has been suggested that IL-18 induces antitumor immunity by breaking the tolerance to MUC1. This further implicates its benefit in cancer therapy since it can induce immunity against the over-expressed self-antigen [99].

The effect of IL-18 as an adjuvant in a prosthetic-specific antigen (PSA) DNA vaccine was demonstrated in a mouse tumor model. Low doses of PSA did not induce protection; however, when the IL-18 plasmid was coadministered, tumor protection was observed. This treatment induced IFN-γ production, enhanced splenocyte activity, and Th1 cell proliferation. Protection was mediated by $CD4^+$ and $CD8^+$ T cells [100].

Since IL-18 has been shown to be involved in cancer progression instead of protection in several reports and IL-18BP is known as a naturally occurring IL-18 regulator, IL-18BP has become another attractive protein used for cancer therapy.

The anticancer effect of IL-18BP in hepatic metastasis has been reported. Injection of IL-18BP prior to intrasplenic injection of B16M cells reduced the number of hepatic metastatic foci and metastatic volume. In addition, reduced intrahepatic retention of B16M cells was observed. VCAM-1 up-regulation in the hepatic microvasculature was abolished. When hepatic sinusoidal endothelium (HSE) cells isolated from IL-18BP-treated mice were assayed for adhesion to B16M cells, the level of adhesion was reduced to that of cells from normal mice. B16M induced melanoma growth factor production from normal HSE. Addition of IL-18BP suppressed the release of this growth factor. The effects of IL-18BP observed suggest that IL-18 promotes growth of melanoma cells and up-regulates VCAM-1 expression on endothelium resulting in tumor cell adhesion and migration. Inhibition of IL-18 effects by IL-18BP may help prevent metastases in cancer therapy.

Interestingly, IL-18 production can be induced by statins, which are compounds that inhibit 3-hydroxy-3-methylglutaryl coenzyme-A (HMG-CoA) reductase and have been used for lowering lipid levels. Moreover, the effect of statins as immunomodulators has been widely studied. Statins can inhibit Ras farnesylation and, thus, are thought to reduce the risk of cancer. Because of its role in cancer risk reduction, the effect of statins on IL-18 production has been investigated. Pravastatin, fluvastatin, and simvastatin induced IL-18 production in human monocytes. This effect was inhibited by mevalonate indicating that inhibition of HMG-CoA reductase results in IL-18 production [101].

The activity of an anticancer drug, 5-fluorouracil (5-FU), has been shown to be involved in IL-18 production. Pancreatic carcinoma cell lines constitutively express IL-18. However, it has been shown in Capan-2, pancreatic tumor cells, that IL-18 secreted from this cell type is an IL-18 precursor with no biological activity. 5-FU is a compound commonly used in pancreatic cancer treatment. This compound induces caspase-1 and caspase-3 activation and subsequent secretion of processed mature IL-18 in Capan-2 cells. Conditioned medium from 5-FU-treated Capan-2 cells induced IFN-γ production by activated T cells in an IL-18-dependent manner. Furthermore, 5-FU significantly increases serum levels of bioactive IL-18 in pancreatic carcinoma patients. These findings demonstrate the mechanism by which a chemotherapeutic agent modulates the immune response [102].

Summary

It has been well-established that IL-18, a pleiotropic cytokine, enhances IFN-γ production, NK cell function, and Th1 cell development. However, it has been shown that IL-18 can also induce Th2 response. IL-18 and IL-12 in the presence of antigen induce development of naïve T cells into Th1 cells. IL-18 on its own induces the Th2 cytokines, IL-4 and IL-13, from T cells, NK cells, basophils, and mast cells. Moreover, naïve T cells can develop into Th2 in the presence of IL-2, IL-18, and antigen. This implicates that the involvement of IL-18 in development of naïve T cells into either Th1 or Th2 cells depends on the cytokine milieu [11, 103–105]. Th2 response and production of factors promoting angiogenesis and metastasis induced by IL-18 could enhance cancer progression instead of eradication. Increased cell adhesion molecule expression is important for interaction between T cells and tumor cells for proper recognition and killing. However, cell adhesion molecule expression induced by IL-18 can also promote tumor metastasis.

Besides inducing IFN-γ production, IL-18 also induces production of other cytokines such as TNF-α, IL-6, and IL-8. TNF-α has been extensively shown to induce tumor progression. It can be produced by various tumors and has been shown to induce tumor cell transformation, proliferation, and angiogenesis [106–119]. IL-6 can act as a growth factor for multiple myeloma, bladder cancer, colorectal cancer, and renal cell carcinoma [120–123]. IL-8 promotes growth and metastasis of various cancers such as melanoma, ovarian cancer, astrocytomas, glioblastoma, and CNS cervical carcinoma metastasis [124–126]. Although IL-18 facilitates the immune response against tumor cells by enhancing IFN-γ production, NK cell activity and Th1 response, its effects on TNF-α, IL-6, and IL-8 production result in promotion of tumor progression.

Cytokines induce immunity to tumor; however, prolonged cytokine production leads to chronic inflammation and cancer promotion [127, 128]. It seems that limited and short-lived expression of cytokines induces conditions favorable to tumor eradication. However, tumor cells utilize various mechanisms to evade destruction by the immune system, such as Th1 response suppression, FasL induction, or apoptosis inhibition. Failed tumor elimination caused by tumor immune evasion or tumor burden may result in chronic inflammation. Continuous secretion of IL-18 from other cells such as endothelial cells, epithelial cells, and tumor cells themselves enhances tumor growth, angiogenesis, metastasis, and even immune evasion. The effect of IL-18 on tumor growth promotion dominates its effect on activating tumor immunity. Under these circumstances, inhibition of IL-18 may be more beneficial than administration of IL-18 and the IL-18 level can instead be used as a marker for cancer progression.

The dual effects of IL-18 as both a Th1 and Th2 response inducer and as a cancer cell destroying and cancer promoting cytokine make the application of this cytokine in cancer therapy more complicated. Further studies on IL-18 biology such as on its regulation by IL-18BP and signal transduction will shed more light on this cytokine for future development of cancer therapy. Cytokine therapy using IL-18 in combination with other cytokines or proteins targeted at activating effector cells is useful to enhance tumor immunity. For intratumoral injection, administration of an IL-18 inhibitor may be more beneficial than of IL-18 (Fig. 6). Experiments

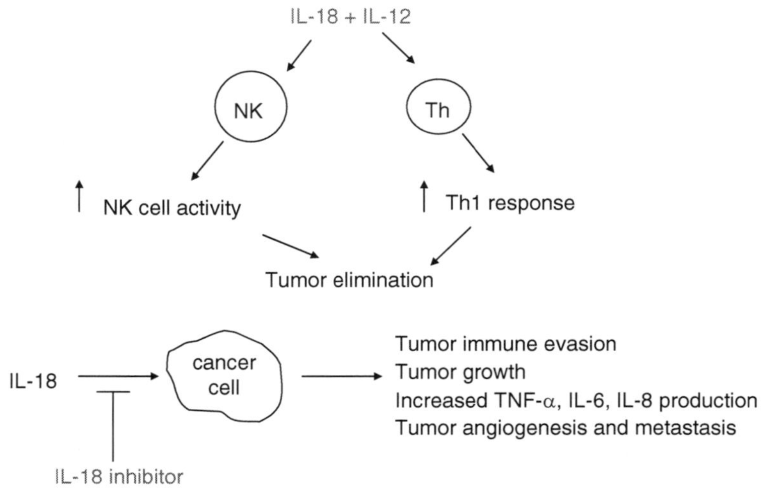

Fig. 6 IL-18 enhances antitumor immunity and IL-18 inhibitor prevents tumor progression. Cancer treatment by providing IL-18 in combination with other stimuli such as IL-12 to enhance effector cell function leads to tumor cell elimination. IL-18 can enhance tumor immune evasion, tumor growth, angiogenesis and metastasis. In addition, it induces other proinflammatory cytokines involved in tumor progression. Cancer therapy using IL-18 inhibitor could prevent tumor progression

investigating the effects of IL-18 and IL-18 inhibitor, such as IL-18BP, on different tumor stages and a follow up of IL-18 levels at different stages should be demonstrated. Tumor stages including IL-18 levels should be considered prior to IL-18 administration for cancer therapy.

Acknowledgment This work is supported by the higher commission of education, Thailand.

References

1. Okamura, H., Tsutsi, H., Komatsu, T., et al. (1995) Nature 378(6552), 88
2. Ushio, S., Namba, M., Okura, T., et al. (1996) J Immunol 156(11), 4274
3. Okamura, H., Nagata, K., Komatsu, T., et al. (1995) Infection and immunity 63(10), 3966
4. Gu, Y., Kuida, K., Tsutsui, H., et al. (1997) Science 275(5297), 206
5. Ghayur, T., Banerjee, S., Hugunin, M., et al. (1997) Nature 386(6625), 619
6. Steele, T. (2002) Leuk Res 26(11), 975
7. Fantuzzi, G, Puren, A. J., Harding, M. W., Livingston, D. J., and Dinarello, C. A. (1998) Blood 91(6), 2118
8. Akita, K., Ohtsuki, T., Nukada, Y., et al. (1997) J Biol Chem 272(42), 26595
9. Lebel-Binay, S., Berger, A., Zinzindohoue, F., Cugnenc, P., Thiounn, N., Fridman, W. H., and Pages, F. (2000) Eur Cytokine Netw 11(1), 15
10. Sugawara, S., Uehara, A., Nochi, T., et al. (2001) J Immunol 167(11), 6568
11. Nakanishi, K., Yoshimoto, T., Tsutsui, H., and Okamura, H. (2001) Cytokine Growth Factor Rev 12(1), 53
12. Pages, F., Berger, A., Henglein, B., et al. (1999) Int J Cancer 84(3), 326
13. Pages, F., Berger, A., Lebel-Binay, S., et al. (2000) Immunol Lett 75(1), 9
14. Cameron, L. A., Taha, R. A., Tsicopoulos, A., Kurimoto, M., Olivenstein, R., Wallaert, B., Minshall, E. M., and Hamid, Q. A. (1999) Eur Respir J 14(3), 553
15. Torigoe, K., Ushio, S., Okura, T., et al. (1997) J Biol Chem 272(41), 25737
16. Parnet, P., Garka, K. E., Bonnert, T. P., Dower, S. K., and Sims, J. E. (1996) J Biol Chem 271(8), 3967
17. Arend, W. P., Palmer, G., and Gabay, C. (2008) Immunol Rev 223, 20
18. Barbulescu, K., Becker, C., Schlaak, J. F., Schmitt, E., Meyer zum Buschenfelde K. H., and Neurath M. F. (1998) J Immunol 160(8), 3642
19. Xu, X., Sun, Y. L., and Hoey, T. (1996) Science 273(5276), 794
20. Sica, A., Dorman, L., Viggiano, V., Cippitelli, M., Ghosh, P., Rice, N., and Young, H. A. (1997) J Biol Chem 272(48), 30412
21. Croston, G. E., Cao, Z., and Goeddel, D. V. (1995) J Biol Chem 270(28), 16514.
22. Adachi, O., Kawai, T., Takeda, K., Matsumoto, M., Tsutsui, H., Sakagami, M., Nakanishi, K., and Akira, S. (1998) Immunity 9(1), 143
23. Kanakaraj, P., Ngo, K., Wu, Y., et al. (1999) J Exp Med 189(7), 1129
24. Novick, D., Kim, S. H, Fantuzzi, G., Reznikov, L. L., Dinarello, C.A., and Rubinstein M. (1999) Immunity 10(1), 127
25. Kim, S. H., Eisenstein, M., Reznikov, L., Fantuzzi, G., Novick, D., Rubinstein, M., and Dinarello, C. A. (2000) Proc Natl Acad Sci USA 97(3), 1190
26. Kim, S. H., Azam, T., Novick, D., Yoon, D. Y., Reznikov, L. L., Bufler, P., Rubinstein, M., and Dinarello, C. A. (2002) J Biol Chem 277(13), 10998
27. Faggioni, R., Cattley, R. C., Guo, J., et al. (2001) J Immunol 167(10), 5913
28. Corbaz, A., ten Hove, T., Herren, S., et al. (2002) J Immunol 168(7), 3608
29. Ludwiczek, O., Kaser, A., Novick, D., Dinarello, C. A., Rubinstein, M., Vogel, W., and Tilg, H. (2002) J Clin Immunol 22(6), 331

30. Mazodier, K., Marin, V., Novick, D., et al. (2005) Blood 106(10), 3483
31. Kumar, S., Hanning, C. R., Brigham-Burke, M. R., et al. (2002) Cytokine 18(2), 61
32. Bufler, P., Azam, T., Gamboni-Robertson, F., Reznikov, L. L., Kumar, S., Dinarello, C. A., and Kim, S. H. (2002) Proc Natl Acad Sci USA 99(21), 13723
33. Munder, M., Mallo, M., Eichmann, K., and Modolell, M. (1998) J Exp Med 187(12), 2103
34. Ahn, H. J., Maruo, S., Tomura, M., et al. (1997) J Immunol 159(5), 2125
35. Kim, S. H., Cho, D., Hwang, S. Y., and Kim, T. S. (2001) Vaccine 19(30), 4107
36. Gillies, S. D., Young, D., Lo, K. M., and Roberts, S. (1993) Bioconjug Chem 4(3), 230
37. Tomura, M., Zhou, X. Y., Maruo, S., et al. (1998) J Immunol 160(10), 4738
38. Hyodo, Y., Matsui, K., Hayashi, N., et al. (1999) J Immunol 162(3), 1662
39. Hashimoto, W., Osaki, T., Okamura, H., Robbins, P. D., Kurimoto, M., Nagata, S., Lotze, M. T., and Tahara, H. (1999) J Immunol 163(2), 583
40. Micallef, M. J., Yoshida, K., Kawai, S., et al. (1997) Cancer Immunol Immunother 43(6), 361
41. Osaki, T., Peron, J. M., Cai, Q., Okamura, H., Robbins, P. D., Kurimoto, M., Lotze, M. T., and Tahara H. (1998) J Immunol 160(4), 1742
42. Kikuchi, T., Akasaki, Y., Joki, T., Abe, T., Kurimoto, M., and Ohno, T. (2000) J Immunother 23(2), 184
43. Lee, J. C., Lee, K. M., Kim, D. W., and Heo, D. S. (2004) J Immunol 172(12), 7335
44. Dasgupta, S., Bhattacharya-Chatterjee, M., O'Malley, B. W., Jr., and Chatterjee, S. K. (2005) J Immunol 175(8), 5541
45. Song, H., Hur, D. Y., Kim, K. E., Park, H, Kim, T, Kim, C. W., Bang, S, and Cho, D. H. (2006) Cell Immunol 242(1), 39
46. Chung, S. W., Cohen, E. P., and Kim, T. S. (2004) Vaccine 22(20), 2547
47. Park, H., Byun, D, Kim, T. S., et al. (2001) Immunol Lett 79(3), 215
48. Ye, Z. B., Ma, T, Li, H, Jin, X. L., and Xu, H. M. (2007) World J Gastroenterol 13(11), 1747
49. Vidal-Vanaclocha, F., Mendoza, L., Telleria, N., et al. (2006) Cancer Metastasis Rev 25(3), 417
50. Whiteside, T. L. (2006) Semin Cancer Biol 16(1), 3
51. Bubenik, J., and Vonka, V. (2003) Immunol Lett 90(2–3), 177
52. Ryan, A. E., Shanahan, F., O'Connell, J., and Houston, A. M. (2005) Cancer Res 65(21), 9817
53. Cho, D., Song, H., Kim, Y. M., et al. (2000) Cancer Res 60(10), 2703
54. Majima, T., Ichikura, T., Chochi, K., et al. (2006) Int J Cancer 118(2), 388
55. Gimbrone, M. A., Jr., Leapman, S. B., Cotran, R. S., and Folkman, J. (1973) J Natl Cancer Inst 50(1), 219
56. Li, C., Shintani, S., Terakado, N., Klosek, S. K., Ishikawa, T., Nakashiro, K., and Hamakawa, H. (2005) Int J Oral Maxillofac Surg 34(5), 559
57. Riedel, K., Riedel, F., Goessler, U. R., Germann, G., and Sauerbier, M. (2007) Arch Med Res 38(1), 45
58. Tello-Montoliu, A., Patel, J. V., and Lip, G. Y. (2006) J Thromb Haemost 4(9), 1864
59. Amin, M. A., Mansfield, P. J., Pakozdi, A., Campbell, P. L., Ahmed, S., Martinez, R. J., and Koch, A. E. (2007) Arthritis Rheum 56(6), 1787
60. Cho, M. L., Jung, Y. O., Moon, Y. M., et al. (2006) Immunol Lett 103(2), 159
61. Kim, J., Kim, C., Kim, T. S., Bang, S. I., Yang, Y., Park, H., and Cho, D. (2006) Biochem Biophys Res Commun 344(4), 1284
62. Alexandrakis, M. G., Passam, F. H., Sfiridaki, K., et al. (2004) Leuk Res 28(3), 259
63. Jung, M. K., Song, H. K., Kim, K. E., Hur, D. Y., Kim, T., Bang, S., Park, H., and Cho, D. H. (2006) Immunol Lett 107(2), 125
64. Kim, K. E., Song, H, Kim, T. S., et al. (2007) Oncogene 26(10), 1468
65. Zhang, B., Wu, K. F., Cao, Z. Y., Rao, Q., Ma, X. T., Zheng, G. G., and Li, G. (2004) Leuk Res 28(1), 91
66. Jiang, D. F., Liu, W. L., Lu, Y. L., Qiu, Z. Y., and He, F. C. (2003) Zhonghua Zhong Liu Za Zhi 25(4), 348
67. Jiang, D., Ying, W., Lu, Y., et al. (2003) Proteomics 3(5), 724
68. Langley, R. R., Carlisle, R., Ma, L., Specian, R. D., Gerritsen, M. E., and Granger, D. N. (2001) Microcirculation 8(5), 335

69. Vidal-Vanaclocha, F., Fantuzzi, G., Mendoza, L., et al. (2000) Proc Natl Acad Sci USA 97(2), 734
70. Amo, Y., Ohta, Y., Hamada, Y., and Katsuoka, K. (2001) Br J Dermatol 145(4), 674
71. Merendino, R. A., Gangemi, S., Ruello, A., Bene, A., Losi, E., Lonbardo, G., and Purello-Dambrosio, F. (2001) Int J Biol Markers 16(2), 126
72. Takada, H., Ohga, S., Mizuno, Y., et al. (1999) Br J Haematol 106(1), 182
73. Gunel, N., Coskun, U., Sancak, B., Hasdemir, O., Sare, M., Bayram, O., Celenkoglu, G., and Ozkan, S. (2003) Am J Clin Oncol 26(4), 416
74. Eissa, S. A., Zaki, S. A., El-Maghraby, S. M., and Kadry, D. Y. (2005) J Egypt Natl Canc Inst 17(1), 51
75. Akahiro, J., Konno, R., Ito, K., Okamura, K., and Yaegashi, N. (2004) Int J Clin Oncol 9(1), 42
76. Tsuboi, K., Miyazaki, T., Nakajima, M., et al. (2004) Cancer Lett 205(2), 207
77. Sozen, S., Coskun, U., Sancak, B., Bukan, N., Gunel, N., Tunc, L., and Bozkirli, I. (2004) Neoplasma 51(1), 25
78. Bukan, N., Sozen, S., Coskun, U., Sancak, B., Gunel, N., Bozkirli, I., and Senocak, C. (2003) Eur Cytokine Netw 14(3), 163
79. Le Page, C., Ouellet, V., Madore, J., Hudson, T. J., Tonin, P. N., Provencher, D. M., and Mes-Masson, A. M. (2006) Int J Cancer 118(7), 1750
80. Diakowska, D., Markocka-Maczka, K., Grabowski, K., and Lewandowski, A. (2006) Exp Oncol 28(4), 319
81. Thong-Ngam, D., Tangkijvanich, P., Lerknimitr, R., Mahachai, V., Theamboonlers, A., and Poovorawan, Y. (2006) World J Gastroenterol 12(28), 4473
82. Tangkijvanich, P., Thong-Ngam, D., Mahachai, V., Theamboonlers, A., and Poovorawan, Y. (2007) World J Gastroenterol 13(32), 4345
83. Asakawa, M., Kono, H., Amemiya, H., Matsuda, M., Suzuki, T., Maki, A., and Fujii, H. (2006) Int J Cancer 118(3), 564
84. Liu, Y., Lin, N., Huang, L., Xu, Q., and Pang, G. (2007) DNA Cell Biol 26(8), 613
85. Nikiteas, N., Yannopoulos, A., Chatzitheofylaktou, A., and Tsigris, C. (2007) Anticancer Res 27(6B), 3849
86. Robertson, M. J., Mier, J. W., Logan, T., et al. (2006) Clin Cancer Res 12(14 Pt 1), 4265
87. Chang, C. Y., Lee, J., Kim, E. Y., Park, H. J., Kwon, C. H., Joh, J. W., and Kim, S. J. (2007) BMC Cancer 7, 87
88. Lagarce, F., Garcion, E., Faisant, N., Thomas, O., Kanaujia, P., Menei, P., and Benoit, J. P. (2006) Int J Pharm 314(2), 179
89. Heuer, J. G., Tucker-McClung, C., and Hock, R. A. (1999) J Immunother 22(4), 324
90. Cho, D., Kim, T. G., Lee, W., et al. (2000) J Invest Dermatol 114(5), 928
91. Yang, J., Jin, G., Liu, X., and Liu, S. (2007) Hum Gene Ther 18(4), 323
92. Li, Q., Carr, A. L., Donald, E. J., Skitzki, J. J., Okuyama, R., Stoolman, L. M., and Chang, A. E. (2005) Cancer Res 65(3), 1063
93. Osaki, T., Hashimoto, W., Gambotto, A., Okamura, H., Robbins, P. D., Kurimoto, M., Lotze, M. T., and Tahara, H. (1999) Gene Ther 6(5), 808
94. Iinuma, H., Okinaga, K., Fukushima, R., Inaba, T., Iwasaki, K., Okinaga, A., Takahashi, I., and Kaneko, M. (2006) J Immunol 176(6), 3461
95. Lian, H., Jin, N., Li, X., et al. (2007) Cancer Immunol Immunother 56(2), 181
96. Lu, J. X., Peng, Y., Meng, Z. F., Jin, L. Q., Lu, Y. S., and Guan, M. X. (2005) Biochem Biophys Res Commun 334(1), 157
97. Lu, J., Peng, Y., Zheng, Z. J., Pan, J. H., Zhang, Y., and Bai, Y. (2008) Cancer Lett 260(1–2), 187
98. Nishio, S., Yamada, N., Ohyama, H., et al. (2008) Cancer Sci 99(1), 113
99. Shi, F. F., Gunn, G. R., Snyder, L. A., and Goletz, T. J. (2007) Vaccine 25(17), 3338
100. Marshall, D. J., Rudnick, K. A., McCarthy, S. G., Mateo, L. R., Harris, M. C., McCauley, C, and Snyder, L. A. (2006) Vaccine 24(3), 244

101. Takahashi, H. K., Weitz-Schmidt, G., Iwagaki, H., Yoshino, T., Tanaka, N., and Nishibori, M. (2006) J Leukoc Biol 80(2), 215
102. Carbone, A., Rodeck, U., Mauri, F. A., et al. (2005) Cancer Biol Ther 4(2), 231
103. Nakanishi, K., Yoshimoto, T., Tsutsui, H., and Okamura, H. (2001) Annu Rev Immunol 19, 423
104. Hoshino, T., Wiltrout, R. H., and Young, H. A. (1999) J Immunol 162(9), 5070
105. Yoshimoto, T., Mizutani, H., Tsutsui, H., et al. (2000) Nat Immunol 1(2), 132
106. Nabors, L. B., Suswam, E., Huang, Y., Yang, X., Johnson, M. J., and King, P. H. (2003) Cancer Res 63(14), 4181
107. Aggarwal, B. B., Schwarz, L., Hogan, M. E., and Rando, R. F. (1996) Cancer Res 56(22), 5156
108. Montesano, R., Soulie, P., Eble, J. A., and Carrozzino, F. (2005) J Cell Sci 118(Pt 15), 3487
109. Duncombe, A. S., Heslop, H. E., Turner, M., Meager, A., Priest, R., Exley, T., and Brenner, M. K. (1989) J Immunol 143(11), 3828
110. Liu, R. Y., Fan, C., Mitchell, S., Chen, Q., Wu, J., and Zuckerman, K. S. (1998) Cancer Res 58(10), 2217
111. Digel, W., Stefanic, M., Schoniger, W., Buck, C., Raghavachar, A., Frickhofen, N., Heimpel, H., and Porzsolt, F. (1989) Blood 73(5), 1242
112. Giri, D. K., and Aggarwal, B. B. (1998) J Biol Chem 273(22), 14008
113. Stifter, G., Heiss, S., Gastl, G., Tzankov, A., and Stauder, R. (2005) Eur J Haematol 75(6), 485
114. Elbaz, O., and Mahmoud, L. A. (1994) Leuk Lymphoma 12(3–4), 191
115. Schmiegel, W., Roeder, C., Schmielau, J., Rodeck, U., and Kalthoff, H. (1993) Proc Natl Acad Sci USA 90(3), 863
116. Wu, S., Boyer, C. M., Whitaker, R. S., Berchuck, A., Wiener, J. R., Weinberg, J. B., and Bast, R. C., Jr. (1993) Cancer Res 53(8), 1939
117. Naylor, M. S., Stamp, G. W., Foulkes, W. D., Eccles, D., and Balkwill, F. R. (1993) J Clin Invest 91(5), 2194
118. Goillot, E., Combaret, V., Ladenstein, R., Baubet, D., Blay, J. Y., Philip, T., and Favrot, M. C. (1992) Cancer Res 52(11), 3194
119. Rosen, E. M., Goldberg, I. D., Liu, D., Setter, E., Donovan, M. A., Bhargava, M., Reiss, M., and Kacinski, B. M. (1991) Cancer Res 51(19), 5315
120. Okamoto, M., Kawamata, H., Kawai, K., and Oyasu, R. (1995) Cancer Res 55(20), 4581
121. Klein, B., Zhang, X. G., Jourdan, M., Content, J., Houssiau, F., Aarden, L., Piechaczyk, M., and Bataille, R. (1989) Blood 73(2), 517
122. Landi, S., Moreno, V., Gioia-Patricola, L., Guino, E., Navarro, M., de Oca, J., Capella, G., and Canzian, F. (2003) Cancer Res 63(13), 3560
123. Angelo, L. S., Talpaz, M., Kurzrock, R. (2002) Cancer Res 62(3), 932
124. Luca, M., Huang, S., Gershenwald, J. E., Singh, R. K., Reich, R., and Bar-Eli, M. (1997) Am J Pathol 151(4), 1105
125. Huang, S., Mills, L., Mian, B., Tellez, C., McCarty, M., Yang, X. D., Gudas, J. M., and Bar-Eli, M. (2002) Am J Pathol 161(1), 125
126. Xu, L., and Fidler, I. J. (2000) Cancer Res 60(16), 4610
127. Dinarello, C. A. (2006) Cancer Metastasis Rev 25(3), 307
128. Aggarwal, B. B., Shishodia, S., Sandur, S. K., Pandey, M. K., and Sethi, G. (2006) Biochem Pharmacol 72(11), 1605

Interleukin-21 and Cancer Therapy

Ian D. Davis, Kresten Skak, Naomi Hunder, Mark J. Smyth, and Pallavur V. Sivakumar

Abstract Interleukin-21 (IL-21) is a pleiotropic cytokine structurally similar to IL-2 and IL-15 but with important distinctions in its biological properties. IL-21 is mainly secreted by activated CD4+ T cells, NKT cells, and follicular T helper (Tfh) cells. The IL-21 receptor is expressed physiologically on lymphoid tissues and peripheral blood mononuclear cells, although expression can be acquired by epithelial, synovial, or transformed cells. The effects of IL-21 signaling include enhancement of adaptive T cell immunity, promotion of antibody production, activation of innate immune responses through NK cells, opposition to immune downmodulation mediated through regulatory T cells, and effects in autoimmunity. IL-21 also has important roles in development of Th17 and Tfh cells. In preclinical models and clinical trials in humans, IL-21 has been shown to mediate anticancer effects either as a single agent or in combination with other strategies such as monoclonal antibodies or tyrosine kinase inhibitors. The biology of IL-21 suggests that it could also be usefully combined with active vaccination, adoptive immunotherapy, or cytotoxic chemotherapy. IL-21 continues to undergo clinical development for a variety of cancer indications.

Introduction

Interleukin-21 (IL-21) is the most recently discovered member of the common γ-chain (γ_c) family of cytokines, which also includes interleukin- (IL)-2, IL-4, IL-7, IL-9, and IL-15. Nuclear magnetic resonance analysis of IL-21 has demonstrated that its structure is similar to the other γ_c-dependent cytokines: an up-up-down-down four-α-helical bundle cytokine [1]. The members of this family all share γ_c as part of a hetero-dimeric or trimeric receptor, where signaling through γ_c is responsible for activation of the JAK/STAT signaling pathway [2, 3]. When IL-21 binds to the IL-21 receptor (IL-21R)/γ_c complex, the primary signaling events are phosphorylation

I.D. Davis (✉)
Ludwig-Austin Joint Medical Oncology Unit, Austin Health, Melbourne, Australia
e-mail: Ian.Davis@ludwig.edu.au

J. Lustgarten et al. (eds.), *Targeted Cancer Immune Therapy*,
DOI 10.1007/978-1-4419-0170-5_3,

of STAT3 and STAT1, but phosphorylation of STAT4 and STAT5 and activation of the PI3/AKT and Ras/MAPK kinase pathways have also been reported to contribute to IL-21 signaling pathways [2, 4–6].

The IL-21R is constitutively expressed at low levels on all lymphocyte subsets and on dendritic cells, with B cells having the highest constitutive expression. Following activation, IL-21R is strongly upregulated on most lymphocytes [7, 8]. In addition, expression of IL-21R has been described on keratinocytes from scleroderma patients [9], synovial fibroblasts and macrophages from rheumatoid arthritis patients [10] and intestinal fibroblasts [11]. The function of IL-21R on these cells is largely unknown, although it has been shown that IL-21 induces expression of matrix metalloproteinase (MMP)-1, MMP-2, MMP-3, and MMP-9 in intestinal fibroblasts [11].

The primary sources of IL-21 are activated CD4$^+$ T cells and activated NKT cells [8, 12]. The nature of the subset of CD4$^+$ T cells producing IL-21 is still disputed. Recent evidence suggests that IL-6, IL-1β as well as IL-21 itself promote IL-21

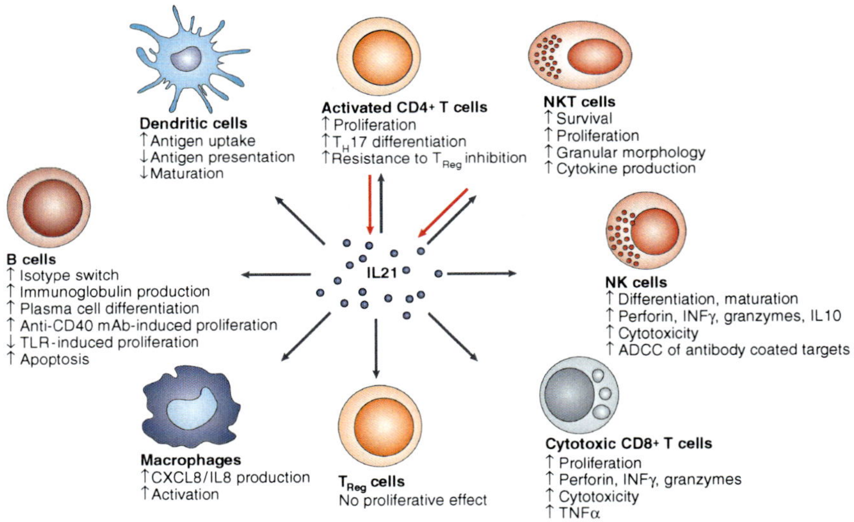

Fig. 1 Pleiotropic immune modulation by IL-21. IL-21 is secreted by activated CD4+ T cells, T follicular helper cells and natural killer T (NKT) cells, and is able to modulate the activity of most lymphocyte subsets. The listed effects on CD4+ T cells and CD8+ T cells have been observed after IL21 stimulation together with T cell receptor (TCR) stimulation or other activating cytokines (IL-2, IL-15), whereas the effects on NK cells also require other activating cytokines or activation through Fc receptors. It has been reported that IL-21 does not have any direct effects on regulatory T (Treg) cells but does suppress FOXP3 in human CD4+ T cells. Other B cell stimulatory agents (cytokines, immunoglobulins, Toll-like receptor (TLR) agonists, CD40 ligation) are also required for the listed effects on B cells, dendritic cells, and macrophages. ADCC, antibody-dependent cellular cytotoxicity; IFNγ, interferon-γ; mAb, monoclonal antibody; TH17, T helper cell 17; TNFα, tumor necrosis factor-α. Reproduced from [58], used with permission

expression. The IL-21-producing cells do not fall into the category of Th1/Th2/Th17 or regulatory T cells (Treg), but rather retain the potential to differentiate further into IL-17- or IL-4-producing cells given the proper stimulus [13].

IL-21 also has effects on regulation of autoimmunity, as described later. This is likely to be highly relevant in the context of cancer, where selective pressure from the immune system resulting in immunoediting shapes the antigenic phenotype of the evolving tumor [14]. An imbalance in the immune response away from immune reactivity and toward active immune suppression would provide a permissive immune environment in which a cancer could flourish.

These data suggest that IL-21 may play a key role in development of adaptive and innate immunity against cancers and may be involved in modulation of immune downregulation. This provides a rational basis for the clinical development of IL-21 as an anticancer reagent, either alone or in combination. This review will summarize the preclinical data supporting this contention and will describe early clinical studies with IL-21 in cancer. The effects of IL-21 are summarised in Fig. 1.

Preclinical Data

Effects of IL-21 on T Cells

As specified earlier, IL-21 is produced by multiple CD4+ T cell subsets as well as NKT cells. Both CD4+ and CD8+ T cell numbers are normal in naïve IL-21- and IL-21R-deficient mice (PVS, unpublished data) [15].

CD4+ T Cells

In vitro, IL-21 drives differentiation of CD4+ T cells to both the Th2 [16] and Th1 subtypes [17]. IL-21R-deficient mice show decreased Th2 responses without a corresponding increased Th1 response after *Schistosoma mansoni* infection [18] and also show reduced activity against a helminth parasite responsive to Th2 cytokines [19]. However, the specific role of IL-21 in differentiation to Th1 vs. Th2 subtypes is as yet unclear. More recently, a role for IL-21 in induction of Th17 responses has been elucidated. Multiple groups have recently shown that IL-21 can be produced by Th17 subset of T cells and that it promotes expansion of this subset in an autocrine manner. In mice, TGF-β together with either IL-6 or IL-21 drive the differentiation of Th17 cells from naïve $CD4^{+}$ T cells [20–23], whereas in humans TGF-β plus IL-21 but not IL-6 induces Th17 cells from naïve, $CD25^{neg}CD45RA^{neg}CD62L^{+}$ $CD4^{+}$ T cells [24]. However, it is controversial if IL-21 is absolutely required for Th17 differentiation/commitment. Evidence for [20, 21] and against [23, 25] the absolute requirement for IL-21 for Th17 commitment has been recently published and more work needs to be done to help elucidate the specific role for IL-21 in this process. Humans and mice may differ in this respect. Interestingly, in addition to driving Th17 differentiation, TGF-β also shuts off autocrine or IL-6-induced IL-21 production [13, 24]. Consistent with these data is the finding that stimulation of naive human CD4⁺ T cells with IL-21 alone lead to induction of the transcription factor, *Tbet*, the critical factor for Th1 differentiation, and IFN-γ secretion, whereas stimulation with IL-21 and TGF-β together inhibited *Tbet* and strongly induced *RORC2* expression, the critical factor for Th17 differentiation in humans [24]. Thus, IL-21 appears to be able to drive both Th1 and Th17 differentiation depending on the context.

Finally, follicular T helper (Tfh) cells have been shown to be a main source of IL-21 [26], and two recent papers suggest a nonredundant role for IL-21 in generation of Tfh and germinal center formation, which is dependent on Tfh cells and independent of Th1, Th2 and Th17 cells [27, 28]. Thus the role of IL-21 in the differentiation of CD4+ T cells is much more complex and important than originally expected, and we are just beginning to understand the function of IL-21 in CD4+ T cell differentiation.

CD8+ T Cells

IL-21 plays a significant role in the activation and differentiation of antigen-specific CD8+ T cells in vitro and in vivo. IL-21-mediated CD8+ T cell activation has been shown to be critical for antitumor responses mediated by IL-21 in multiple preclinical tumor models. IL-21 has minimal effects on proliferation of naïve and memory CD8+ T cells by itself but in combination with IL-7 or IL-15 leads to enhanced proliferation of these cells [29]. IL-21 also seems to have effects on CD8+ T cells that differ from those of IL-2 and IL-15. IL-2 and IL-15 induce an effector phenotype in CD8+ T cells, which correlates with a corresponding decrease in CD28 and CD62L expression, while IL-21 sustains CD28 expression on CD8+ T cells [29, 30]. Similar observations have been reported in naïve human CD8+ T cells where IL-21 lead to the proliferation and accumulation of CD28+ cytotoxic antigen-specific CD8+ T cells when stimulated with DC/tumor antigen. This population also showed a tenfold higher affinity for antigen [31]. In contrast, IL-21 induced proliferation and cytotoxic function in memory CD8+ T cells from HIV-infected patient samples [32], suggesting that IL-21 may have differential effects on antigen-specific naïve and memory CD8+ T cells. It has recently been demonstrated that IL-2 and IL-21 mediate opposing effects on antigen-induced CD8+ T cell differentiation [33]. IL-2 and IL-15 promoted expression of CD44, granzyme B expression and cytotoxic function in naïve CD8+ T cells, while IL-21 suppressed this effect. However, IL-21-primed CD8+ T cells were more effective killers when transferred in vivo into tumor-bearing mice. The IL-21-stimulated CD8+ T cells had a distinct gene expression profile, with increased expression of L-selectin, a homing and trafficking molecule. These data suggest that IL-21 may confer differential effects on CD8+ T cells depending differentiation status of cells, and nature of costimulus. However, it is clear that IL-21 has physiological significance in expanding and activating CD8+ T cells as IL-21R-deficient mice show lower numbers and cytolytic activity in antigen-specific CD8+ T cells when immunized with vaccinia virus expressing the HIV antigen gp160 [29].

T Regulatory Cells

Treg are a population of CD4+CD25+FoxP3+IL-7R^{lo} cells that have profound suppressive effects on T cell proliferation and function [34] and that are involved in constitutive suppression of autoimmunity. Multiple recent studies have shown that IL-21 antagonizes development of TGFβ-induced Foxp3 generation that normally leads to development of Tregs [20, 35]. Furthermore, a three to fourfold increase in FoxP3+ T cells have been in IL-21-deficient mice [21]. Treg express IL-21R [36] and IL-21 has effects on Treg that contrast sharply to those of other γ_c cytokines such as IL-2 and IL-15. In contrast to IL-2, IL-21 does not enhance the proliferation of Treg [37, 38]. IL-21 allows CD4+ T helper cells to become resistant to the suppressive effects of Treg without directly reversing the function of CD4+CD25+ Treg [36]. Furthermore, IL-21 may render CD4+CD25– T cells resistant to suppressive effects of Tregs [36] In contrast, IL-2, IL-7, and IL-15 have direct effects on Treg, either by enhancing their proliferation or by reversing their anergic effects [36]. These data suggest IL-21 may negatively regulate Treg development and function and thereby promote a shift in immune regulation toward an activated and hence anticancer response.

Effects of IL-21 on NK Cells and NKT Cells

In contrast to IL-15, IL-21 is not required for the development of NK cells as evidenced by IL-21R gene-deficient mice, which have normal number of NK cells [39]. Nevertheless, IL-21 has important effects on NK cells, including increased production of IFN-γ and IL-10, increased cytolytic activity and changes in expression pattern of NK cell markers, leading to increased NK cell-mediated tumor killing in vivo [40–42]. Importantly, IL-21 is able to augment NK cell-mediated antibody-dependent cellular cytotoxicity (ADCC). These observations provide justification for clinical trials in combination with monoclonal antibodies (discussed later).

NKT cells express the receptor for IL-21, and the effect of this cytokine on NKT cell function has only recently been studied [12]. IL-21, particularly in combination with IL-2, IL-15, or the glycolipid antigen α-galactosylceramide (α-GC), increases the proliferation of NKT cells. Furthermore, IL-21 enhances NKT cell cytokine production, granular morphology including granzyme B expression, and some inhibitory NK cell receptors. Furthermore, NKT cells may be capable of autocrine IL-21-mediated stimulation, since they are potent producers of this cytokine following in vitro stimulation via CD3 and CD28 in conjunction with IL-12, and also following in vivo stimulation with α-GC. The influence of IL-21 in NKT cell-dependent immune responses should be the subject of future investigations.

Effects of IL-21 on B Cells

IL-21 plays a critical role in B cell function and immunoglobulin (Ig) production, both of which may have consequences for autoimmunity and cancer therapy. IL-21 induces proliferation of naïve B cells when stimulated with either T cell derived costimulus (anti-CD40) or BCR (anti-IgM) but induces apoptosis when B cells are stimulated with TLR-ligands such as LPS or CpG oligodeoxynucleotides [7, 8, 43, 44]. The molecular mechanisms by which these occur have recently been reviewed [45]. Expansion of polyclonally activated naïve B cells (a response not specific for antigen) is thus inhibited by IL-21, whereas a productive antigen-specific response is promoted by IL-21. Although no defects in B cell development are seen in IL-21 or IL-21R-deficient mice, naïve and immunized IL-21 gene deficient mice show markedly reduced IgG1 and increased IgE [15]. IL-21 enhances IgG production by human B cells and can have a positive or negative effect on IgE production depending on the stimulus [46]. IL-21 also has potent effects on differentiation of B cells into plasma cells. This has been demonstrated by over-expressing IL-21 in mice [44] and by driving differentiation of human B cells in vitro by activation through the B cell receptor or through CD40 [47]. Some of the observed effects on B cells in IL-21 or IL-21R-deficient mice may be due to the deficiency of Tfh cells in these mice, which results in lack of germinal center formation and thus has a strong impact on B cell differentiation and isotype switching [27, 28]. The generation of mice with B cell or T cell specific IL-21R gene targeting shall reveal the relative contribution of the direct effect of IL-21 on B cells and the indirect effects through Tfh cells on the B cell phenotype.

These effects have consequences for both autoimmunity and cancer. In autoimmune disease models, IL-21 overexpression is associated with increased serum IgG [44, 48, 49], and blocking IL-21 using an IL-21 antagonist reduces IgG levels and disease severity [49, 50]. In contrast, IL-21 induces growth arrest and/or apoptosis of multiple B cell lymphoma cell lines and primary tumor cells in vitro, suggestive of a direct antitumor effect against these malignancies [51–55]. Furthermore, IL-21 also induces antitumor Ig production in some tumor models leading to enhanced antitumor effects [56, 57] and as explained earlier, IL-21 is a potent mediator of ADCC against multiple tumor targets.

Animal Tumor Studies

IL-21 Monotherapy

The antitumor effect of IL-21 has been broadly investigated in mouse tumor models using a variety of different IL-21 sources: recombinant mouse IL-21, delivery of IL-21-encoding plasmids, and IL-21-transfected tumor lines. Antitumor effects of IL-21 have been demonstrated both on solid established subcutaneous tumors, on lung and liver metastasis from intravenously injected tumors, and on disseminated tumors. IL-21 has antitumor effects as monotherapy, but shows enhanced efficacy when used in combination with several other therapies (reviewed in [58]).

Moderate tumor growth inhibition after administration of IL-21 was demonstrated in mice bearing established subcutaneous RenCa renal cell carcinomas and B16 melanomas. This antitumor effect was dependent on $CD8^+$ T cells but was largely independent of NK cells, as shown by depletion studies and the use of β_2-microglobulin gene targeted ($CD8^+$ T cell deficient) mice [59]. Similarly, a tumor growth reduction and prolonged survival was observed after IL-21 plasmid injection in mice bearing MCA205 fibrosarcoma and B16 melanoma [60]. In another model using intravenous injection of B16 melanoma cells, IL-21 plasmid injection significantly decreased formation of lung and liver metastasis. This effect was shown to be dependent on NK cells and perforin, but independent of B and T lymphocytes and IFN-γ [40]. These studies illustrate that IL-21 can mediate antitumor effects through both NK cells and $CD8^+$T cells.

Several studies have demonstrated powerful antitumor effects of IL-21 when expressed by tumor cells. IL-21-transfected melanoma [61], fibrosarcoma [61], mammary cancer [62], bladder cancer [63], renal cell carcinoma [64], glioma [65], colon cancer [66], and neuroblastoma [67] generally had unaltered growth characteristics in vitro but were completely rejected in vivo. In some of these studies, rechallenge with the parental tumor line in mice that had previously rejected the IL-21-transfected tumor showed that immunological memory toward the tumor line had formed and the parental tumor cells were rejected [62–65]. Injection of IL-21-transfected tumor cells also induced a "bystander" response (elimination of nontransfected cells) when coinjected with parental tumor cells, and even when IL-21-transfected gliomas were injected into established intra-cranial gliomas most tumors were completely rejected [65].

In another model, adoptive transfer to mice of TCR-transgenic OT-I $CD8^+$ T cells (recognizing an H-$2K^b$ restricted ovalbumin peptide) was performed followed by challenge with intraperitoneal injection of the ovalbumin-expressing thymoma line, E.G7 [68]. The mice were subsequently treated with IL-2, IL-15, IL-21 or vehicle. Interestingly, both IL-2 and IL-21 strongly enhanced the number of OT-I cells at the peak of the response, but IL-21 and to less extent IL-15 was superior in generating long-lived memory responses, and only IL-21-treated mice showed long-term (60 days) survival [68]. A comparison of the effects of the same three cytokines on markers of maturation on TCR-transgenic pmel-1 T cells following in vitro stimulation with cognate antigen was recently performed [33]. Surprisingly, in contrast to IL-2 and IL-15, IL-21 suppressed acquisition of cytolytic effector T cell characteristics, but when the cells subsequently were transferred into mice bearing B16 and vaccinated, the IL-21 cultured cells had superior antitumor responses compared with cells cultured in IL-2 or IL-15. These data suggest that IL-21 has a unique ability to promote long-term survival of $CD8^+$ T cells and preserve the ability of $CD8^+$ T cells to become potent effector cells given the right stimulus; properties that are supposed to be vital for successful cancer immunotherapy.

IL-21 Combination Therapies

Rituximab is a monoclonal antibody specific for the CD20 molecule expressed on most B cell non-Hodkgin's lymphomas [69]. Preclinical studies indicated that a major mechanism of action of rituximab was through enhancement of ADCC [70] and that this can be enhanced by IL-21 in murine models of lymphoma [54]. In vitro studies of human CLL cells have demonstrated that the majority of CLL patients have surface IL-21 receptor-alpha, and that IL-21 can induce apoptosis of these cells through upregulation of proapoptotic proteins [54]. In addition, IL-21 enhances the ADCC functions of NK cells against rituximab-coated CLL cells in vitro. Data similar to that for rituximab has been demonstrated for trastuzumab (monoclonal antibody specific for EGFR type 2 [Her2/neu/c-erbB2]) and for cetuximab (monoclonal antibody specific for EGFR type 1). IL-21 has been tested in models using trastuzumab-coated breast cancer cells and cetuximab-coated EGFR+ tumor cell lines [41, 71].

Apart from enhancing ADCC activity, IL-21 has also shown enhanced antitumor efficacy in preclinical tumor models with antibodies that induce tumor cell death or costimulate T cell activation. Induction of tumor cell apoptosis by agonistic mAb against DR5 (TRAILR), combined with delayed IL-21 treatment, suppressed tumor growth and preestablished tumor metastases [72]. This was shown to be due to enhanced CTL activity and establishment of tumor-specific memory response. Furthermore, sequentially combining TrimAb (a cocktail of antibodies against TRAILR, CD40, and CD137) with recombinant IL-21 also significantly improved the antitumor activity against very advanced disease in preclinical tumor models [73].

Human Clinical Trials

IL-21 Monotherapy

Recombinant human IL-21 (rIL-21) administered intravenously as a single agent has undergone testing in phase 1 and 2 clinical trials in Australia and the United States [74–77, 77A]. These trials involved patients with metastatic melanoma or RCC and were designed to assess the safety and efficacy of rIL-21 in these conditions, to investigate two different drug administration schedules, and to determine the biological effects of rIL-21 in humans.

rIL-21 has mild toxicity and is generally well tolerated. The most common adverse events were fatigue, fever, nausea, and headache, occurring in about 50% of patients. Other common adverse events included influenza-like symptoms, chills, vomiting, rash, pruritus, myalgia, and anorexia, overall occurring in about 25% of patients. Significantly, capillary leak syndrome has not been observed even at dose levels above the maximum tolerated intravenous dose of 30 μg/kg in either treatment schedule. Clinical responses were observed in subjects with melanoma (one complete response, one partial response, 20 stable disease, 27 progressive disease), and in subjects with renal cell carcinoma (4 partial responses, 13 stable disease, 2 progressive disease). Other treatment regimens are now being tested including an ongoing study of subcutaneous dosing (Eudract No. 2006–000376–32).

The effects of rIL-21 therapy on the immune system have been assessed by analysis of blood samples from patients treated with IL-21 [76]. Unfortunately, no analysis of tumor infiltrating lymphocytes or tumor draining lymph nodes was performed; nevertheless, these data provide some interesting insight into the in vivo activity of rIL-21. Biomarkers of rIL-21 activity included assessment of leukocyte subsets, phosphorylation of STAT3, ex vivo cytotoxicity, expression of effector molecules in enriched CD8+ T cells and CD56+NK cells by quantitative RT-PCR, and gene array profiling of CD8+ T cells. rIL-21 showed detectable biological effects in vivo at all dose levels, including as low as 1 μg/kg/dose. A transient decrease in circulating lymphocytes was observed following rIL-21 dosing in the "5+9" dosing regimen (5 days of daily dosing followed by 9 days rest), with complete recovery during the resting periods, suggesting that rIL-21 causes redistribution of lymphocytes rather than apoptosis. By contrast, monocytes were increased in numbers during treatment cycles, and increased expression of the high affinity FcγRIII on monocytes was observed [77A], suggesting that rIL-21 enhances the ability of monocytes to elicit ADCC. A dose-dependent upregulation of soluble CD25 (IL-2Rα) in serum was consistently observed during dosing periods. sCD25 is cleaved from activated lymphocytes and is supposed to be a marker of T cell and NK cell activation. rIL-21 also induced the upregulation of mRNA expression of the effector proteins granzyme A and B and perforin in isolated CD8+ T cells; proteins that are important for the cytolytic activity of cytotoxic T lymphocytes. Furthermore, mRNA expression of IFN-γ and the homing molecule CXCR3 was also upregulated in CD8+ T cells, and the percentage of CD8+ T cells expressing the lymph node homing molecules, CD62L and CCR7, was augmented. Finally, NK cell cytotoxicity was increased after rIL-21 therapy. Together these data confirm the preclinical observations, showing that administration of rIL-21 to humans induces activation of CD8+ T cells and NK cells in vivo, which may be important for the antitumor effect of rIL-21.

IL-21 Combination Therapies (Fig. 2)

Monoclonal antibodies – Rituximab. A Phase I study was initiated to determine safety and tolerability of this combination in patients with indolent CD20+ B cell non-Hodgkin's lymphoma (NHL) who had relapsed after previous rituximab therapy [78, 79]. Twenty-one patients were enrolled from US study centers, and treated with a fixed weekly dose of rituximab (375 mg/m^2) in combination with a weekly dose of rIL-21 (30, 100, or 150 μg/kg, iv). Subjects without progressive disease after the first 4-week course were eligible for a repeat course. Subjects enrolled in the study were heavily pretreated, with a median of 3 prior therapies (range 1–10). NHL subtypes represented in the study included chronic lymphocytic leukemia and small lymphocytic leukemia (CLL/SLL, $n = 11$), follicular lymphoma ($n = 9$) and marginal zone lymphoma ($n = 1$). During the initial dose escalation in the first 9 patients, retreatment at 150 μg/kg was associated with grade 3 nausea, vomiting, and diarrhea in one patient, and grade 2 edema in another, thus 100 μg/kg was selected as the dose for the subsequent 12 patients treated in the expansion cohort. Overall the combination therapy was well tolerated in the outpatient setting, with the most common adverse events consisting of flu-like symptoms and transient cytopenias (neutropenia and thrombocytopenia). One subject with preexisting cardiac disease, who was treated at 100 μg/kg, suffered a myocardial infarction while on study and subsequently died following stent rethrombosis. Overall best response as determined by Cheson criteria included 2 complete responses, 1 complete response unconfirmed, 5 partial responses, 11 stable disease, and 2 unevaluable subjects. Although the overall response rate was 38%, 11 of 13 evaluable patients had tumor shrinkage at some point on study. The two confirmed complete responses occurred in CLL/SLL patients, one of whom was shown by highly sensitive flow cytometry to have cleared the bone marrow, a result that is rarely seen with rituximab alone. In light of the encouraging results seen in CLL patients in the Phase 1 clinical study and the in vitro data, further studies of rIL-21 in combination with antibodies or chemotherapy in CLL may be of interest.

Antibodies to epidermal growth factor receptor (EGFR) family members. rIL-21 is currently being evaluated in a Phase I trial in combination with cetuximab for metastatic colon cancer (European Clinical Trials database number 2006–004231–30). Enrollment is ongoing.

Tyrosine kinase inhibitors (TKIs). Until 2005, the only FDA-approved systemic therapy for metastatic renal cell carcinoma (mRCC) was IL-2, which induces tumor responses in a small fraction of patients with a considerable level of toxicity. This disease was an early focus of the rIL-21 development program due to previous success of immunotherapy in mRCC, strong preclinical data, and encouraging results from phase 1 rIL-21 monotherapy studies. However, as the treatment landscape changed for mRCC with the approval of the vascular endothelial growth factor (VEGF) receptor TKIs sorafenib and sunitinib [80], considerable interest was generated for a strategy combining immunotherapy with the new anti-angiogenic agents.

Recently, we have described the antitumor effects of these TKIs in combination with rIL-21 in a murine RCC model (PVS et al., manuscript in preparation). Concurrent combination therapies of IL-21 with either sorafenib or sunitinib significantly inhibited tumor growth. Effects of the combination therapy were significantly better than with either monotherapy alone. In vitro analysis revealed that pharmacological concentrations of the TKIs did not inhibit IL-21 receptor expression or intracellular STAT3 signaling in various subsets of immune cells. Furthermore, the TKIs did not inhibit the effects of IL-21 on $CD4^+$ and $CD8^+$ T cell proliferation, ADCC or mixed lymphocyte reaction assays, indicating that neither sunitinib nor sorafenib counteracted the function of IL-21 on lymphocytes. It is conceivable that treatment with TKIs makes tumor cells more sensitive to immunotherapy, either directly or by stressing the cells via an anti-angiogenic effect. Furthermore, the anti-angiogenic effects of the TKIs might "normalize" the tumor vasculature, and thereby facilitate immune cell infiltration.

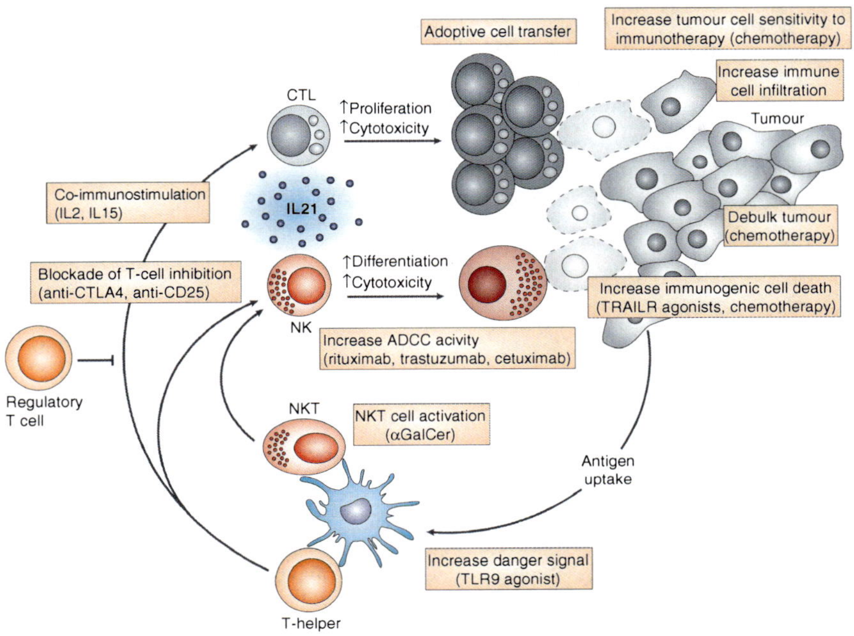

Fig. 2 Potential combination strategies with IL-21 therapy. IL-21 has pleiotropic effects on both natural killer (NK) cells and cytotoxic T lymphocytes (CTLs) with subsequent antitumor activity. Complete eradication of the tumor probably requires combination therapy. Potential combination strategies include costimulation with other immune therapies, therapies that induce immunogenic cell death or increase the "danger signal" from the tumor, therapies that debulk the tumor, or therapies that make the tumor cells more sensitive to immune therapy. *α-GalCer* α-galactosylceramide, *ADCC* antibody-dependent cellular cytotoxicity, *CTLA4* cytotoxic T lymphocyte antigen 4, *TLR9* Toll-like receptor 9, *TRAILR* tumor necrosis factor (TNF)-related apoptosis-inducing ligand receptor. Reproduced from [58], used with permission

To explore this combination strategy further, a phase 1/phase 2 study was initiated in the United States and Canada to study the safety and efficacy of the combination of rIL-21 and sorafenib in metastatic RCC [81, 82]. Nineteen patients with up to one prior systemic therapy for mRCC were enrolled in the phase 1 dose escalation portion of the study, with 30 additional subjects planned for the Phase 2 group. Patients received treatment with sorafenib 400 mg orally twice daily plus rIL-21 intravenously (10, 30, 40, or 50 μg/kg) on days 1–5 and 15–19 of each 6-week treatment course. The maximum tolerated dose for rIL-21 in combination with sorafenib was determined to be 30 μg/kg, iv; dose-limiting toxicity consisted of grade 3 diffuse rash in 3 patients, accompanied by hand-foot syndrome. Of the 14 evaluable patients in the dose escalation group, best responses on study included 2 confirmed partial responses and 11 subjects with stable disease, and 1 subject with progressive disease by RECIST. Twelve of the 14 patients had tumor shrinkage of 6–53%, confirmed by an independent radiologic review. Median progression free survival in the 14 evaluable subjects was 40 weeks, with a disease control rate (partial response plus stable disease) at 24 weeks of 77%. No pharmacokinetic interaction between rIL-21 and sorafenib was evident, and sorafenib did not appear to diminish rIL-21 associated immune activation as assessed by induction of soluble CD25. Enrollment of second and third-line treatment subjects into the phase 2 part of the study is ongoing. A phase 1 study to explore the combination of subcutaneous rIL-21 with sunitinib for first-line therapy of patients with metastatic RCC was initiated in Europe by Novo Nordisk, although results are not yet available (European Clinical Trials database number 2006–005751–16).

Future Strategies

Chemotherapy

Immunotherapy has traditionally but incorrectly been considered incompatible with cytotoxic chemotherapy. This misconception arose due to the cytostatic and cytotoxic effects of most chemotherapeutics on proliferating cells, and the induction of leukopenia after chemotherapy. However, more recently this view is being changed as chemotherapy may also augment antitumor immunity: most chemotherapeutics induce tumor necrosis and apoptosis, which may cause local inflammatory responses and generation of adaptive immunity toward tumor antigens. Also, homeostatic expansion of lymphocytes following chemotherapy may enhance antitumor immunity, and certain chemotherapeutics, especially cyclophosphamide, may preferentially deplete Tregs, allowing preferential expansion of tumor-reactive effector T cells. These considerations have been extensively reviewed [83, 84]. Combination chemotherapy and immunotherapy has been used for good effect in metastatic melanoma [85].

To date, little has been published about IL-21 in combination with chemotherapy. Our own studies in animal tumor models suggest that an additive antitumor effect can be obtained when IL-21 is combined with oxaliplatin, 5-fluorouracil, and pegylated liposomal doxorubicin, whereas irinotecan or dacarbazine administration ablated the effect of IL-21 (KS and PVS, unpublished data). The best effect was obtained when IL-21 administration was postponed 1 week relative to chemotherapy, suggesting that the adverse effect of chemotherapy on immune function may initially inhibit immune activation by IL-21, but this effect is reversible. Thus, we believe that IL-21 can be successfully combined with chemotherapy in the clinic if careful consideration is given to scheduling. IL-21 is currently being tested in ovarian cancer in combination with pegylated liposomal doxorubicin (clinicaltrials.gov identifier NCT00523380).

Vaccines and Adoptive Cell Therapy

Vaccination as a preventive strategy in cancer has recently proven successful with the approval of two vaccines against human papilloma virus, the main cause of cervical cancer, and several therapeutic vaccines against various cancers are being tested clinically [86, 87]. Animal studies with IL-21 suggest that IL-21 may be useful as a vaccine adjuvant to enhance and prolong $CD8^+$ T cell responses. Several studies have shown that injection of live or irradiated, IL-21-transfected tumor cells can be used as a vaccine against the parental cell line [61–64]. Other studies have used vaccination combined with adoptive transfer of tumor-specific $CD8^+$ T cells to show enhanced antitumor effect against B16 tumors when the mice subsequently received IL-21 [29, 88]. An additional benefit was obtained when IL-21 was given in combination with IL-2 or IL-15. Thus, the rationale for using IL-21 to enhance vaccine efficacy is sound. In addition to the effects on $CD8^+$ T cells, IL-21 may also enhance antigen-specific B cell and antibody responses, which may further add to the effect [65, 89].

Also for adoptive cell therapy (ACT) there is ample evidence to assume that IL-21 may be used in vitro to enhance proliferation of antigen-stimulated $CD8^+$ T cells [8, 31, 90], yet maintaining them in a state where they retain the full potential to become potent effector cells in vivo [33], as described earlier (see "Effects on T cells" and "Animal tumor studies"). Although ACT of autologous, in vitro stimulated $CD8^+$ T cells is not likely to be a commercial blockbuster, it has generated some of the highest response rates ever seen in stage IV melanoma patients [91].

Immune Modulation Such as Anti-CTLA-4 or Treg Depletion

Although few published data are available yet in animal models, it is possible that further enhancement of the clinical efficacy of IL-21 may be achieved by combining it with interventions aimed at reducing the immunosuppressive activity of T cell surface molecules such as CTLA-4 or cellular mediators of immunosuppression such as Treg [62, 92–96]. Although appealing, the risk of clinically severe autoimmunity will need careful consideration [93, 97–103].

Summary

IL-21 has many biological features that make it attractive as a potential anticancer agent, including biological potency even at low doses, favorable effects on both innate and adaptive immunity, inhibition of immunosuppressive mechanisms, and acceptable toxicity. Clinical responses have been observed in humans using rIL-21 as a single agent in phase 1 and 2 clinical trials, which is highly encouraging. The strong preclinical data supporting combination therapies is now also being translated to the clinic and the results of these and further clinical strategies are awaited with interest.

Acknowledgments IDD is supported in part by a Victorian Cancer Agency Clinician Researcher Fellowship and is an Australian National Health and Medical Research Council Honorary Practitioner Fellow. MJS is supported by a NH&MRC Senior Principal Research Fellowship and Program Grant.

References

1. Bondensgaard, K., Breinholt, J., Madsen, D., Omkvist, D. H., Kang, L., Worsaae, A., Becker, P., Schiodt, C. B., and Hjorth, S. A. (2007) J Biol Chem 282, 23326
2. Asao, H., Okuyama, C., Kumaki, S., Ishii, N., Tsuchiya, S., Foster, D., and Sugamura, K. (2001) J Immunol 167, 1
3. Habib, T., Senadheera, S., Weinberg, K., and Kaushansky, K. (2002) Biochemistry 41, 8725
4. Brenne, A. T., Ro, T. B., Waage, A., Sundan, A., Borset, M., and Hjorth-Hansen, H. (2002) Blood 99, 3756
5. Strengell, M., Matikainen, S., Siren, J., Lehtonen, A., Foster, D., Julkunen, I., and Sareneva, T. (2003) J Immunol 170, 5464
6. Zeng, R., Spolski, R., Casas, E., Zhu, W., Levy, D. E., and Leonard, W. J. (2007) Blood 109, 4135
7. Jin, H., Carrio, R., Yu, A., and Malek, T. R. (2004) J Immunol 173, 657
8. Parrish-Novak, J., Dillon, S. R., Nelson, A., Hammond, A., Sprecher, C., Gross, J. A., Johnston, J., Madden, K., Xu, W., West, J., Schrader, S., Burkhead, S., Heipel, M., Brandt, C., Kuijper, J. L., Kramer, J., Conklin, D., Presnell, S. R., Berry, J., Shiota, F., Bort, S., Hambly, K., Mudri, S., Clegg, C., Moore, M., Grant, F. J., Lofton-Day, C., Gilbert, T., Rayond, F., Ching, A., Yao, L., Smith, D., Webster, P., Whitmore, T., Maurer, M., Kaushansky, K., Holly, R. D., and Foster, D. (2000) Nature 408, 57
9. Distler, J. H., Jüngel, A., Kowal-Bielecka, O., Michel, B. A., Gay, R. E., Sprott, H., Matucci-Cerinic, M., Chilla, M., Reich, K., Kalden, J. R., Muller-Ladner, U., Lorenz, H. M., Gay, S., and Distler, O. (2005) Arthritis Rheum 52, 856
10. Jüngel, A., Distler, J. H., Kurowska-Stolarska, M., Seemayer, C. A., Seibl, R., Forster, A., Michel, B. A., Gay, R. E., Emmrich, F., Gay, S., and Distler, O. (2004) Arthritis Rheum 50, 1468
11. Monteleone, G., Caruso, R., Fina, D., Peluso, I., Gioia, V., Stolfi, C., Fantini, M. C., Caprioli, F., Tersigni, R., Alessandroni, L., MacDonald, T. T., and Pallone, F. (2006) Gut 55, 1774
12. Coquet, J. M., Kyparissoudis, K., Pellicci, D. G., Besra, G., Berzins, S. P., Smyth, M. J., and Godfrey, D. I. (2007) J Immunol 178, 2827
13. Suto, A., Kashiwakuma, D., Kagami, S., Hirose, K., Watanabe, N., Yokote, K., Saito, Y., Nakayama, T., Grusby, M. J., Iwamoto, I., and Nakajima, H. (2008) J Exp Med 205, 1369
14. Dunn, G. P., Bruce, A. T., Ikeda, H., Old, L. J., and Schreiber, R. D. (2002) Nat Immunol 3, 991
15. Ozaki, K., Spolski, R., Feng, C. G., Qi, C.-F., Cheng, J., Sher, A., Morse, H. C., III, Liu, C., Schwartzberg, P. L., and Leonard, W. J. (2002) Science 298, 1630
16. Wurster, A. L., Rodgers, V. L., Satoskar, A. R., Whitters, M. J., Young, D. A., Collins, M., and Grusby, M. J. (2002) J Exp Med 196, 969
17. Strengell, M., Sareneva, T., Foster, D., Julkunen, I., and Matikainen, S. (2002) J Immunol 169, 3600
18. Pesce, J., Kaviratne, M., Ramalingam, T. R., Thompson, R. W., Urban, J. F., Cheever, A. W., Young, D. A., Collins, M., Grusby, M. J., and Wynn, T. A. (2006) J Clin Invest 116, 2044
19. Frohlich, A., Marsland, B. J., Sonderegger, I., Kurrer, M., Hodge, M. R., Harris, N. L., and Kopf, M. (2007) Blood 109, 2023
20. Korn, T., Bettelli, E., Gao, W., Awasthi, A., Jager, A., Strom, T. B., Oukka, M., and Kuchroo, V. K. (2007) Nature 448, 484
21. Nurieva, R., Yang, X. O., Martinez, G., Zhang, Y., Panopoulos, A. D., Ma, L., Schluns, K., Tian, Q., Watowich, S. S., Jetten, A. M., and Dong, C. (2007) Nature 448, 480
22. Zhou, L., Ivanov, I., Spolski, R., Min, R., Shenderov, K., Egawa, T., Levy, D. E., Leonard, W. J., and Littman, D. R. (2007) Nat Immunol 8, 967
23. Coquet, J. M., Chakravarti, S., Smyth, M. J., and Godfrey, D. I. (2008) J Immunol 180, 7097
24. Yang, L., Anderson, D. E., Baecher-Allan, C., Hastings, W. D., Bettelli, E., Oukka, M., Kuchroo, V. K., and Hafler, D. A. (2008) Nature 454, 350
25. Sonderegger, I., Kisielow, J., Meier, R., King, C., and Kopf, M. (2008) Eur J Immunol 38, 1833
26. Chtanova, T., Tangye, S. G., Newton, R., Frank, N., Hodge, M. R., Rolph, M. S., and Mackay, C. R. (2004) J Immunol 173, 68

27. Vogelzang, A., McGuire, H. M., Yu, D., Sprent, J., Mackay, C. R., and King, C. (2008) Immunity 29, 127
28. Nurieva, R. I., Chung, Y., Hwang, D., Yang, X. O., Kang, H. S., Ma, L., Wang, Y. H., Watowich, S. S., Jetten, A. M., Tian, Q., and Dong, C. (2008) Immunity 29, 138
29. Zeng, R., Spolski, R., Finkelstein, S. E., Oh, S., Kovanen, P. E., Hinrichs, C. S., Pise-Masison, C. A., Radonovich, M. F., Brady, J. N., Restifo, N. P., Berzofsky, J. A., and Leonard, W. J. (2005) J Exp Med 201, 139
30. Alves, N. L., Arosa, F. A., and van Lier, R. A. (2005) J Immunol 175, 755
31. Li, Y., Bleakley, M., and Yee, C. (2005) J Immunol 175, 2261
32. White, L., Krishnan, S., Strbo, N., Liu, H., Kolber, M. A., Lichtenheld, M. G., Pahwa, R., and Pahwa, S. (2007) Blood 109, 3873
33. Hinrichs, C. S., Spolski, R., Paulos, C. M., Gattinoni, L., Kerstann, K. W., Palmer, D. C., Klebanoff, C. A., Rosenberg, S. A., Leonard, W. J., and Restifo, N. P. (2008) Blood 111, 5326
34. Shevach, E. M. (2006) Immunity 25, 195
35. Fantini, M. C., Rizzo, A., Fina, D., Caruso, R., Becker, C., Neurath, M. F., MacDonald, T. T., Pallone, F., and Monteleone, G. (2007) Eur J Immunol 37, 3155
36. Peluso, I., Fantini, M. C., Fina, D., Caruso, R., Boirivant, M., MacDonald, T. T., Pallone, F., and Monteleone, G. (2007) J Immunol 178, 732
37. Antony, P. A., and Restifo, N. P. (2005) J Immunother 28, 120
38. Ahmadzadeh, M., Antony, P. A., and Rosenberg, S. A. (2007) J Immunother 30, 294
39. Kasaian, M. T., Whitters, M. J., Carter, L. L., Lowe, L. D., Jussif, J. M., Deng, B., Johnson, K. A., Witek, J. S., Senices, M., Konz, R. F., Wurster, A. L., Donaldson, D. D., Collins, M., Young, D. A., and Grusby, M. J. (2002) Immunity 16, 559
40. Brady, J., Hayakawa, Y., Smyth, M. J., and Nutt, S. L. (2004) J Immunol 172, 2048
41. Roda, J. M., Parihar, R., Lehman, A., Mani, A., Tridandapani, S., and Carson, W. E., III (2006) J Immunol 177, 120
42. Skak, K., Frederiksen, K. S., and Lundsgaard, D. (2008) Immunology 123, 575
43. Mehta, D. S., Wurster, A. L., Whitters, M. J., Young, D. A., Collins, M., and Grusby, M. J. (2003) J Immunol 170, 4111
44. Ozaki, K., Spolski, R., Ettinger, R., Kim, H. P., Wang, G., Qi, C. F., Hwu, P., Shaffer, D. J., Akilesh, S., Roopenian, D. C., Morse, H. C., III, Lipsky, P. E., and Leonard, W. J. (2004) J Immunol 173, 5361
45. Spolski, R., and Leonard, W. J. (2008) Annu Rev Immunol 26, 57
46. Wood, N., Bourque, K., Donaldson, D. D., Collins, M., Vercelli, D., Goldman, S. J., and Kasaian, M. T. (2004) Cell Immunol 231, 133
47. Ettinger, R., Sims, G. P., Fairhurst, A. M., Robbins, R., da Silva, Y. S., Spolski, R., Leonard, W. J., and Lipsky, P. E. (2005) J Immunol 175, 7867
48. Vinuesa, C. G., Cook, M. C., Angelucci, C., Athanasopoulos, V., Rui, L., Hill, K. M., Yu, D., Domaschenz, H., Whittle, B., Lambe, T., Roberts, I. S., Copley, R. R., Bell, J. I., Cornall, R. J., and Goodnow, C. C. (2005) Nature 435, 452
49. Herber, D., Brown, T. P., Liang, S., Young, D. A., Collins, M., and Dunussi-Joannopoulos, K. (2007) J Immunol 178, 3822
50. Young, D. A., Hegen, M., Ma, H. L., Whitters, M. J., Albert, L. M., Lowe, L., Senices, M., Wu, P. W., Sibley, B., Leathurby, Y., Brown, T. P., Nickerson-Nutter, C., Keith, J. C., Jr., and Collins, M. (2007) Arthritis Rheum 56, 1152
51. de Totero, D., Meazza, R., Zupo, S., Cutrona, G., Matis, S., Colombo, M., Balleari, E., Pierri, I., Fabbi, M., Capaia, M., Azzarone, B., Gobbi, M., Ferrarini, M., and Ferrini, S. (2006) Blood 107, 3708
52. Akamatsu, N., Yamada, Y., Hasegawa, H., Makabe, K., Asano, R., Kumagai, I., Murata, K., Imaizumi, Y., Tsukasaki, K., Tsuruda, K., Sugahara, K., Atogami, S., Yanagihara, K., and Kamihira, S. (2007) Cancer Lett 256, 196
53. de Totero, D., Meazza, R., Capaia, M., Fabbi, M., Azzarone, B., Balleari, E., Gobbi, M., Cutrona, G., Ferrarini, M., and Ferrini, S. (2008) Blood 111, 517

54. Gowda, A., Roda, J., Hussain, S. R., Ramanunni, A., Joshi, T., Schmidt, S., Zhang, X., Lehman, A., Jarjoura, D., Carson, W. E., Kindsvogel, W., Cheney, C., Caligiuri, M. A., Tridandapani, S., Muthusamy, N., and Byrd, J. C. (2008) Blood 111, 4723
55. Jahrsdorfer, B., Blackwell, S. E., Wooldridge, J. E., Huang, J., Andreski, M. W., Jacobus, L. S., Taylor, C. M., and Weiner, G. J. (2006) Blood 108, 2712
56. Bolesta, E., Kowalczyk, A., Wierzbicki, A., Eppolito, C., Kaneko, Y., Takiguchi, M., Stamatatos, L., Shrikant, P. A., and Kozbor, D. (2006) J Immunol 177, 177
57. Iuchi, T., Teitz-Tennenbaum, S., Huang, J., Redman, B. G., Hughes, S. D., Li, M., Jiang, G., Chang, A. E., and Li, Q. (2008) Cancer Res 68, 4431
58. Skak, K., Kragh, M., Hausman, D., Smyth, M. J., and Sivakumar, P. V. (2008) Nat Rev Drug Discov 7, 231
59. Søndergaard, H., Frederiksen, K. S., Thygesen, P., Galsgaard, E. D., Skak, K., Kristjansen, P. E., Odum, N., and Kragh, M. (2007) Cancer Immunol Immunother 56, 1417
60. Wang, G., Tschoi, M., Spolski, R., Lou, Y., Ozaki, K., Feng, C., Kim, G., Leonard, W. J., and Hwu, P. (2003) Cancer Res 63, 9016
61. Ma, H.-L., Whitters, M. J., Konz, R. F., Senices, M., Young, D. A., Grusby, M. J., Collins, M., and Dunussi-Joannopoulos, K. (2003) J Immunol 171, 608
62. Comes, A., Rosso, O., Orengo, A. M., Di Carlo, E., Sorrentino, C., Meazza, R., Piazza, T., Valzasina, B., Nanni, P., Colombo, M. P., and Ferrini, S. (2006) J Immunol 176, 1750
63. Furukawa, J., Hara, I., Nagai, H., Yao, A., Oniki, S., and Fujisawa, M. (2006) J Urol 176, 1198
64. Kumano, M., Hara, I., Furukawa, J., Oniki, S., Nagai, H., Miyake, H., and Fujisawa, M. (2007) J Urol 178, 1504
65. Daga, A., Orengo, A. M., Gangemi, R. M., Marubbi, D., Perera, M., Comes, A., Ferrini, S., and Corte, G. (2007) Int J Cancer 121, 1756
66. Ugai, S., Shimozato, O., Kawamura, K., Wang, Y. Q., Yamaguchi, T., Saisho, H., Sakiyama, S., and Tagawa, M. (2003) Cancer Gene Ther 10, 187
67. Croce, M., Meazza, R., Orengo, A. M., Fabbi, M., Borghi, M., Ribatti, D., Nico, B., Carlini, B., Pistoia, V., Corrias, M. V., and Ferrini, S. (2008) Cancer Immunol Immunother 57, 1625
68. Moroz, A., Eppolito, C., Li, Q., Tao, J., Clegg, C. H., and Shrikant, P. A. (2004) J Immunol 173, 900
69. Cvetkovic, R. S., and Perry, C. M. (2006) BioDrugs 20, 253
70. Dall'Ozzo, S., Tartas, S., Paintaud, G., Cartron, G., Colombat, P., Bardos, P., Watier, H., and Thibault, G. (2004) Cancer Res 64, 4664
71. Roda, J. M., Joshi, T., Butchar, J. P., McAlees, J. W., Lehman, A., Tridandapani, S., and Carson, W. E., III (2007) Clin Cancer Res 13, 6419
72. Smyth, M. J., Hayakawa, Y., Cretney, E., Zerafa, N., Sivakumar, P., Yagita, H., and Takeda, K. (2006) J Immunol 176, 6347
73. Smyth, M. J., Teng, M. W. L., Sharkey, J., Westwood, J. A., Haynes, N. M., Yagita, H., Takeda, K., Sivakumar, P. V., and Kershaw, M. H. (2008) Cancer Res 68, 3019
74. Davis, I. D., Skrumsager, B. K., Cebon, J., Nicholaou, T., Barlow, J. W., Moller, N. P. H., Skak, K., Lundsgaard, D., Frederiksen, K. S., Thygesen, P., and McArthur, G. A. (2007) Clin Cancer Res 13, 3630
75. Thompson, J. A., Curti, B. D., Redman, B. G., Bhatia, S., Weber, J. S., Agarwala, S. S., Sievers, E. L., Hughes, S. D., DeVries, T. A., and Hausman, D. F. (2008) J Clin Oncol 26, 2034
76. Frederiksen, K. S., Lundsgaard, D., Freeman, J. A., Hughes, S. D., Holm, T. L., Skrumsager, B. K., Petri, A., Hansen, L. T., McArthur, G. A., Davis, I. D., and Skak, K. (2008) Cancer Immunol Immunother 57, 1439
77. Davis, I. D., Brady, B., Kefford, R., Millward, M. J., Skrumsager, B. K., Mouritzen, U., Kristjansen, P. E., and McArthur, G. A. (2008) J Clin Oncol 26, 3042
77A. Davis, I. D., Brady, B., Kefford, R. F., Millward, M., Cebor, J., Skrumsager, B. K., Mouritzen, U., Hansen, L. T., Skak, K., Lundsgaard, D., Frederiksen, K. S., Kristjansen, P. E., McArthur, G. (2009) Clin Cancer Res 15, 2123

78. Timmerman, J. M., Byrd, J. C., Andorsky, D. J., Siadak, M. F., DeVries, T., Hausman, D. F., and Pagel, J. M. (2007) ASH Annual Meeting Abstracts 110: 2577
79. Timmerman, J. M., Byrd, J. C., Andorsky, D. J., Siadak, M. F., DeVries, T. A., Hausman, D. F., and Pagel, J. M. (2008) J Clin Oncol 26, 8554
80. Pezaro, C., and Davis, I. D. (2008) Curr Med Chem 15, 1166
81. Bhatia, S., Curti, B. D., Gordon, M. S., Quinn, D. I., DeVries, T. A., Hunder, N. H., and Thompson, J. A. (2007) Mol Cancer Therapeut 6, 3354S
82. Bhatia, S., Curti, B. D., Gordon, M. S., Quinn, D. I., Thompson, J.A., DeVries, T. A., Dodds, M. G., Hunder, N. N., and Hausman, D. F. (2008) J Clin Oncol 26, 16008
83. Lake, R. A., and Robinson, B. W. (2005) Nat Rev Cancer 5, 397
84. Zitvogel, L., Apetoh, L., Ghiringhelli, F., and Kroemer, G. (2008) Nat Rev Immunol 8, 59
85. Ives, N. J., Stowe, R. L., Lorigan, P., and Wheatley, K. (2007) J Clin Oncol 25, 5426
86. Davis, I. D., Jefford, M., Parente, P., and Cebon, J. (2003) J Leukoc Biol 73, 3
87. Nicholaou, T., Ebert, L., Davis, I. D., Robson, N., Klein, O., Maraskovsky, E., Chen, W., and Cebon, J. (2006) Immunol Cell Biol 84, 303
88. He, H., Wisner, P., Yang, G., Hu, H. M., Haley, D., Miller, W., O'Hara, A., Alvord, W. G., Clegg, C. H., Fox, B. A., Urba, W. J., and Walker, E. B. (2006) J Transl Med 4, 24
89. Nakano, H., Kishida, T., Asada, H., Shin-Ya, M., Shinomiya, T., Imanishi, J., Shimada, T., Nakai, S., Takeuchi, M., Hisa, Y., and Mazda, O. (2006) J Gene Med 8, 90
90. Li, Y., and Yee, C. (2008) Blood 111, 229
91. Rosenberg, S. A., Restifo, N. P., Yang, J. C., Morgan, R. A., and Dudley, M. E. (2008) Nat Rev Cancer 8, 299
92. Kirkwood, J. M., Tarhini, A. A., Panelli, M. C., Moschos, S. J., Zarour, H. M., Butterfield, L. H., and Gogas, H. J. (2008) J Clin Oncol 26, 3445
93. Ribas, A. (2006) J Natl Compr Canc Netw 4, 687
94. Peggs, K. S., Quezada, S. A., Korman, A. J., and Allison, J. P. (2006) Curr Opin Immunol 18, 206
95. Barnett, B., Kryczek, I., Cheng, P., Zou, W., and Curiel, T. J. (2005) Am J Reprod Immunol 54, 369
96. Litzinger, M. T., Fernando, R., Curiel, T. J., Grosenbach, D. W., Schlom, J., and Palena, C. (2007) Blood 110, 3192
97. Beck, K. E., Blansfield, J. A., Tran, K. Q., Feldman, A. L., Hughes, M. S., Royal, R. E., Kammula, U. S., Topalian, S. L., Sherry, R. M., Kleiner, D., Quezado, M., Lowy, I., Yellin, M., Rosenberg, S. A., and Yang, J. C. (2006) J Clin Oncol 24, 2283
98. Sanderson, K., Scotland, R., Lee, P., Liu, D., Groshen, S., Snively, J., Sian, S., Nichol, G., Davis, T., Keler, T., Yellin, M., and Weber, J. (2005) J Clin Oncol 23, 741
99. Ribas, A., Camacho, L. H., Lopez-Berestein, G., Pavlov, D., Bulanhagui, C. A., Millham, R., Comin-Anduix, B., Reuben, J. M., Seja, E., Parker, C. A., Sharma, A., Glaspy, J. A., and Gomez-Navarro, J. (2005) J Clin Oncol 23, 8968
100. Maker, A. V., Phan, G. Q., Attia, P., Yang, J. C., Sherry, R. M., Topalian, S. L., Kammula, U. S., Royal, R. E., Haworth, L. R., Levy, C., Kleiner, D., Mavroukakis, S. A., Yellin, M., and Rosenberg, S. A. (2005) Ann Surg Oncol 12, 1005
101. Maker, A. V., Attia, P., and Rosenberg, S. A. (2005) J Immunol 175, 7746
102. Attia, P., Phan, G. Q., Maker, A. V., Robinson, M. R., Quezado, M. M., Yang, J. C., Sherry, R. M., Topalian, S. L., Kammula, U. S., Royal, R. E., Restifo, N. P., Haworth, L. R., Levy, C., Mavroukakis, S. A., Nichol, G., Yellin, M. J., and Rosenberg, S. A. (2005) J Clin Oncol 23, 6043
103. Phan, G. Q., Yang, J. C., Sherry, R. M., Hwu, P., Topalian, S. L., Schwartzentruber, D. J., Restifo, N. P., Haworth, L. R., Seipp, C. A., Freezer, L. J., Morton, K. E., Mavroukakis, S. A., Duray, P. H., Steinberg, S. M., Allison, J. P., Davis, T. A., and Rosenberg, S. A. (2003) Proc Natl Acad Sci USA 100, 8372

IL-24 in Regulation of Antitumor Immune Response and in Signaling

Sita Aggarwal, William Hansel, and Rajasree Solipuram

Abstract In cancer therapy, cytokines are generally used to increase immunity. Cytokines are either proteins or glycoproteins, which are secreted by immune cells. It is now known that the tumor microenvironment secretes a mixture of cytokines that plays an important role in carcinogenesis. In chronic inflammation, cytokines released at the site of a tumor facilitate tumor growth, instead of promoting antitumor immunity. In 1995, a protein called melanoma differentiation-associated gene-7 (MDA-7), also known as suppressor of tumorigenicity-16 (ST-16), was discovered; it was renamed as interlukine-24 because of its cytokine-like properties and was found to inhibit the growth and proliferation in melanoma cells. The rat counterpart of IL-24 was named as mob-5 or C49a. The murine counterpart was named as FISP. Ectopic expression of MDA-7/IL-24 by means of a replication defective adenovirus (Ad-MDA-7/IL-24) results in growth suppression, inhibits angiogenesis and apoptosis not only in melanoma cells but also in numerous other cancer cell types such as glioblastoma, carcinomas of breast, colon, lung, ovarian and prostate sparing normal epithelial and fibroblasts. Therefore, this article reviews anti-cytokine therapies of MDA-7/IL-24 being pursued in cancer and more details about signaling pathways associated with MDA-7/IL-24 in cancer.

Introduction

Melanoma differentiation-associated gene-7 (*MDA-7*) was first discovered in 1995 by subtraction hybridization of cDNA libraries of induced differentiated melanoma cells [1]. Because of structural homology to members of the interleukin (IL)-10 cytokine, chromosomal localization, and cytokine like properties, MDA-7 was renamed as IL-24 [2–6]. MDA-7/IL-24 is a secreted nuclear protein of predicted

S. Aggarwal (✉)
William Hansel Cancer Prevention Laboratory, Pennington Biomedical Research Center, Louisiana State University System, Baton Rouge, LA 70808, USA
e-mail: sita.aggarwal@pbrc.edu

J. Lustgarten et al. (eds.), *Targeted Cancer Immune Therapy*,
DOI 10.1007/978-1-4419-0170-5_4,

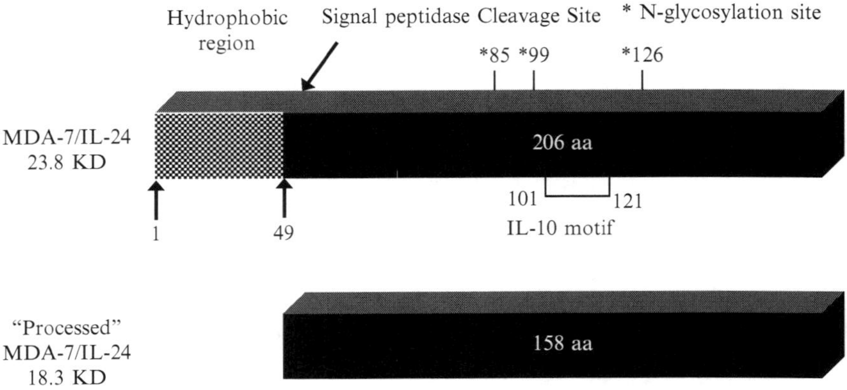

Fig. 1 MDA-7/IL-24 protein: The human melanoma differentiation-associated gene-7/interleukin-24 (*MDA-7/IL-24*), encodes a protein of 206 amino acids with a predicted molecular mass of 23.8 kDa comprising *N*-glycosylation sites at positions 85, 99, and 126; an IL-10 signature motif from position 101–121; a hydrophobic region of signal peptide (1–49 amino acids); a signal peptidase cleavage site between amino acids 49 and 50. The processed mature form of MDA-7/IL-24 protein is composed of 158 amino acids with a predicted molecular mass of 18.3 kDa

size of 23.8 kDa, which is composed of an IL-10 signature motif at amino acids 101–121 shared by other members of the IL-10 family of cytokines [7, 8]. MDA-7/IL-24 is a glycosylated protein and in addition to proTh1 cytokine activity, possesses anti-antigenic properties mediated through IL-22R [9, 10]. It contains a consensus signal sequence and a proteolytic cleavage site, which is then processed to remove the hydrophobic region [6, 11] (Fig. 1). The location of MDA-7/IL-24 has been shown to be important, and it has divergent effects. Intracellular MDA-7/IL-24 has been shown to have a cytotoxic effect in lung cancer cells [12]. Like most other apoptosis-inducing cytokines, including members of tumor necrosis factor (TNF) superfamily [13], it has been shown that *MDA-7/IL-24* regulates the immune system by inducing various inflammatory cytokines, such as TNF, IL-1, and IL-6 [9, 14]. In early studies, *MDA-7/IL-24* gene transfer by adenovirus was shown to suppress proliferation and colony formation in melanoma cells but not in normal cells. MDA-7/IL-24 expression is lost during tumor progression, in correlation with tumor invasion and metastasis [11, 15]. Later, it was found that MDA-7/IL-24 not only induces tumor cell death in melanoma cells but also in a wide variety of tumors such as fibrosarcoma, breast carcinoma, lung cancer, ovarian cancer, pancreatic cancer, prostate cancer, malignant cancer, and colon cancer. The tumor suppressing property of MDA-7/IL-24 is now very well established and does not depend on the status of other tumor suppressor genes, such as *p53*, *Ras*, and *Rb* or apoptosis regulating genes such as *bax* or *caspases* in tumor cells [16–20]. Surprisingly, the cytotoxicity of MDA-7/IL-24 is selective for tumor cell killing and its overexpression in various normal cells that include normal human epithelial cells, melanocytes, astrocytes, or fibroblasts did not affect their growth and viability [21]. The *in vitro* results were further confirmed by *in vivo* animal models with human breast, lung, and colorectal

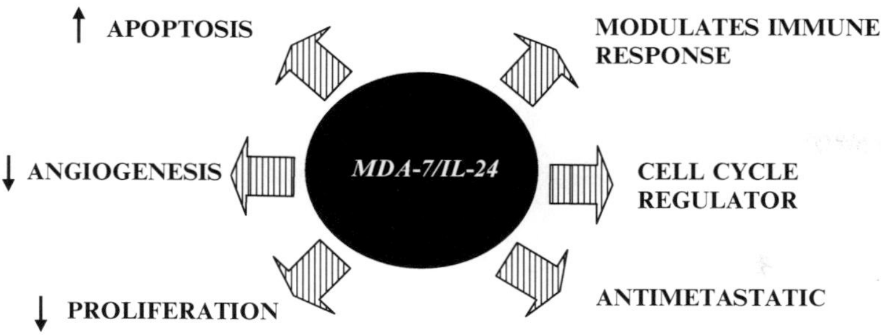

Fig. 2 Pleotropic effect of *MDA-7/IL-24* in cancer cells

carcinoma and glioma xenografts [19, 20, 22, 23]. Looking at the remarkable multiple antitumor properties of MDA-7/IL-24, Fisher called it a "Magic Bullet" for cancer (Fig. 2) [24]. Its properties include induction of apoptosis in cancer cells, decreased angiogenesis in cancer cells, inhibition of metastases of cancer cells, modulation of immune system, and inhibition of tumor cell proliferation without having any effect on normal cell proliferation. Further investigation of underlying molecular mechanisms involving MDA-7/IL-24 induction of apoptosis in various cancer cells are in process. Some studies indicate that Bax, double-stranded RNA-dependent protein kinase (PKR), growth arrest and DNA damage family genes (GADD) have roles [25–27]. MDA-7/IL-24 has recently been tested on cancer patients in Phase I clinical trials. Thus the present chapter reviews the signaling pathways activated during apoptosis, angiogenesis, and metastases of cancer cells by *MDA-7/IL-24* in different cancer cell types and also discusses clinical reports on *Ad-MDA-7/IL-24* administration in patients in Phase I clinical trials.

MDA-7 as a Cytokine

The human *MDA-7* gene is located on chromosome 1q31–32 and belongs to the IL-10 family [3, 18, 28]. Homology of *MDA-7* with *IL-10* family members varies between 15 and 40%, because of its limited homology with *IL-10*, *MDA-7* was redesignated as *IL-24* [2, 29]. IL-10 signals through class II cytokine receptors and it shares the receptor IL-10Rβ chain with IL-22 [30–32]. Also, IL-10 signals through IL-10R as a dimer of IL-10R1/IL-10R2 on the cell surface. Human IL-10R (hIL-10) is species specific and binds only to hIL-10 [4, 33]. Although IL-10 and IL-24 belong to same family, IL-10 and MDA-7/IL-24 have different effects. IL-10 suppresses the immune response and inflammation [34], while MDA-7/IL-24 modulates the immune response [35]. Unlike *IL-10*, *MDA-7* mediates signal through two types of IL-20R complexes. As shown in Fig. 3, these include the IL-20Rβ subunit with IL-20Rα (type I IL-20R1 complex) and the IL-20Rβ subunit with the IL-22R subunit (type II IL–20R2 complex). Type I is shared by IL-19,

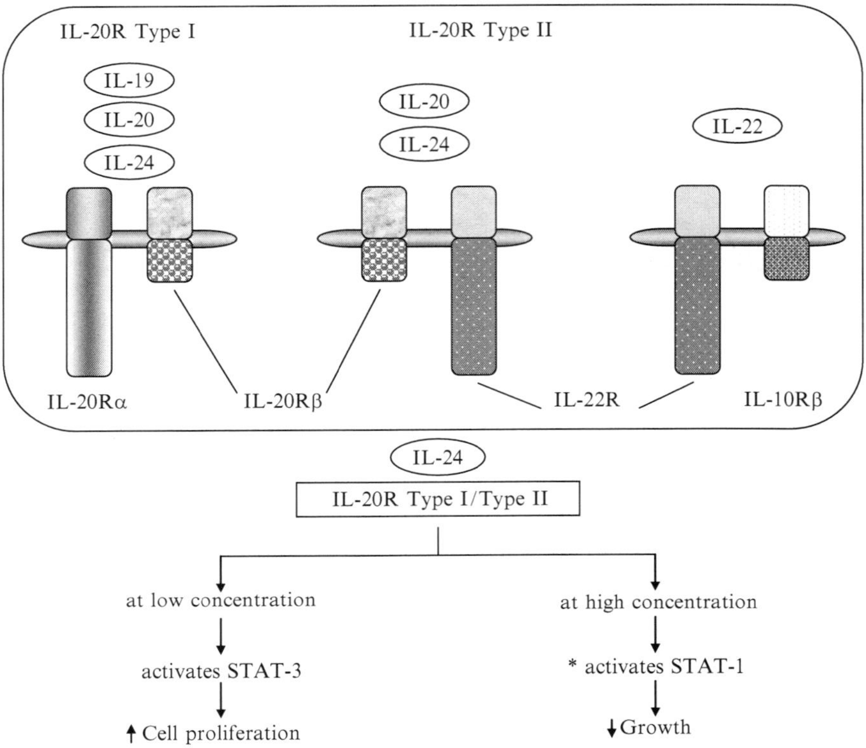

Fig. 3 IL-22R and IL-20R complexes and signaling pathways associated with them

IL-20, and MDA-7/IL-24, while type II is shared by IL-20 and MDA-7/IL-24 [36]. IL-20R1 and IL-20R2 are ubiquitously expressed in mouse tissues [37], while their expression is limited in human keratinocytes and are found in very low levels in peripheral blood mononuclear cells (PBMCs), bone marrow, and the spleen [38]. The exact tissue distribution profile of these receptors is not yet known. Low levels of expression of MDA-7/IL-24 can be upregulated in PBMCs and in T cells ($CD4^+$ and memory cells) by treating them with lipopolysaccrides (LPS) [9] and by anti-CD3 mAb [39], respectively. No expression was observed in natural killer cells or B cells before and after stimulation. The expression of MDA-7/IL-24 was increased in the cells committed to T1 cell differentiation [39]. This expression of MDA-7/IL-24 in PBMCs is regulated at the posttranscriptional level through stabilization of MDA-7/IL-24 mRNA [40]. Treatment of PBMCs with MDA-7/IL-24 induces the expression of secondary cytokines such as IL-6, interferon-gamma (INF-γ), TNF-α, IL-β, IL-12, and granulocyte macrophage-colony stimulating factor (GM-CSF) [9]. However, treatment of PBMCs with MDA-7/IL-24 did not stimulate the proliferative functions [39]. These secondary cytokines may activate the antitumor response [9, 35]. MDA-7/IL-24 alone does not activate the nuclear transcription factor – kappa

B (NF-κB) but significantly upregulates the effect of another cytokine, a TNF-α-induced NF-κB activation and TNF-α-induced NF-κB regulated gene expression [41] in a receptor-independent manner. In another study, it was shown that MDA-7/IL-24 activates NF-κB via the activation of PKR [42]. The expression of MDA-7/IL-24 was lost as the tumor progresses, which explains the ineffective immune response within the tumor [35]. The distribution of IL-20R1 and IL-20R2 expression was tumor cell line specific [38, 43]. Further, binding of MDA-7/IL-24 to its receptor complexes leads to the activation of signal pathways in a concentration-dependent manner [44]. At lower concentrations, MDA-7/IL-24 activates the signal transducer and activation of transcript 3 (STAT-3) and promotes cellular proliferation [36, 44]. At higher concentrations MDA-7/IL-24 activates STAT-1 and leads to cell growth inhibition (Fig. 3) [44]. Furthermore, the expression of IL-20R1 and IL-20R2 was higher in tumor cells as well as in tumor blood vessels in case of tumor tissues from lung cancer patients. In normal tissues, the expression of receptor complexes was restricted to mononuclear cells [44]. Intratumoral administration of *Ad-MDA-7/IL-24* induces the production of INF-γ, TNF-α, and IL-6 in the serum of patients [45]. Also, a marked increase was reported in $CD3^{+}CD8^{+}$ T cells after treatment [45]. In summary, the methods by which *MDA-7/IL-24* modulates immunity is still not understood, and additional experiments are needed to determine which of the receptor chains serve as actual ligand-binding components in various cell types.

MDA-7/IL-24 Induced Apoptosis in Cancer Cells

In normal cells, apoptosis is initiated in response to developmental cues, cell stress, changes in growth factor signaling, and signaling from oncogenes. Cancer cells, however, are often able to bypass this mechanism and escape apoptosis, which is a key hallmark of cancer and is critical for cancer development and tumor cell survival [46–48]. Therefore, methods that promote apoptosis in cancer cells are useful therapeutics. One of them is gene transfer induced apoptosis. Adenoviral (Ad)-mediated overexpression of the *Ad-MDA-7/IL-24* induces apoptosis in a wide range of cancer cells [19, 20, 22, 23]. Several signaling pathways that promote apoptotic mechanisms via *Ad-MDA-7/IL-24* have been reported. In initial studies of human melanoma cells, *Ad-MDA-7/IL-24* induced apoptosis via the p38 mitogen-activated protein kinase (MAPK) pathway [27]. Ad-MDA-7/IL-24 increased the expression at both mRNA and protein levels of GADD-inducible genes, such as GADD153, GADD45α, and GADD34 and the selective (MAPK) pathway inhibitor, SB203580 inhibited *Ad-MDA-7/IL-24* induced apoptosis [27]. Subsequently, findings were confirmed in malignant glioma and prostate carcinomas [24, 27]. In lung cells, *Ad-MDA-7/IL-24* induced apoptosis was through the activation of PKR and its downstream targets. This is followed by phosphorylation of the α-subunit of eukaryotic translation initiation factor 2 (eIF-2α) and the release of cytochrome c from mitochondria [26, 49]. Interestingly, the same group reported that there was also a direct interaction between PKR and MDA-7/IL-24 [50]. Although MDA-7/IL-24 protein binds to

IL-20 and IL-22 receptor complexes to mediate its action, it has been shown in one study that specific inhibitors of tyrosine kinase or JAK/STAT activation pathways do not alter *Ad-MDA-7/IL-24*-induced apoptotic activity [5]. There is no correlation between the expressions of receptor complexes with the apoptotic activity of *Ad-MDA-7/IL-24* in various cancer cells [51]. In the context of ovarian cancer, activation of both the mitochondrial intrinsic pathway [52] and the extrinsic pathways [53] were involved in *Ad-MDA-7/IL-24*-induced apoptosis. The mitochondrial extrinsic pathway involves the activation of transcription factors, such as c-Jun and activating transcription factor 2 (AP-2), and immediate death inducer down stream targets, such as Fas ligand (FasL), and its cognate receptor Fas. As a result of Fas-FasL association, activation of NF-κB, Fas-associated factor 1, Fas-associated death domain, and caspase-8 takes place and induces apoptosis [53, 54]. Activation of the intrinsic pathway involves the disruption of mitochondrial potential and activation of downstream capase-9 and caspase-3 via cytochrome c release [54]. In human pancreatic cancer cells, *Ad-MDA-7/IL-24* induces apoptosis via the Wnt/PI3K pathways [55]. Also, the same group identified a novel bystander mechanism of apoptosis by MDA-7/IL-24 in pancreatic cancer that functions via IL-20 receptors and activates STAT-3 [55]. Genetically, complex cancers such as pancreatic cancer have been shown to develop innate resistance to *MDA-7/IL-24*-induced apoptosis, because of a diminished capacity to convert MDA-7/IL-24 mRNA into protein. This limitation can be overcome by a combinatorial approach [56]. The combination of an *Ad-MDA-7/IL-24* with pharmacologic and genetic agents to simultaneously block several downstream signaling pathways was found to increase apoptosis in cancer cells [56, 57]. For example, using the pharmacologic agents PD98059 or U1026 eliminates the MDA-7/IL-24 mRNA translational block in mutant K-*ras* pancreatic cancer cells resulting in protein production and apoptosis [57]. This concept was further supported by another study showing that transfection of mutant K-ras pancreatic carcinoma cells with an antisense K-ras expression vector and *Ad-MDA-7/IL-24* inhibits colony formation in vitro [58]. The use of arsenic trioxide, *N*-(4-hydroxyphenyl) retinamide, NSC656240, or 17-allyl-amino-17-demethoxygeldanamycin in combination with *Ad-MDA-7/IL-24* induces apoptosis in vitro in cancer cells [59]. Further, these combination studies also showed the suppression of tumorigenesis *in vivo* in nude mice models [56, 58]. Additionally, in ovarian cancer cells, apoptosis can be enhanced by combination treatments with ionizing radiation (IR) and with *Ad-MDA-7/IL-24* [60]. Prostate tumors develop resistance to radiation therapy due to the overexpression of antiapoptotic genes such as bcl-x_L and *bcl-2* genes, and the combination of IR and *Ad-MDA-7/IL-24* increases the therapeutic benefit of *MDA-7/IL-24* gene [61]. This radiosensitizing process of *MDA-7/IL-24* involves c-Jun NH_2-terminal kinase (JNK) kinase activation pathway in prostate cancer [61], malignant gliomas [23], and nonsmall cell lung carcinomas [62]. Recently, another novel pathway of *MDA-7/IL-24* in regulating apoptosis has been reported showing that *MDA-7/IL-24* induces the secretion of endogenous INF-β and TRAIL/FasL activation [63]. Yet another possibility of developing resistance to MDA-7/IL-24-induced apoptosis due to the activation of NF-κB [13] and the use of NF-κB inhibitors with combination of MDA-7/IL-24 to modulate the apoptotic activity in the cancer cells may be

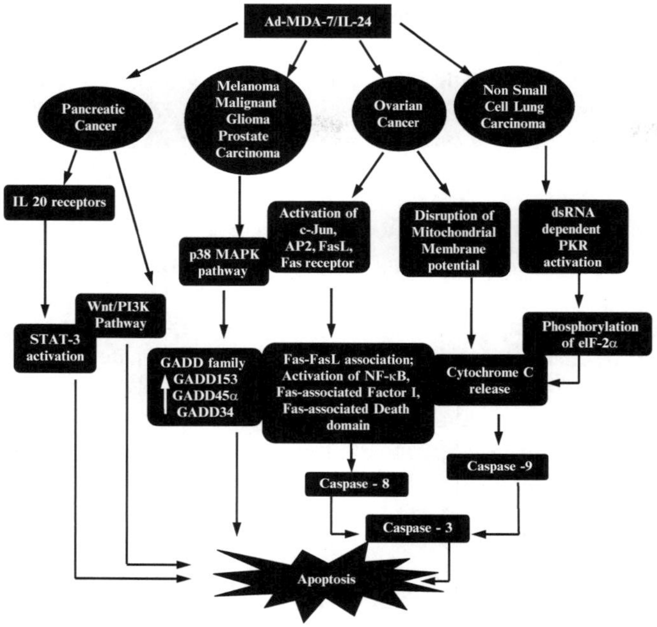

Fig. 4 *Ad-.MDA-7/IL-24* induced signaling pathways promote apoptosis in different cancer cell lines

beneficial. For example, recently it was shown that curcumin, a potent NF-κB inhibitor, improves the radiation therapy in human colorectal cancer xenografts in nude mice [64]. We also showed that MDA-7/IL-24 increases the activation of TNF-induced NF-κB in A293 cells stably transfected with *MDA-7* [41]. Activation of NF-κB is dependent on cell type [65] and the possibility that MDA-7/IL-24 activates NF-κB in only a few cancer cell lines needs to be explored. The present data supports the idea that *MDA-7/IL-24* affects multiple but distinct signaling pathways in various cancer cells that promote apoptosis as shown in Fig. 4.

MDA-7/IL-24 Inhibits Angiogenesis in Cancer Cells

Growing new blood vessels from existing ones – a process called angiogenesis – plays an important role in expanding tumor size. In addition, cancer cells escape through the new blood vessels into the circulation and metastasize [66]. Cancer cells stimulate angiogenic factors such as vascular endothelial growth factor (VEGF), basic fibroblastic growth factor (bFGF), epidermal growth factor (EGF), angiopoetin, integrins, IL-8, and platelet-derived endothelial cell growth factor (PD-ECGF) [67]. The degree of angiogenesis is directly related to the aggressiveness of the tumor [68, 69]. Therefore, selective inhibition of angiogenesis is a good strategy and numerous antiangiogenic agents including MDA-7/IL-24 are currently in various phases of clinical trial. In the nude mice model, Saeki et al. showed that an inhibition of tumor growth was due to *Ad-MDA-7/IL-24* treatment [20]. VEGF has previously been shown to bind VEGFR1 and VEGFR2 [70, 71]. The binding of VEGF to VEGFR2 activates cell survival pathways such as AKT and ERK1/ERK2 [72, 73]. However, the molecular mechanism by which *Ad-MDA-7/IL-24* inhibits VEGF is unknown. In 2003, it was reported that *MDA-7/IL-24* was a potent inhibitor of angiogenesis, and this effect was mediated by secreted MDA-7/IL-24 affecting endothelial cells through interactions with the IL-20/IL-22 receptor complexes [10]. Apoptosis was prevented by secreted MDA-7/IL-24 protein in the cancer cells such as A549 nonsmall cell carcinoma that lack functional IL-20/IL-22 receptors [74]. However, in animals treated with the combination of radiation and *Ad-MDA-7/IL-24* secreted MDA-7, which inhibits angiogenesis by sensitizing endothelial cells to ionizing radiation without affecting normal cells [19]. Further, Inoue et al. showed that MDA-7 protein inhibits tumor angiogenesis directly as well as indirectly. One study showed that MDA-7/IL-24 purified protein directly inhibits endothelial cell differentiation *in vivo* without affecting cell proliferation, and this effect was restricted to receptor positive cells [10]. In the same study, it has been reported that MDA-7/IL24 protein inhibited VEGF and FGF-induced endothelial cell migration [10]. One possible explanation was the activation of STAT-1 [75] and another was the inhibition of the PI3/AKT pathway [76, 77]. Intratumoral administration of MDA-7/IL24 in nanoparticles resulted in reduced vascularization [44, 78]. Another study showed that the direct inhibition of VEGF expression by MDA-7 protein involves c-Src kinase/STAT-3 signaling pathway, which was confirmed by showing that *Ad-MDA-7/IL-24* inhibited VEGF in Src(+/+), but not in Src(−/−) mouse embryo fibroblasts, and in indirect *Ad-MDA-7/IL-24* involves VEGF/VEGFR2 signaling [79]. Recently, the same group showed that the combination of bevacizumab, a humanized monoclonal antibody against VEGF, and MDA-7 resulted in decreased cell survival, apoptosis of lung cancer cells, and tumor regression in *in vivo* subcutaneous lung tumor xenografts [80]. In conclusion, MDA-7/IL-24 mediates its antiangiogenic function via a direct mechanism in the tumor cells containing functional IL-20/IL-22 receptors and an indirect mechanism in cancer cells lacking functional IL-20/IL-22 receptors.

MDA-7/IL-24 in Tumor Metastases and Invasion

A number of studies suggested that MDA-7/IL-24 also plays a role in tumor invasion and metastases. An initial study showed that MDA-7/IL-24 expression and melanoma tumor invasion are inversely correlated [11]. A further study supported the idea, showing that *MDA-7/IL-24* inhibited the migration of vascular smooth muscle cells [81]. MDA-7/IL-24 inhibited expression of the signaling molecules p85PI3K, pFAK, matrix metalloproteinase-2 (MMP-2), and MMP-9, which were previously shown to be candidates in tumor invasion and metastases [82–84]. One of the signaling pathways associated with tumor invasion and metastasis is the Wnt signaling pathway [55]. On the one hand, in the absence of Wnt signaling, β-catenin is bound with E-cadherin, regulating cell-cell adhesion. β-catenin is also sequestered in a complex with axin, APC, and glycogen synthase kinase-3β, which phosphorylates it on Ser/Thr residues, targeting it for proteosomal-dependent degradation. On the other hand, in the presence of Wnt, the E-cadherin is down regulated in tumor cell surfaces, and this loss of E-cadherin expression leads to the disassociation of cells and results in cell migration [55]. Further, β-catenin uncouples from the degradation complex and translocates to the nucleus, where its binds Lef/Tcf transcription factors, thus activating target genes involved in metastases and invasion. Ramesh et al. [77] showed that MDA-7 inhibits tumor metastases in a nude mouse model. In conclusion, the results from *in vitro* and *in vivo* studies confirm the anti-metastatic property of *MDA-7/IL-24*.

Clinical Evaluation of *MDA-7/IL-24*

A number of gene therapy-based drugs have been tested and have shown promise in Phase I/II clinical trials. For example, *Ad-p53* gene transfer has shown some promise in clinics in patients with advanced recurrent head and neck squamous cell carcinoma, recurrent glioma, lung cancer, and paclitaxel resistant ovarian cancer [85–88]. But there are some limitations with gene therapy. First, adenovirus vector-mediated gene delivery prevents repeated dosing because of its immune modulating properties [89]. Second, systemic therapy with the *Ad-gene* for the treatment of disseminated cancers is not feasible [90]. Third, the cytotoxic effects of therapeutic genes are limited to the tumor cells expressing the therapeutic protein, and to a lesser extent to adjacent tumor cells with no cytotoxic effects on distant tumor cells [91–94]. In an attempt to overcome these limitations of gene therapy, *MDA-7/IL-24* was initially associated with a nonreplicative adenoviral vector deleted in the E1 region (INGN 241) [1, 22]. The results from preclinical and clinical studies are summarized in Table 1. The initial studies were done in five melanoma human tumor samples, and it was found that MDA-7/IL-24 protein expression was decreased in the advanced melanomas [15]. The expression of MDA-7/IL-24 was absent in 14 out of 15 cases of lymphnode metastases [15]. This study was further strengthened by looking at the expression of MDA-7/IL-24 protein in a larger sample of 41 primary melanomas and 41 metastasis cases. Significant differences were found when comparing primary tumors to paired metastases. Decrease in MDA-7/IL-24 expression in primary melanomas facilitates progression to invasive and metastatic stages [11]. In contrast, another study with 183 nonsmall cell lung cancer patients found no significant correlation in MDA-7/IL-24 expression and patient survival or between MDA-7/IL-24 status and any patient characteristic including pathologic stage. In these studies, these authors found that MDA-7/IL-24-high adenocarcinoma showed a significantly higher incidence of apoptotic

Table 1 Summary of results from preclinical and clinical studies

Reference	Number of cases	Type of cancer	Results
[15]	5 15	Primary melanoma Lymph node metastases	MDA-7 levels were low in primary melanomas, declined with increasing tumor depth and increasing clinical stage and were virtually absent in lymph node metastases
[11]	41	Primary tumor and metastases from cutaneous melanoma	Inverse correlation between endogenous MDA-7, protein expression, and melanoma progression
[95]	183	Pathologic-stage I-IIIA nonsmall cell lung cancer	MDA-7/IL-24 status was a significant prognostic factor in lung adenocarcinoma, not in lung squamous cell carcinoma
[96]	28	Advanced carcinoma Resectable Solid tumors	MDA-7/IL24 administration was well tolerated; MDA-7 DNA and RNA were detectable in 100% of the injected lesions, with the highest concentrations found at the site of injection. Apoptosis in the injected lesions was correlated significantly with MDA-7 protein expression; "bystander" killing effect mediated by MDA-7
[45]	22	Advanced cancer	Significantly higher elevations of IL-6 and TNF-α and marked increases of CD3+CD8+ T cells were observed. Apoptosis occurred in large volume of tumor, tumor-regulating and immune-activating events were observed

tumor cell death than MDA-7/IL-24 low adenocarcinoma. MDA-7/IL-24 expression was a significant factor to predict a favorable prognosis in adenocarcinoma but not in squamous cell carcinoma [95]. A Phase I clinical trial was conducted to test the tolerance and safety of administration of INGN 241 in patients with advanced melanoma. INGN 241 was found to be safe and well tolerated in patients with metastatic melanoma and solid tumor patients when *Ad-MDA-7/IL-24* was administered intratumorally as a single injection [45, 96]. These studies included 28 patients with resectable solid tumors and 22 patients with advance carcinoma. MDA-7/IL-24 was expressed in tumor cells that were undergoing apoptosis. These studies confirmed the activation of the host immune response by detecting serum cytokines such as TNF-α, IL-6, IFN-γ, and GM-CSF and found an increased number of CD8 positive T cells with no change in CD4 positive T cells [45, 96]. The studies are consistent with previous findings that expression of MDA-7/IL-24 protein induces apoptosis in tumor cells and elicits tumor-regulatory and immune-activating events.

Summary

It is clear that *Ad-MDA-7/IL-24* administration induces apoptosis in cancer cells but not in normal cells. Because of its remarkable selection for cancer cells, *MDA-7/IL-24* has progressed from the "bench to the bedside." Very few preclinical and clinical studies have been conducted to assess the clinical significance of MDA-7/IL-24, and more studies are clearly needed.

Acknowledgments This research was supported by the Hansel/Downey Research Fund and the Pennington Biomedical Research Foundation. We also thank Cathy Huey and Jiveshwar Kumar, M.D. for a careful reading and editing of the manuscript.

References

1. Jiang, H., Lin, J. J., Su, Z. Z., Goldstein, N. I., and Fisher, P. B. (1995) Oncogene 11, 2477
2. Chada, S., Sutton, R. B., Ekmekcioglu, S., Ellerhorst, J., Mumm, J. B., Leitner, W. W., Yang, H. Y., Sahin, A. A., Hunt, K. K., Fuson, K. L., Poindexter, N., Roth, J. A., Ramesh, R., Grimm, E. A., and Mhashilkar, A. M. (2004) Int Immunopharmacol 4, 649
3. Huang, E. Y., Madireddi, M. T., Gopalkrishnan, R. V., Leszczyniecka, M., Su, Z., Lebedeva, I. V., Kang, D., Jiang, H., Lin, J. J., Alexandre, D., Chen, Y., Vozhilla, N., Mei, M. X., Christiansen, K. A., Sivo, F., Goldstein, N. I., Mhashilkar, A. B., Chada, S., Huberman, E., Pestka, S., and Fisher, P. B. (2001) Oncogene 20, 7051
4. Kotenko, S. V., Krause, C. D., Izotova, L. S., Pollack, B. P., Wu, W., and Pestka, S. (1997) EMBO J 16, 5894
5. Sauane, M., Gopalkrishnan, R. V., Lebedeva, I., Mei, M. X., Sarkar, D., Su, Z. Z., Kang, D. C., Dent, P., Pestka, S., and Fisher, P. B. (2003) J Cell Physiol 196, 334
6. Jiang, H., Su, Z. Z., Lin, J. J., Goldstein, N. I., Young, C. S., and Fisher, P. B. (1996) Proc Natl Acad Sci USA 93, 9160
7. Pestka, S., Krause, C. D., Sarkar, D., Walter, M. R., Shi, Y., and Fisher, P. B. (2004) Annu Rev Immunol 22, 929
8. Sauane, M., Gopalkrishnan, R. V., Sarkar, D., Su, Z. Z., Lebedeva, I. V., Dent, P., Pestka, S., and Fisher, P. B. (2003) Cytokine Growth Factor Rev 14, 35
9. Caudell, E. G., Mumm, J. B., Poindexter, N., Ekmekcioglu, S., Mhashilkar, A. M., Yang, X. H., Retter, M. W., Hill, P., Chada, S., and Grimm, E. A. (2002) J Immunol 168, 6041
10. Ramesh, R., Mhashilkar, A. M., Tanaka, F., Saito, Y., Branch, C. D., Sieger, K., Mumm, J. B., Stewart, A. L., Boquoi, A., Dumoutier, L., Grimm, E. A., Renauld, J. C., Kotenko, S., and Chada, S. (2003) Cancer Res 63, 5105
11. Ellerhorst, J. A., Prieto, V. G., Ekmekcioglu, S., Broemeling, L., Yekell, S., Chada, S., and Grimm, E. A. (2002) J Clin Oncol 20, 1069
12. Sieger, K. A., Mhashilkar, A. M., Stewart, A., Sutton, R. B., Strube, R. W., Chen, S. Y., Pataer, A., Swisher, S. G., Grimm, E. A., Ramesh, R., and Chada, S. (2004) Mol Ther 9, 355
13. Aggarwal, B. B. (2003) Nat Rev Immunol 3, 745
14. Liao, Y. C., Liang, W. G., Chen, F. W., Hsu, J. H., Yang, J. J., and Chang, M. S. (2002) J Immunol 169, 4288
15. Ekmekcioglu, S., Ellerhorst, J., Mhashilkar, A. M., Sahin, A. A., Read, C. M., Prieto, V. G., Chada, S., and Grimm, E. A. (2001) Int J Cancer 94, 54
16. Lebedeva, I. V., Sarkar, D., Su, Z. Z., Kitada, S., Dent, P., Stein, C. A., Reed, J. C., and Fisher, P. B. (2003) Oncogene 22, 8758

17. Lebedeva, I. V., Su, Z. Z., Chang, Y., Kitada, S., Reed, J. C., and Fisher, P. B. (2002) Oncogene 21, 708
18. Mhashilkar, A. M., Schrock, R. D., Hindi, M., Liao, J., Sieger, K., Kourouma, F., Zou-Yang, X. H., Onishi, E., Takh, O., Vedvick, T. S., Fanger, G., Stewart, L., Watson, G. J., Snary, D., Fisher, P. B., Saeki, T., Roth, J. A., Ramesh, R., and Chada, S. (2001) Mol Med 7, 271
19. Nishikawa, T., Ramesh, R., Munshi, A., Chada, S., and Meyn, R. E. (2004) Mol Ther 9, 818
20. Saeki, T., Mhashilkar, A., Swanson, X., Zou-Yang, X. H., Sieger, K., Kawabe, S., Branch, C. D., Zumstein, L., Meyn, R. E., Roth, J. A., Chada, S., and Ramesh, R. (2002) Oncogene 21, 4558
21. Lebedeva, I. V., Washington, I., Sarkar, D., Clark, J. A., Fine, R. L., Dent, P., Curiel, D. T., Turro, N. J., and Fisher, P. B. (2007) Proc Natl Acad Sci USA 104, 3484
22. Su, Z. Z., Madireddi, M. T., Lin, J. J., Young, C. S., Kitada, S., Reed, J. C., Goldstein, N. I., and Fisher, P. B. (1998) Proc Natl Acad Sci USA 95, 14400
23. Yacoub, A., Mitchell, C., Lebedeva, I. V., Sarkar, D., Su, Z. Z., McKinstry, R., Gopalkrishnan, R. V., Grant, S., Fisher, P. B., and Dent, P. (2003) Cancer Biol Ther 2, 347
24. Fisher, P. B. (2005) Cancer Res 65, 10128
25. Cao, X. X., Mohuiddin, I., Chada, S., Mhashilkar, A. M., Ozvaran, M. K., McConkey, D. J., Miller, S. D., Daniel, J. C., and Smythe, W. R. (2002) Mol Med 8, 869
26. Pataer, A., Vorburger, S. A., Barber, G. N., Chada, S., Mhashilkar, A. M., Zou-Yang, H., Stewart, A. L., Balachandran, S., Roth, J. A., Hunt, K. K., and Swisher, S. G. (2002) Cancer Res 62, 2239
27. Sarkar, D., Su, Z. Z., Lebedeva, I. V., Sauane, M., Gopalkrishnan, R. V., Valerie, K., Dent, P., and Fisher, P. B. (2002) Proc Natl Acad Sci USA 99, 10054
28. Saeki, T., Mhashilkar, A., Chada, S., Branch, C., Roth, J. A., and Ramesh, R. (2000) Gene Ther 7, 2051
29. Lebedeva, I. V., Sauane, M., Gopalkrishnan, R. V., Sarkar, D., Su, Z. Z., Gupta, P., Nemunaitis, J., Cunningham, C., Yacoub, A., Dent, P., and Fisher, P. B. (2005) Mol Ther 11, 4
30. Dumoutier, L., Van Roost, E., Colau, D., and Renauld, J. C. (2000) Proc Natl Acad Sci USA 97, 10144
31. Kotenko, S. V., Izotova, L. S., Mirochnitchenko, O. V., Esterova, E., Dickensheets, H., Donnelly, R. P., and Pestka, S. (2001) J Biol Chem 276, 2725
32. Xie, M. H., Aggarwal, S., Ho, W. H., Foster, J., Zhang, Z., Stinson, J., Wood, W. I., Goddard, A. D., and Gurney, A. L. (2000) J Biol Chem 275, 31335
33. Liu, Y., Wei, S. H., Ho, A. S., de Waal Malefyt, R., and Moore, K. W. (1994) J Immunol 152, 1821
34. Moore, K. W., de Waal Malefyt, R., Coffman, R. L., and O'Garra, A. (2001) Annu Rev Immunol 19, 683
35. Sarkar, D., Su, Z. Z., Lebedeva, I. V., Sauane, M., Gopalkrishnan, R. V., Dent, P., and Fisher, P. B. (2002) Biotechniques Suppl, 30
36. Dumoutier, L., Leemans, C., Lejeune, D., Kotenko, S. V., and Renauld, J. C. (2001) J Immunol 167, 3545
37. Blumberg, H., Conklin, D., Xu, W. F., Grossmann, A., Brender, T., Carollo, S., Eagan, M., Foster, D., Haldeman, B. A., Hammond, A., Haugen, H., Jelinek, L., Kelly, J. D., Madden, K., Maurer, M. F., Parrish-Novak, J., Prunkard, D., Sexson, S., Sprecher, C., Waggie, K., West, J., Whitmore, T. E., Yao, L., Kuechle, M. K., Dale, B. A., and Chandrasekher, Y. A. (2001) Cell 104, 9
38. Parrish-Novak, J., Xu, W., Brender, T., Yao, L., Jones, C., West, J., Brandt, C., Jelinek, L., Madden, K., McKernan, P. A., Foster, D. C., Jaspers, S., and Chandrasekher, Y. A. (2002) J Biol Chem 277, 47517
39. Wolk, K., Kunz, S., Asadullah, K., and Sabat, R. (2002) J Immunol 168, 5397
40. Poindexter, N. J., Walch, E. T., Chada, S., and Grimm, E. A. (2005) J Leukoc Biol 78, 745
41. Aggarwal, S., Takada, Y., Mhashilkar, A. M., Sieger, K., Chada, S., and Aggarwal, B. B. (2004) J Immunol 173, 4368
42. Kumar, A., Haque, J., Lacoste, J., Hiscott, J., and Williams, B. R. (1994) Proc Natl Acad Sci USA 91, 6288
43. Gopalkrishnan, R. V., Sauane, M., and Fisher, P. B. (2004) Int Immunopharmacol 4, 635

44. Inoue, S., Shanker, M., Miyahara, R., Gopalan, B., Patel, S., Oida, Y., Branch, C. D., Munshi, A., Meyn, R. E., Andreeff, M., Tanaka, F., Mhashilkar, A. M., Chada, S., and Ramesh, R. (2006) Curr Gene Ther 6, 73
45. Tong, A. W., Nemunaitis, J., Su, D., Zhang, Y., Cunningham, C., Senzer, N., Netto, G., Rich, D., Mhashilkar, A., Parker, K., Coffee, K., Ramesh, R., Ekmekcioglu, S., Grimm, E. A., van Wart Hood, J., Merritt, J., and Chada, S. (2005) Mol Ther 11, 160
46. Ashkenazi, A. (2002) Nat Rev Cancer 2, 420
47. Ghobrial, I. M., Witzig, T. E., and Adjei, A. A. (2005) CA Cancer J Clin 55, 178
48. Hanahan, D., and Weinberg, R. A. (2000) Cell 100, 57
49. Pataer, A., Chada, S., Hunt, K. K., Roth, J. A., and Swisher, S. G. (2003) J Thorac Cardiovasc Surg 125, 1328
50. Pataer, A., Vorburger, S. A., Chada, S., Balachandran, S., Barber, G. N., Roth, J. A., Hunt, K. K., and Swisher, S. G. (2005) Mol Ther 11, 717
51. Lebedeva, I. V., Emdad, L., Su, Z. Z., Gupta, P., Sauane, M., Sarkar, D., Staudt, M. R., Liu, S. J., Taher, M. M., Xiao, R., Barral, P., Lee, S. G., Wang, D., Vozhilla, N., Park, E. S., Chatman, L., Boukerche, H., Ramesh, R., Inoue, S., Chada, S., Li, R., De Pass, A. L., Mahasreshti, P. J., Dmitriev, I. P., Curiel, D. T., Yacoub, A., Grant, S., Dent, P., Senzer, N., Nemunaitis, J. J., and Fisher, P. B. (2007) Int J Oncol 31, 985
52. Leath, C. A., III, Kataram, M., Bhagavatula, P., Gopalkrishnan, R. V., Dent, P., Fisher, P. B., Pereboev, A., Carey, D., Lebedeva, I. V., Haisma, H. J., Alvarez, R. D., Curiel, D. T., and Mahasreshti, P. J. (2004) Gynecol Oncol 94, 352
53. Gopalan, B., Litvak, A., Sharma, S., Mhashilkar, A. M., Chada, S., and Ramesh, R. (2005) Cancer Res 65, 3017
54. Shanker, M., Gopalan, B., Patel, S., Bocangel, D., Chada, S., and Ramesh, R. (2007) Cancer Lett 254, 217
55. Chada, S., Bocangel, D., Ramesh, R., Grimm, E. A., Mumm, J. B., Mhashilkar, A. M., and Zheng, M. (2005) Mol Ther 11, 724
56. Lebedeva, I. V., Su, Z. Z., Sarkar, D., Gopalkrishnan, R. V., Waxman, S., Yacoub, A., Dent, P., and Fisher, P. B. (2005) Oncogene 24, 585
57. Lebedeva, I. V., Sarkar, D., Su, Z. Z., Gopalkrishnan, R. V., Athar, M., Randolph, A., Valerie, K., Dent, P., and Fisher, P. B. (2006) Cancer Res 66, 2403
58. Su, Z., Lebedeva, I. V., Gopalkrishnan, R. V., Goldstein, N. I., Stein, C. A., Reed, J. C., Dent, P., and Fisher, P. B. (2001) Proc Natl Acad Sci USA 98, 10332
59. Pataer, A., Chada, S., Roth, J. A., Hunt, K. K., and Swisher, S. G. (2008) Cancer Biol Ther 7, 103
60. Emdad, L., Sarkar, D., Lebedeva, I. V., Su, Z. Z., Gupta, P., Mahasreshti, P. J., Dent, P., Curiel, D. T., and Fisher, P. B. (2006) J Cell Physiol 208, 298
61. Su, Z. Z., Lebedeva, I. V., Sarkar, D., Emdad, L., Gupta, P., Kitada, S., Dent, P., Reed, J. C., and Fisher, P. B. (2006) Oncogene 25, 2339
62. Kawabe, S., Nishikawa, T., Munshi, A., Roth, J. A., Chada, S., and Meyn, R. E. (2002) Mol Ther 6, 637
63. Ekmekcioglu, S., Mumm, J. B., Udtha, M., Chada, S., and Grimm, E. A. (2008) Cytokine 43, 34
64. Kunnumakkara, A. B., Diagaradjane, P., Guha, S., Deorukhkar, A., Shentu, S., Aggarwal, B. B., and Krishnan, S. (2008) Clin Cancer Res 14, 2128
65. Bonizzi, G., Piette, J., Merville, M. P., and Bours, V. (1997) J Immunol 159, 5264
66. Folkman, J. (1971) N Engl J Med 285, 1182
67. McCarty, M. E., and Ellis, L. M. (2002) Cancer Biol Ther 1, 127
68. Folkman, J., and D'Amore, P. A. (1996) Cell 87, 1153
69. Hanahan, D., and Folkman, J. (1996) Cell 86, 353
70. Ferrara, N. (2002) Semin Oncol 29, 10
71. Ferrara, N., Gerber, H. P., and LeCouter, J. (2003) Nat Med 9, 669
72. Gerber, H. P., McMurtrey, A., Kowalski, J., Yan, M., Keyt, B. A., Dixit, V., and Ferrara, N. (1998) J Biol Chem 273, 30336
73. Guo, D., Jia, Q., Song, H. Y., Warren, R. S., and Donner, D. B. (1995) J Biol Chem 270, 6729

74. Chada, S., Mhashilkar, A. M., Ramesh, R., Mumm, J. B., Sutton, R. B., Bocangel, D., Zheng, M., Grimm, E. A., and Ekmekcioglu, S. (2004) Mol Ther 10, 1085
75. Yu, H., and Jove, R. (2004) Nat Rev Cancer 4, 97
76. Mhashilkar, A. M., Stewart, A. L., Sieger, K., Yang, H. Y., Khimani, A. H., Ito, I., Saito, Y., Hunt, K. K., Grimm, E. A., Roth, J. A., Meyn, R. E., Ramesh, R., and Chada, S. (2003) Mol Ther 8, 207
77. Ramesh, R., Ito, I., Gopalan, B., Saito, Y., Mhashilkar, A. M., and Chada, S. (2004) Mol Ther 9, 510
78. Ramesh, R., Ito, I., Saito, Y., Wu, Z., Mhashikar, A. M., Wilson, D. R., Branch, C. D., Roth, J. A., and Chada, S. (2004) DNA Cell Biol 23, 850
79. Inoue, S., Branch, C. D., Gallick, G. E., Chada, S., and Ramesh, R. (2005) Mol Ther 12, 707
80. Inoue, S., Hartman, A., Branch, C. D., Bucana, C. D., Bekele, B. N., Stephens, L. C., Chada, S., and Ramesh, R. (2007) Mol Ther 15, 287
81. Chen, J., Chada, S., Mhashilkar, A., and Miano, J. M. (2003) Mol Ther 8, 220
82. Barnett, S. F., Bilodeau, M. T., and Lindsley, C. W. (2005) Curr Top Med Chem 5, 109
83. Folgueras, A. R., Pendas, A. M., Sanchez, L. M., and Lopez-Otin, C. (2004) Int J Dev Biol 48, 411
84. Schaller, M. D. (2004) J Cell Biol 166, 157
85. Clayman, G. L., el-Naggar, A. K., Lippman, S. M., Henderson, Y. C., Frederick, M., Merritt, J. A., Zumstein, L. A., Timmons, T. M., Liu, T. J., Ginsberg, L., Roth, J. A., Hong, W. K., Bruso, P., and Goepfert, H. (1998) J Clin Oncol 16, 2221
86. Lang, F. F., Bruner, J. M., Fuller, G. N., Aldape, K., Prados, M. D., Chang, S., Berger, M. S., McDermott, M. W., Kunwar, S. M., Junck, L. R., Chandler, W., Zwiebel, J. A., Kaplan, R. S., and Yung, W. K. (2003) J Clin Oncol 21, 2508
87. Roth, J. A., Nguyen, D., Lawrence, D. D., Kemp, B. L., Carrasco, C. H., Ferson, D. Z., Hong, W. K., Komaki, R., Lee, J. J., Nesbitt, J. C., Pisters, K. M., Putnam, J. B., Schea, R., Shin, D. M., Walsh, G. L., Dolormente, M. M., Han, C. I., Martin, F. D., Yen, N., Xu, K., Stephens, L. C., McDonnell, T. J., Mukhopadhyay, T., and Cai, D. (1996) Nat Med 2, 985
88. Wolf, J. K., Bodurka, D. C., Gano, J. B., Deavers, M., Ramondetta, L., Ramirez, P. T., Levenback, C., and Gershenson, D. M. (2004) Gynecol Oncol 94, 442
89. Yang, Y., Li, Q., Ertl, H. C., and Wilson, J. M. (1995) J Virol 69, 2004
90. Niidome, T., and Huang, L. (2002) Gene Ther 9, 1647
91. Das, S., Nama, S., Antony, S., and Somasundaram, K. (2005) Cancer Gene Ther 12, 417
92. Davies, M. A., Lu, Y., Sano, T., Fang, X., Tang, P., LaPushin, R., Koul, D., Bookstein, R., Stokoe, D., Yung, W. K., Mills, G. B., and Steck, P. A. (1998) Cancer Res 58, 5285
93. Fujiwara, T., Grimm, E. A., Mukhopadhyay, T., Cai, D. W., Owen-Schaub, L. B., and Roth, J. A. (1993) Cancer Res 53, 4129
94. Ji, L., Fang, B., Yen, N., Fong, K., Minna, J. D., and Roth, J. A. (1999) Cancer Res 59, 3333
95. Ishikawa, S., Nakagawa, T., Miyahara, R., Kawano, Y., Takenaka, K., Yanagihara, K., Otake, Y., Katakura, H., Wada, H., and Tanaka, F. (2005) Clin Cancer Res 11, 1198
96. Cunningham, C. C., Chada, S., Merritt, J. A., Tong, A., Senzer, N., Zhang, Y., Mhashilkar, A., Parker, K., Vukelja, S., Richards, D., Hood, J., Coffee, K., and Nemunaitis, J. (2005) Mol Ther 11, 149

IL-28 and IL-29 in Regulation of Antitumor Immune Response and Induction of Tumor Regression

Muneo Numasaki

Abstract Type III interferons (IFNs), also known as IFN-λs, are recently described as a novel group of the cytokine family that shares with type I IFNs the same Jak/STAT intracellular signaling pathway driving the expression of a common set of IFN-stimulated genes despite the distinct receptor system usage from type I IFNs. Accordingly, type III IFNs exhibit multiple common biological features with type I IFNs including antiviral activity and antitumor activity in more restricted cell types. Early in vitro studies using human neuroendocrine and colorectal tumor cell lines displayed that, like type I IFNs, type III IFNs can exert direct biological effects on tumor cell growth and functions, such as an induction of apoptosis, by multiple mechanisms. Subsequently, an ensemble of studies based on the use of genetically modified murine tumor cells producing IFN-λ2 (IL-28A) or the in vivo delivery of naked plasmid DNA provided important information on the host-mediated antitumor mechanisms induced by locally produced IL-28A. Of note, these studies have revealed the immunomodulatory functions of type III IFNs, including biological effects on polymorphonuclear neutrophils, NK cells, and T cells, which mainly contribute to type III IFN-induced in vivo antitumor immunity. IFN-γ is partially involved in type III IFN-induced antitumor activity. Additionally, IL-12 enhances type III IFN-mediated antitumor action in the presence or absence of IFN-γ. On the whole, these findings provide clear evidence that type III IFNs have bioactivities to elicit antitumor immune response and indicate the possibility for the application of type III IFNs to cancer immunotherapy.

Introduction

Type I interferons (IFNs), namely IFN-α/β, were originally discovered due to its powerful antiviral activity [1, 2]. Type I IFNs were later shown to have pleiotropic biological activities in addition to their well-known ability to inhibit viral replication.

M. Numasaki (✉)
Department of Nutrition Physiology, Pharmaceutical Sciences, Josai University, 1-1 Keyakidai, Sakato, Saitama, 350-0295, Japan
e-mail: Numasaki77@aol.com

J. Lustgarten et al. (eds.), *Targeted Cancer Immune Therapy*,
DOI 10.1007/978-1-4419-0170-5_5, © Springer Science+Business Media, LLC 2009

They modulate innate and acquired immune responses, cell growth, and apoptosis [3]. Type I IFN forms a vast multigenic family [4]. The human genome carries 13 genes coding for closely related IFN-α subtypes [5]. In addition, they contain genes coding for IFN-β, IFN-κ [6], IFN-ε/τ [7], and IFN-ω [8]. In spite of this remarkable variability, all type I IFN subtypes appear to bind the same heterodimeric receptor [4]. Type I IFNs have been used for the clinical treatment of several malignancies, including renal cell carcinoma, melanoma, Kaposi's sarcoma, hairy cell leukemia, and chronic myeloid leukemia. For a long time, it was thought that the direct inhibitory effects on tumor cell growth and functions were the major mechanisms involved in the antitumor response observed in type I IFN-treated patients [9]. Actually, type I IFNs are able to directly inhibit the proliferation of tumor cells in vitro and in vivo, and exert other direct effects on tumor cells including downregulation of oncogene expression, induction of tumor suppressor genes, and enhancement of major histocompatibility complex (MHC) class I expression, which can enhance immune recognition [10]. In addition to the direct effects on tumor cells, type I IFNs exert multiple biological effects on host immune cells, especially T cells and dendritic cells, that can play a central role in the overall antitumor response [11].

Intriguingly, the multigenic type I IFN system cohabits with the seemingly redundant type III IFN system discovered more recently. Type III IFN (IFN-λ or IL-28A/B or IL-29) is structurally and genetically close to the members of the IL-10 family of cytokines but displays type I IFN-like biological activity [12, 13]. In humans, three genes encode for three members of this new family, IL-28A, IL-28B, and IL-29. Among these molecules, only IL-29 is glycosylated [12, 13]. In the mouse system, the *IL-29* gene is a pseudogene. *IL-28A* and *IL-28B* genes encode glycosylated protein [14].

Type III IFN expression has been shown to depend on the same triggers (viral infection or toll-like receptor (TLR) ligands) [12, 13, 15–20] and signal transduction pathway as those inducing type I IFN expression. Type I and type III IFNs bind distinct heterodimeric receptors [12, 13]. The type I IFN receptor is made of the ubiquitously expressed IFNAR1 and IFNAR2c subunits [21]. The type III IFN receptor is made of the IL-10Rβ subunit, which is widely expressed and shared by other IL-10-related cytokines, and of the IL-28 receptor (IL-28R) subunit, which is specific to type III IFNs and responsible for signal transduction [12, 13, 21]. Although type I and type III IFN receptors are unrelated, they trigger strikingly similar responses, mostly through the activation of several latent transcriptional factors of the signal transducer and activator of transcription (STAT) family including STAT1, STAT2, STAT3, STAT4, and STAT5 [12, 22, 23]. In particular, type III IFN receptor engagement leads to the phosphorylation of STAT1 and STAT2 and the formation of the interferon-stimulated gene factor 3 (ISGF3) transcription complex, which is composed of STAT1, STAT2, and IFN regulatory factor (IRF) 9/p48 [12], and to the induction of myxovirus resistance protein A (MxA) and 2'-5' oligoadenylate synthetase 1 (OAS1), which mediate the antiviral effects of type I IFNs [12, 24]. Type I and type III IFNs also lead to activation of the mitogen-activated protein (MAP) kinases JNK and p38, but not ERK [24]. Accordingly, type III IFNs have been shown to elicit biological activities including antiviral, antiproliferative, and immunomodulatory properties, similar to those of type I IFNs. Therefore, despite the structural difference and the utilization of a distinct receptor system, type III IFNs seem to be functionally related to type I IFNs.

In the first part of this chapter, we will summarize the current knowledge on the novel IFN family member and in the last part, we will review studies from several laboratories, including our group, displaying the antitumor activity of type III IFNs with the usage of genetically modified tumor cells in murine tumor models.

Type III IFN-Encoding Genes

In late 2002, two groups independently reported the identification of a small family of interferon-like cytokines through computational analyses of the human genome sequence database [12, 13]. The three family members were designated alternatively as IFN-λ1, IFN-λ2, and IFN-λ3, or IL-29, IL-28A, and IL-28B, respectively. The genes encoding IL-28A, IL-28B, and IL-29 are located on the same genomic contig, which is from chromosomal region 19q13.13 [12, 13]. This chromosomal location differs from the type I and type II IFN families clustered on chromosome 9 and 12, respectively. The genes encoding type III IFNs are composed of multiple exons, 5 for IL-29, and 6 for IL-28A and IL-28B, resembling the structural organization of genes encoding IL-10-related cytokines [12, 13]. This is in clear contrast to type I IFNs, which are encoded within a single exon. At amino acid level, IL-28A has an 81–96% identity to IL-28B and IL-29, 11–13% identity to IL-10, and 15–19% identity to IFN-γ and IL-22 [12, 13].

Mouse type III IFN-encoding genes were mapped to chromosome 7A3. This region has a similar organization as the human type III IFN locus [14]. Two genes colinear with the human IL-28A and IL-28B genes are intact and are predicted to encode functional proteins, which are designated as mouse IL-28A and IL-28B in accordance with the corresponding human genes [14]. Mouse IL-28A and IL-28B have higher sequence identity to human IL-28A and IL-28B than to IL-29 [14]. In contrast to the IL-28A and IL-28B genes, the mouse IL-29 gene has lost the entire exon 2 and acquired the stop codon within exon 1, resulting in a pseudogene in all murine strains studied [14]. Both mouse IL-28A and IL-28B possess a site for N-linked glycosylation (Asn105-Met-Thr in IL-28A and Asn107-Asp-Ser in IL-28B) [14].

Sources and Regulation of Type III IFNs Production

Like type I IFNs, type III IFN mRNAs expression can be detected in low amounts in libraries from a wide range of human tissues, including blood, brain, lung, ovary, pancreas, pituitary, placenta, prostate, and testis by RT-PCR analysis [25]. This in fact may serve as a natural surveillance system for the innate immune function, as is the case with type I IFNs. The 5′ regulatory regions of these genes reportedly bear a number of sequence elements involved in the transcriptional regulation of the type I IFN genes. This observation is borne out by the fact that a multitude of biological stimuli trigger type III IFN production: (a) viral infection, (b) double-stranded nucleic acids such as the double-stranded RNA (dsRNA) produced during viral replication, (c) TLR ligands.

Type III IFNs have been primarily discovered as antiviral cytokines [12, 13]. Viruses are in fact the primary natural inducers of type III IFNs. There have been many reports that infection of encephalomyocarditis virus (EMCV) [13], Sindbis virus [12], Dengue virus [12], Torque Teno virus (TTV) [26], respiratory syncytial virus [27], herpes simplex virus type-2 [20], or vesicular stomatitis virus (VSV) [12] leads to transcriptional activation of IL-28A, IL-28B, and IL-29 variously in human peripheral mononuclear cells, monocyte-derived dendritic cells (MDDCs), bronchial epithelial cells, and a number of human cell lines. Among them, monocyte-derived DC and plasmacytoid DC appear to be the major cellular sources of type III IFNs [20]. Many other pathogenic microbes and their products can also elicit type III IFN production and release. Endotoxin, which is a lipopolysaccharide (LPS) component of Gram-negative bacteria cell walls, is a potent type III IFN inducer [17].

Double-stranded RNA (dsRNA) is frequently used as a replicative intermediate by viruses. Both natural and synthetic dsRNAs have been observed to function as efficient inducers of type III IFNs. Of the synthetic, double-stranded polynucleotides, homopolymer pair poly-riboinosinic-ribocytidilic acid (polyI:C) is the most active and has been used for induction of type I and type III IFNs production [13].

Although type III IFNs differ genetically and structurally from type I IFNs and use their own specific receptor, the expression of type III and type I IFNs is regulated in a similar fashion in virus-infected cells exhibiting both early and late phases of IFN induction [15]. However, type III IFN genes are under a more complex regulation than type I IFN genes, since type III IFN genes have a higher number of regulatory elements on their promoters [15]. Type III IFN gene promoters have several putative IFN-stimulated response elements (ISRE) and NF-κB binding sites [28]. The promoter sequences of IL-28A and IL-28B genes are almost identical, whereas the promoter of IL-29 is somewhat different from the IL-28A/B promoters [28]. Namely, NF-κB and multiple IFN regulatory factor (IRF) family members induce the expression of *IL-29* gene [28]. In contrast to IL-29, IL-28A/B genes are predominantly regulated by an IRF family member IRF7 [28]. Therefore, the IL-29 gene is mainly regulated by virus-activated IRF3 and IRF7, resembling that of the IFN-β gene, whereas IL-28A/B gene expression is mainly controlled by IRF7, resembling those of IFN-α genes [28]. Viral infection serves to activate IRF3, which is expressed broadly and constitutively at high level in cells, via specific serine phosphorylation events, leading to the synthesis and release of IFNs, predominantly IL-29 and IFN-β. In paracrine fashion, these newly released IFNs are free to act on neighboring cells. The binding of IFNs to the respective specific receptor induces the expression of another transcriptional activator, IRF7, in a STAT1-dependent manner. When cells expressing other IRF7 are in turn infected with viruses, IRF7 is phosphorylated, and the cells respond by expressing other type III and type I genes, such as IL-29, IL-28A/B, IFN-α, and INF-β.

Type III Interferon Receptor Subunit IL-28 Receptor

Type III IFNs act through a cell surface receptor, which is composed of the newly identified IL-28R and IL-10Rβ with both chains apparently required for full binding affinity [12, 13]. At the time of its discovery, IL-10Rβ has been already known as the second chain of the IL-10 [29], IL-22 [30], or IL-26 receptor [31], formerly known as the class II cytokine receptor (CRF2)-9. IL-28R belongs to members of the class II cytokine receptor family, which are tripartite single-pass transmembrane proteins defined by structural similarities in the extracellular domain including the ligand-binding residues [33, 34]. In accordance with the CRF2 characteristics, both transmembrane chains have an extracellular moiety containing two tandem fibronectin III domains, a structural motif in the immunoglobulin fold superfamily, with several amino acid positions conserved within this receptor family [33, 34]. Like IL-10, IL-22, and IL-26, the binding of type III IFNs to IL-28R induces a conformational change that enables IL-10Rβ to interact with the newly formed ligand-receptor complex [35].

The human IL-28R-encoding gene is located on chromosomoe 1p36.11, near the *IL22RA1* locus, whereas the IL-10R2-encoding gene is located on 21q22.11, near the *IFNAR1*, *IFNAR2*, and *IFNGR2* loci [12, 13, 36]. The first exon of the human IL-28R-encoding gene contains 5-UTR and the signal peptide [12, 13]. The transmembrane moieties are predicted to be encoded by sequences derived from exon 6 of the corresponding genes [12, 13]. The longer intracellular moiety of IL-28R (predicted 271 aa vs. 79 aa in the IL-10Rβ) contains three tyrosine residues, which are potential targets for phosphorylation [12, 13]. Dumoutier et al. indicated two tyrosines, Tyr^{343} and Tyr^{517}, of human IL-28R can independently mediate STAT2 activation by type III IFNs [23]. This work also showed that when both tyrosines 343 and 517 were mutated to phenylalanine, antiviral and antiproliferative activities of type III IFNs were completely abolished [23]. The extracellular domains of IL-28R and IL-10Rβ contain four putative N-linked glycosylation sites [12, 13].

The murine genes encoding IL-28R and IL-10Rβ are located on chromosome 4D3 and 16C4 [14]. The mouse IL-28R chain is ~67% similar to its human counterpart [14]. Although the mouse and human IL-28R sequences are similar, only two of three tyrosine residues of the human receptor intracellular domain are conserved in the mouse orthologue [14]. The mouse receptor contains three additional tyrosine residues [14]. The Tyr^{341}-based motif of mouse IL-28R (YLERP) shows similarities with that surrounding Tyr^{343} of human IL-28R (YLERP). In addition, the COOH-terminal amino acid sequence of mouse IL-28R containing Tyr^{533} (YLVRstop) is similar to the COOH-terminal amino acid sequence of human IL-28R containing Tyr^{517} (YMARstop). Therefore, both the mouse and human IL-28R chains contain similar docking sites for STAT2 recruitment and activation. Human IL-28R has a stretch of negatively charged residues close to the end of the intracellular domain. This region in the mouse IL-28R is significantly altered by a short insertion and substitution of several amino acid residues, resulting in a longer and more negatively charged region in the mouse receptor [14].

Several research groups including our own have examined the expression of the type III IFN receptor complex components. The IL-10Rβ chain is ubiquitously expressed, which can be explained by its function as part of several cytokine receptors. The one notable exception is the brain, where the IL-10Rβ chain seems to be expressed at a very low level [37]. Therefore, the expression of the IL-28R chain should determine whether a cell is responsible to the type III IFNs or not [12, 13]. The near relation of type III IFNs to type I IFNs and IL-10 initially suggested extensive effects of type III IFNs on various cell populations. Actually, Sheppard et al. observed at first that, using northern blot analysis, various organs variably express the major IL-28R transcript and therefore contain putative target cells in humans [13]. These organs include the adrenal gland and kidney, and those from the digestive (stomach, small intestine, colon, and liver), respiratory (lung) and immune (spleen and thymus) systems, with the highest expression found in the pancreas, thyroid, skeletal muscle, heart, prostate, and testis [13]. Interestingly, most IL-28R mRNA-expressing tissues form outer body barriers and contain epithelial cells [38]. These quantitative results are in line with the data published by Kotenko et al. [9]. A pattern similar to that obtained in tissues using northern blot analysis was found in corresponding hematopoietic (HL-60 promyelocytic leukemia, K-562 erythroleukemia, MOLT-4 T-cell leukemia and Raji B-cell leukemia) and non-hematopoietic (HeLa S3 cervical adenocarcinoma, Caco-2, SW480, HCT116, SW480 and DLD-1 colorectal adenocarcinoma, A549 alveolar cell carcinoma, LK-1 lung adenocarcinoma and G-361 melanoma) cell lines [12, 39, 40].

At present, it is thought that the surface expression of IL-28R is more restricted relative to the type I IFN receptor, although detailed information regarding the expression level and cell distribution of the type III IFN specific receptor IL-28R is relatively limited. Therefore, whereas type I IFN signaling is observed for a broad spectrum of cell types, type III IFN signaling is generally weaker and more restrictive, which is correlated with a low expression of the IL-28R subunit of the type III IFN receptor. Actually, at the cellular level, B cell lymphoma Raji and hepatoma HepG2 cells respond well to type III IFNs. On the contrary, in HT1080 fibrosarcoma, Sw13 adrenal carcinoma cells and MCF-7 breast cancer cells, all of which respond to type I IFNs, no significant response to type III IFNs was observed [25]. Furthermore, in humans, primary bronchial epithelial cells and primary gastric epithelial cells are responsive to type III IFNs, whereas primary fibroblasts and umbilical vein endothelial cells do not express IL-28R, and therefore are not responsive to type III IFNs (14 and our unpublished observations).

In the mouse, IL-28R mRNA has been found in keratinocytes and lung fibroblasts [14, 41]. In immune systems, our studies using RT-PCR did not detect any expression of IL-28R mRNA in primary spleen cells from C57BL/6 mice [38, 41]. Moreover, we could not detect any IL-28R expression in resting primary immune cells such as B and T cells [41]. Lasfar et al. also observed that primary lymphocytes and macrophages, the major players in specific antitumor immunity, are found to be unresponsive to type III IFNs [14]. In accordance with the results obtained with primary immune cell subpopulations, corresponding cell lines (EL4 and P815) expressed IL-10Rβ but not IL-28R [42]. Conversely, Siebler et al. reported the opposite finding that the IL-28R mRNA is expressed in primary murine CD4 T cells [43]. In the case of NK cells, Murakami's group demonstrated the mRNA expression of IL-28R [42]. In general, tissues that are mainly composed of epithelia such as intestine, skin, or lung are the most responsive to type III IFNs. These data indicate that a key difference between the type I and type III IFN systems could be the cell specificity of their respective receptor expression.

Type III IFN-Induced Signal Transduction

Signaling induced by a cytokine binding to type II cytokine receptor, whose extracellular parts commonly consist of tandem fibronectin type III domains and cytoplasmic domain is associated with a tyrosine kinase of the Janus kinase (Jak) family, is known to occur primarily via the Jak/STAT pathway. Both IL-28R and IL10Rβ subunits are necessary to form a functional type III IFN receptor. The formation of the IL-28R-IL-10Rβ ternary complex initiates signaling events by activating the transduction elements bound to the intracytoplasmic part of the two chains composed of functional type III IFN receptor. Type III IFNs induce the activation of a Jak/STAT signaling pathway leading to tyrosine phosphorylation of STAT1, STAT2, STAT3, STAT4, and STAT5 [12, 13, 22, 23, 44]. In structure, IL-28R is most closely related at the sequence level with the soluble class II cytokine receptor IL-22Rα2, whereas a second type III IFN receptor chain IL-10Rβ is commonly utilized by IL-10, IL-22, and IL-26 [33]. IL-10, IL-22, and IL-26 can stimulate STAT3 phosphorylation, and IL-22 and IL-26 have been shown to phosphorylate STAT1. But only the type III IFN family induces the tyrosine phosphorylation of STAT2. The characteristics to be able to phosphorylate STAT1, STAT2, and STAT3 are common to the type III IFN family and the type I IFNs. Thus, STAT2 activation has been, at present, restricted to type I IFNs and type III IFNs. From studies of IL-10 and IL-22 signal transduction, it is known that its short (82 amino acids) intracytoplasmic part binds the tyrosine kinase Tyk2 but does not provide STAT recruitment sites [45]. Jak1 was shown to be critical in mediating IFN-induced STAT phosphorylation [22]. Thus, it is likely that, as is true for the type I IFN receptor system, Jak1 and Tyk2 are the two tyrosine kinases associated with the type III IFN receptor subunit and mediating STAT activation. STAT2 is specifically recruited in the ISGF3 transcription factor that translocates to the nucleus and drives the expression of the gene family carrying an ISRE sequence in their promoter (Fig. 1). ISGF3 is formed by dimerization of STAT1 and STAT2 via SH2 phosphotyrosine interactions and association of the heterodimer with IRF9. Type III IFNs induce the formation of both ISGF3 and STAT1 homodimers, which are able to recognize ISRE and GAS sequences [12, 14, 23]. Among the IFN-induced genes, suppressor of cytokine signaling (SOCS)1 and SOCS3 are

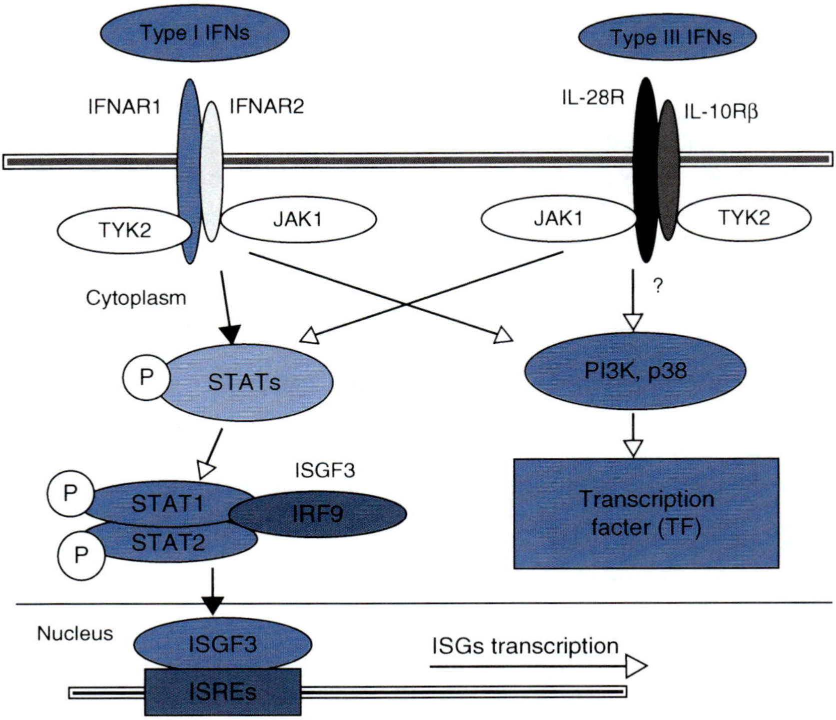

Fig. 1 Signaling pathways induced by type I IFNs and type III IFNs. Type I IFNs binding to their receptor complex induces Jak1 and Tyk2 activation and phosohorylation of STAT1 and STAT2. The phosphorylated STAT1 and STAT2 complex with IRF9 forms the ISGF3, which enters the nucleus, binds the ISRE and initiates ISGs transcription. Additionally, type I IFNs also activate the PI3K and p38 pathways to stimulate transcription of relevant genes. Similarly, type III IFNs activate the Jak-STAT pathway. However, it is currently unknown whether type III IFNs activate the PI3K and p38 pathways

involved in the negative regulation of type III IFN signaling [46, 47]. Overexpression of SOCS1 in hepatic cell lines inhibits type III signaling as well [46]. Additionally, type I IFNs can activate a variety of signaling molecules and cascades, which may operate in concert with or independently of STATs. Similarly, type III IFNs were shown to activate Erk 1/2 and Akt in an intestinal epithelial cell line [39].

Antitumor Effects of Type III IFN

Type I IFNs represent the cytokines exhibiting the longest record of use in clinical oncology [48]. These cytokines have been used in over 40 countries for the treatment of more than 14 types of cancer [48]. Even though today some new anticancer drugs have replaced type I IFN in the treatment of certain hematological malignancies such as hairy cell leukemia and chronic myeloid leukemia, these cytokines are still widely used in the treatment of patients with specific types of tumor including renal cell carcinoma and metastatic melanoma [49, 50]. As mentioned earlier in this chapter, there are similarities in biological activities between type I IFN and type III IFN. Therefore, based on the functional similarity with type I IFNs, it would be anticipated that type III IFNs would also have antitumor activities.

As expected, early studies using human intestinal epithelial cell lines, neuroendocrine cell lines, and glioblastoma cell lines revealed that type III IFNs can elicit direct antiproliferative effects like type I IFNs [39, 40, 47]. It is well-known that type I IFNs can exert a direct growth-inhibitory effect on a wide variety of tumor cells in vitro and in vivo [49, 50]. This type I IFN-induced growth-inhibitory effect is mediated by multiple mechanisms. Both protein kinase R (PKR) and ribonuclease L (RNaseL), which are antiviral proteins, are also integral mediators of the antiproliferative function of type I IFNs [51, 52]. Both mediate the antiproliferative function via inhibiton of protein synthesis. Namely, PKR phosphorylates a number of cellular targets including the eukaryotic translation initiation factor, eIF2a, which leads to a generalized inhibition of protein synthesis. RNaseL also cleaves single-stranded RNAs, including mRNA, and contributes to the inhibition of protein synthesis [53].

In vitro studies using multiple human cell lines including B cell lymphoma, hepatoma, neuroendocrine, and colorectal tumor cell lines provided the evidence that type III IFNs can induce the 2′, 5′-OAS in these cells [12, 23, 39]. Our studies also displayed that type III IFNs significantly suppressed the in vitro growth of human non-small cell lung cancer (NSCLC) cell lines and markedly upregulated the mRNA expression of 2′,5′-OAS in these cell lines (unpublished data). Therefore, 2′,5′-OAS could at least in part contribute to the antiproliferative effect of type III IFNs. Brand et al. reported that mRNA levels of PKR in intestinal epithelial cell lines remained unchanged after type III IFN treatment [39]. We obtained the same result in human respiratory epithelial cell lines (unpublished data). In contrast, in hepatoma and B cell lines, type IIII IFNs mediated PKR gene induction [54]. Collectively, PKR appears to be involved in the type III IFN-induced antiproliferative effect in a limited range of cell types.

Type I IFNs can also exert a more direct negative regulatory effect on the cell cycle by specifically upregulating the expression of a number of cyclin-dependent kinase inhibitors (CKIs). Type I IFNs specifically enhance the levels of the CKI, $p21^{Waf1/Cip1}$, which plays a crucial regulatory role in the progression from the G1 to S phase [55]. Type I IFNs also increase the exression of another CKI $p15^{Ink4b}$ that can complex specifically with Cdk4 [56]. A third protein, $p27^{Kip1}$, that preferentially binds to cyclinE/Cdk2 complexes, and dissociates the retinoblastoma gene product (pRb) and the related pocket proteins (p107 and p130) is concomitantly suppressed [57]. Rb and the related pocket proteins, in their nonphosphorylated forms, interact strongly with the E2F family of transcription factors, inhibiting their activity [58]. Phosphorylation of Rb (and p107 or p130) normally releases E2F transcription factors, and permits transition from the G1 to S phase.

In the case of type III IFNs, our studies using several human NSCLC lines demonstrated the elevated mRNA expression of $p21^{Waf1/Cip1}$ and, to a lesser extent, $p27^{Kip1}$, but not $p15^{Ink4b}$, after type III IFN treatment, and that knockdown of $p21^{Waf1/Cip1}$ with a $p21^{Waf1/Cip1}$-specific double-stranded small inhibitory RNA (p21-siRNA) oligonucleotide largely attenuated the observed antiproliferative effect, suggesting the major role of $p21^{Waf1/Cip1}$ in the growth-inhibitory function of type III IFNs (unpublished data). Analysis of cell cycle distribution showed type III IFN treatment of NSCLC lines resulted in an accumulation of cell numbers in the G1 phase in a dose-dependent manner (unpublished data). This increase of the G1 population was accompanied by the reduction of S and G2 populations. Finally, our findings indicated that type III IFNs can induce cell cycle arrest at the G1 phase. These data are in line with the results published earlier by Sato et al. [42].

Another important mechanism, by which type III IFNs exert a growth-inhibitory effect, was demonstrated by Zitzmann's research group [47]. They observed that type III IFNs significantly suppressed the growth of human neuroendocrine BON1 tumor cells, but did not result in a significant accumulation of this tumor cell in the G1 phase after type III IFN treatment [47]. Moreover, the same group indicated that incubation with type III IFN significantly increased the amount of cleaved caspase-3- and poly(ADP-ribose)polymerase (PARP)-product in BON1 tumor cells [47]. In this case, treatment with type III IFN resulted in induction of apoptosis rather than in the interference of cell cycle progression in BON1 tumor cells. Moreover, Sato et al. reported that type III IFNs upregulated surface expression of FAS, dephosphorylated Rb and activated both caspase-3 and caspase-7 in B16 melanoma cells, suggesting the promotion of apoptosis [42]. In contrast, our studies using NSCLC lines displayed that type III IFNs could not induce apoptosis by measuring DNA fragmentation and surface Annexin V expression (unpublished data). In addition, Brand et al. indicated that type III IFNs did not influence FAS ligand-induced apoptosis but decreased cell proliferation in human intestinal epithelial cells [24].

Induction of apoptosis in tumor cells is a well-known direct function of type I IFNs. Type I IFNs can mediate apoptosis through multiple pathways and multiple molecules. These include TNF-alpha-related apoptosis inducing ligand (TRAIL/Apo2L) [59], Fas/FasL [60], XIAP associated factor-1 (XAF-1) [61], caspase-3 [62], caspase-7 [63], caspase-8 [64], PKR [60], 2′,5′-OAS [65], death activating protein kinases (DAP kinase) [61], phospholipid scramblase [61], galectin 9 [61], IFN regulatory factors (IRFs) [61], promyelocytic leukemia gene (PML) [61], and regulators of IFN induced death (RIDs) [61]. In contrast, there are few articles available describing the relation between type III IFNs and apoptosis. Therefore, at this point, in the case of type III IFNs, the precise mechanisms responsible for the induction of apoptosis in tumor cells remain largely to be elucidated.

One of the important mechanisms of antitumor activities of type I IFNs is inhibition of tumor-induced angiogenesis [66]. Type I IFNs can inhibit a number of steps in the angiogenic process. Type I IFNs can inhibit FGF-induced endothelial proliferation [67]. Type I IFNs have been shown to be cytostatic to human dermal microvascular endothelial cells [68], and to human capillary endothelial cells [69]. Type I IFNs can also inhibit the endothelial cell migration step of angiogenesis [70].

Moreover, Type I IFNs can affect the expression of several angiogenic factors, including vascular endothelial growth factor (VEGF) [71], bFGF [72], IL-8 [73], and collagenase type IV [74]. Indeed, systemic therapy with the use of recombinant type I IFNs produces antiangiogenic effects in vascular tumors, including hemangioma [75], Kaposi's sarcoma [76], melanoma [77], and bladder carcinoma [78].

In contrast to type I IFNs, there have been no reports available demonstrating type III IFNs possess antiangiogenic activities. One of the key differences reported between type I and type III IFN system is in the expression of their respective receptor subunits. For example, vascular endothelial cells express IFNAR1, IFNAR2, and IL-10Rβ, but not IL-28R, on the cell surface [14]. Therefore, vascular endothelial cells appear to be, in general, unresponsive to type III IFNs. In addition, type III IFN treatment upregulated, not suppressed, the secretion of proangiogenic cytokine IL-8, which promotes tumor angiogenesis, from human colon cancer cells [24]. Additionally, exposure of human macrophages to type III IFN IL-29 significantly induces IL-8 production [79]. In contrast, Pekarek et al. reported that, using human peripheral blood mononuclear cells, type III IFN member IL-29 elevated the expression of mRNA for three chemokines, monokine induced IFN-γ (MIG), IFN-γ inducible protein 10 (IP-10), and IFN-γ inducible T cell α chemoattractant (I-TAC) in the absence of other stimuli [80]. These factors are members of the ELR^- subfamily of CXC chemokunes and display potent inhibitory effects on angiogenesis. Taken collectively, it is now unknown whether type III IFNs possess antiangiogenic properties like type I IFNs.

Several laboratories including ours carried out an ensemble of studies where the mouse type III IFN IL-28A gene was transduced into different types of mouse tumor cells and the in vivo behavior of genetically modified cells constitutively releasing IL-28A was evaluated after injection into immunocompetent syngeneic mice [14, 41, 42]. In these experiments, a gene therapy approach was introduced to investigate whether type III IFNs may possess antitumor actions instead of systemic therapy because cytokine gene therapy has many advantages in comparison with systemic administration of cytokine. Systemic administration of cytokines at pharmacologic doses results in a high concentration of cytokines in the circulation and often in suboptimal levels in tissues at the site of tumors. In contrast, cytokine gene transfer allows the localized expression of the cytokine at the targeted sites, avoiding deleterious side effects and resembling the paracrine mode of action of cytokines, which are produced in high amounts at the site of tumors and act on the immune system by providing transient signals between cells to generate effector responses.

Ahmed et al. investigated whether the constitutive expression of IL-28A at the tumor site may affect the in vivo tumorigenicity of B16 menanoma cells, which are responsive to type III IFNs and characterized as a low immunogenicity [14]. This study provided the initial evidence that the tumorigenicity of B16 cells producing IL-28A in syngeneic immunocompetent mice was highly impaired or completely abolished and that the inhibition of tumor establishment was dependent on the amount of IL-28A released by the genetically modified tumor cells [14]. Fifty percent of mice injected with B16 clone producing 100–150 ng of IL-28A for 24 h/10^6 cells developed tumors, whereas 100% of animals injected with B16 clone releasing 1–5 ng of IL-28A developed tumors. When the B16 clone, which produced IL-28A but was resistant to IL-28A treatment, was used to examine whether the antitumor effect of IL-28A was due to direct action on B16 cells or mediated by a host response, type III IFN-unresponsive B16 clone expressing IL-28A displayed reduced tumorigenicity and repressed the growth of parental B16 cells in vivo to a level comparable to IL-28A-responsive B16 cells, providing the evidence that host-defense mechanisms play a major role in mediating type III IFN-induced antitumor activity in vivo [14]. In this tumor model, only ~10% mice, which rejected B16 melanoma cells producing IL-28A, survived the subsequent parental B16 tumor challenge, suggesting the failure of development of a strong long-lasting immune memory [14]. Taken together with the findings that tumor-infiltrating immune cells were not detected in tumor tissues from B16 cells secreting IL28A and mouse primary lymphocytes and macrophages are unresponsive to type III IFNs, it was proposed as one of the possible mechanisms that IL-28A produced by genetically modified B16 cells could affect neighboring keratinocytes and other tumor stromal cells, and could inhibit their tumor-supportive function, leading to the reduced tumorigenicity in the B16 melanoma tumor model [14].

The antitumor therapeutic potential of type III IFN gene transfer into experimental tumors was also evaluated in animal models by another group using various approaches, comprising both the use of genetically modified cells and the in vivo delivery of type III IFN gene via injection of naked plasmid DNA. Sato et al. reported the antitumor activity of type III IFN IL-28A using the two different experimental tumor models [42]. They demonstrated that subcutaneous injection of IL-28A-secreting either B16 cells or Colon26 cells into syngeneic immunocompetent mice resulted in host-dependent growth suppression of the genetically-modified tumor cells, mostly mediated by NK cells [42]. Subsequently, mice injected intravenously with B16 cells secreting IL-28A exhibited fewer lung metastases than mice inoculated with control B16 cells [42]. In addition, targeting of Colon26 liver metastatic lesions by hydrodynamic gene delivery of plasmid DNA encoding mouse IL-28A lead to marked reduction of liver metastatic foci along with survival advantages [42]. By studying the in vivo turnover of different lymphocyte subsets in mice injected with IL-28 plasmid DNA, the number of NK and NKT cells in the liver markedly increased [42]. In contrast, B16 lung metastases were not successfully treated by hydrodynamic injection of IL-28A expression plasmid, indicating that the local delivery of type III IFNs to target sites is necessary for the control of metastatic tumor growth, and that type III IFN-induced systemic cytotoxic T cell (CTL) response is relatively weak in this tumor model [42].

Despite the type III IFN-resistant phenotype, induction of antitumor response following type III IFN IL-28A gene transfer was subsequently confirmed in the MCA205 tumor model [41]. In vivo growth of MCA205 producing IL-28A was efficiently inhibited by an IL-28A-elicited host-mediated immune response [41]. In this tumor model, the tumorigenic behavior of MCA205 cells producing either type I IFN IFN-α or type III IFN IL-28A was compared after subcutaneous injection. It was found that IFN-α-secreting MCA205 cells were rejected efficiently compared with IL-28A-producing MCA205 cells, which exhibited only a delay of tumor growth [41]. This finding suggested that the potency of the antitumor activity of IL-28A might be slightly lower than that of IFN-α, although MCA205 cells releasing IL-28A secreted approximately threefold less cytokine than did MCA205 cells producing IFN-α [41]. IFN-α showed direct biological effects on MCA205 cells, including enhancement of the MHC class I antigen expression, whereas IL-28A failed, suggesting that IFN-α, but not IL-28A, can directly influence the immunogenicity of MCA205 cells.

In regard to the cellular antitumor mechanisms of IL-28A, the findings in mice selectively depleted of various immune cell populations indicated that CD8 T cells play an important role in IL-28A-mediated antitumor immunity in the MCA205 tumor model because the protective effect was partially abolished in CD8 T cell-depleted animals [41]. This finding is in clear contrast with the result obtained in the B16 melanoma tumor model, in which depletion of CD8 T cells had no consequence on the tumor growth rate [42]. Additionally, in the MCA205 tumor model, local secretion of IL-28A by tumor cells induced more powerful tumor-specific cytotoxic T cells against parental cells [41]. This is consistent with the observed dense infiltration of CD8 T cells into tumor tissues from MCA205 cells producing IL-28A. However, primary mouse CD8 T cells are not expressing IL-28R on the cell surface and are found to be unresponsive to IL-28A treatment [41]. This characteristic of type III IFNs is in clear contrast with that of type I IFNs, which can directly act on T cells [81]. Therefore, the detailed mechanisms that underlie this CD8 T cell-dependent antitunor action by type III IFNs are currently unknown and will require further experimental analyses. In contrast, the expression of mRNA for IL-28R is clearly detected in Con A-stimulated mouse T cells, suggesting that the activated mouse CD8 T cells might possess the ability to respond to type III IFNs [41]. However, IL-28 does not have ability to directly enhance the cytotoxic activity of CTLs [41]. A recent report by Jordan et al. indicated that type III IFN IL-29 influences the cytokine production by Con A-stimulated human T cells, which is isolated from peripheral blood mononuclear cells [79]. IL-28A also displayed the biological function to induce chemokine secretion by mouse lung fibroblasts [41]. Taken together, one possible mechanism, by which IL-28A elicits CD8 T cell responses, is proposed that IL-28A first stimulates CD8 T cells indirectly through induction of other cytokines and chemokines by surrounding cells including stromal fibroblasts and keratinocytes, and subsequently acts on activated T cells directly [41].

In the tumor model of MCA205, a slower growth rate of tumors secreting IL-28A in CD4 T cell-depleted mice than in control mice was consistently observed, implicating that CD4 T cells inhibit the IL-28A-induced antitumor response [41]. Both CD4 T cells and CD8 T cells have been described to be important for the efficient induction of antitumor cellular immunity [82, 83]. This unexpected finding that CD4 T cells are not required for the antitumor activity of IL-28A is not in agreement with the notion that CD4 T cell help is necessary for the full activation of naive CD8 T cells [84]. However, a similar inhibitory effect of CD4 T cells has been previously reported in IL-12- or IL-23-transduced CT26 tumor model [85, 86]. These findings may be possibly explained by taking into account the $CD4^{+}CD25^{+}$ T regulatory cells [87]. With regard to the relation between type III IFNs and $CD4^{+}CD25^{+}$ T regulatory cells, Mennechet et al. reported that IL-28A promotes the generation of partially mature dendritic cells (DCs), which displays a tolerogenic phenotype [88]. Namely, type III IFN-matured DCs with the ability to migrate to lymph nodes express high levels of MHC class I and II, but low levels of costimulatory molecules [88]. These type III IFN-treated DCs specifically induced IL-2-dependent proliferation of a $CD4^+CD25^+Foxp3^+$ T regulatory cell population in culture, which is thought, in general, to result in suppression of the antitumor immune response [87]. Therefore, type III IFN-treated DCs can stimulate the proliferation of preexisting $CD4^+CD25^+$ T regulatory cells in the presence of IL-2 and inhibit efficient antitumor immunity. Of particular interest, these findings provide other important evidence that type I IFNs and type III IFNs can exert different biologic effects on DC differentiation, phenotype, and function.

The finding that, in the MCA205 tumor model, IL-28A-elicited antitumor response was partially abrogated in NK cell-depleted mice strongly implied that NK cells play an important role in the antitumor activity of IL-28A [41]. This finding is consistent with the result demonstrated by Sato et al. using the tumor model of B16 melanoma [42]. However, the surprising finding is that IL-28A is unable to enhance NK cell cytolytic activity both in vitro and in vivo [41]. This biological feature of type III IFNs on NK cells is in sharp contrast with type I IFNs, which markedly promote NK cell-mediated cytotoxicity in culture and in vivo [89]. In addition, on the one hand, IL-28A does not have capability to directly stimulate the growth of NK cells in culture [41]. On the other hand, administration of IL-28A into SCID mice significantly expanded the splenic NK cells depending on the dose of injection and expression of IL-28A in the liver increased the hepatic NK cells [41, 42]. In the case of type I IFNs, exposure to type I IFNs is associated with NK cell blastogenesis and proliferation, but not IFN-γ expression in vivo [90]. The immunoregulatory effect of type I IFNs to elicit the expression of IL-15 in mouse cell populations has been proposed to contribute to the induction of NK cell proliferation [91]. In contrast, the detailed mechanisms for type III IFN-induced proliferation of NK cells in vivo remain largely unknown [41, 42]. Nonetheless, type III IFNs appear to augment the NK cell-mediated antitumor activity in vivo via increasing the total number of NK cells [41]. Another possible explanation of underlying mechanisms is that IL-28A, like IL-21 [92], could enhance the cytolytic activity of NK cells previously activated by stimulators such as other cytokines and chemokines, but could not induce cytotoxic activity in resting NK cells.

Polymorphonuclear neutrophils contribute, in some way, to the suppression of tumor growth in the MCA205 tumor model as shown by the fact that treatment with a monoclonal antibody (mAb) against Gr-1 partially abrogated the IL-28A-elicited tumor growth suppression [41]. Polymorphonuclear neutrophils can be frequently involved in the generation of a CD8 T cell-mediated antitumor response [93]. Notably, evidence that polymorphonuclear neutrophils may be important for the induction of an antitumor immunity has already been suggested [93], and a specific role for polymorphonuclear neutrophils in the development of CD8 T cell-mediated antitumor responses was also demonstrated [94]. However, little is known about the biological effects of type III IFNs on this cell population. Especially, the direct biological activity of type III IFNs on polymorphonuclear neutrophils remains largely to be elucidated. In contrast, type III IFNs appear to be able to positively regulate the expression of several chemokines, which subsequently activates polymorphonuclear neutrophils. This was first demonstrated in the human in culture systems using peripheral mononuclear cells [80]. Indeed, type III IFN IL-29 induces IL-8 secretion from human peripheral mononuclear cells, especially macrophages, suggesting that type III IFNs have capabilities to stimulate polymorphonuclear neutrophils indirectly via induction of chemokines including IL-8 [80].

The fact that MCA205 cells secreting IL-28A were significantly more tumorigenic in IFN-γ KO mice than in syngeneic immunocompetent mice indicated that IFN-γ is involved in IL-28A-mediated antitumor response [41]. Type II IFN IFN-γ is a pleiotropic cytokine that can act on both tumor cells and host immunity [95, 96]. IFN-γ directly inhibits proliferation of some tumor cells and indirectly suppresses tumor growth in vivo by activating NK cells and macrophages and inducing angiostatic chemokines such as MIG and IP-10 with consequent inhibition of tumor angiogenesis [97, 98]. Nevertheless, abrogation of IFN-γ could not completely attenuate the antitumor action of IL-28A, indicating that IFN-γ-independent pathways are also involved in IL-28A-mediated antitumor activity [41]. In contrast, based on the finding obtained from the animals treated with neutralizing anti-IL-12 p40 mAb, IL-12 is not involved in type III IFN-mediated antitumor activity [41]. Now, little is known about the relation between type III IFNs and IL-12 expression. In contrast to the IFN-γ promotion of IL-12 expression, type I IFNs can negatively regulate IL-12 expression in DCs and monocytes [99]. Because type III IFNs display overlapping biological activities with type I IFNs, type III IFNs may also have the ability to down-regulate IL-12 expression, like type I IFNs [41]. In addition, other cytokines including IL-17 and IL-23 are also not required for the IL-28A-induced antitumor activity [41].

IFN-γ is partially involved in type III IFN-mediated antitumor action, whereas a wide range of doses of IL-28A exert no direct effects on the release of IFN-γ by NK cells and CD8 T cells stimulated with or without anti-mouse CD3 mAb in culture [41]. In contrast, IL-28A induces IFN-γ release by primary CD4 T cells stimulated with anti-mouse CD3 mAb or costimulated with anti-mouse CD3 mAb plus anti-mouse CD28 mAb [43]. This biological effect of IL-28A on IFN-γ secretion appears to be dose-dependent [43]. In addition, this ability of IL-28A to induce IFN-γ secretion by CD4 T cells is T-bet dependent [43]. However, in contrast with IL-12, daily administration of IL-28A into C57BL/6 mice for three consecutive days could not induce measurable serum IFN-γ levels in vivo [41]. Therefore, the pathway from type III IFNs to IFN-γ expression in the mouse remains to be largely elucidated.

In human systems, with regard to the induction of IFN-γ secretion, a recent report by Jordan et al. described that type III IFN IL-29 treatment induced a modest elevation of released IFN-γ in T cells, following stimulation with Con A or in a mixed-lymphocyte reaction (MLR) [79]. Thus, there is a readily accessible and functional pathway from type III IFNs to IFN-γ expression in humans that does not appear to be fully operational in the mouse system. In the case of type I IFNs, there are positive effects on human T cell IFN-γ expression following stimulation with particular molecules including polyI:C [100].

Combination therapy with local production of IL-28A by genetically modified tumor cells and systemic administration of IL-12 protein has a synergistic antitumor effect without apparent deleterious side effects, suggesting possible advantages in this combined therapy [41]. IL-28A secretion or administration of IL-12 rejected none, whereas the combination of two manipulations resulted in rejection of MCA205 cells in 40% of mice and dramatically delayed tumor growth in the remainder [41]. The presence of protective antitumor immunity in the surviving mice indicates that the effectiveness of this combination strategy extends beyond initial rejection of MCA205 cells secreting IL-28A to the development of protective long-lasting immunity, which is specific for the initial MCA205 tumor [41]. Studies with lymphocyte subset ablation and using IFN-γ KO mice indicated that rejection of MCA205 tumor cells brought about by the synergistic effects of IL-28A and IL-12 is mediated by systemic antitumor response that is dependent on the presence of both NK cells and CD8 T cells, but not CD4 T cells, and involves IFN-γ [41]. As mentioned earlier, type III IFNs themselves appear to have, if any, a limited capability to stimulate IFN-γ secretion in mouse systems, whereas type III IFN IL-28 significantly enhances the IL-12-mediated IFN-γ secretion by CD4 T cells stimulated with anti-mouse CD3 mAb in vitro, and increases serum IFN-γ concentration and the total number of spleen cells when compared with IL-12 alone in C57BL/6 mice [41, 43]. This biological effect of type III IFN on IL-12-induced IFN-γ expression is common with type I IFN. It has been reported that there is a modest type I IFN effect on IL-12 induction of IFN-γ production by mouse cells in culture [101]. Thus, the enhancement of the antitumor effect by combination therapy with type III IFN IL-28A and IL-12 appears to be, at least in part, dependent on increased IFN-γ production [41].

A surprising finding was that the enhancement of the antitumor effect of IL-28A by systemic treatment with IL-12 protein is found even in IFN-γ KO mice (41). This finding provided the evidence that IL-12 is able to enhance the antitumor action of type III IFN through IFN-γ-independent pathways [41]. Of interest, there have been lots of reports describing that the antitumor effect of systemic administration of IL-12 protein into mice is largely abrogated in IFN-γ KO mice [102]. On the contrary, in IFN-γ KO mice, IL-12 produced by genetically modified tumor cells is able to induce production of other mediators, instead of IFN-γ, including GM-CSF by both CD4 T cells and CD8 T cells and IL-15 by nonlymphoid cells, which are critically involved in the IL-12-induced antitumor activity in IFN-γ KO mice in the C26 tumor model [103, 104]. Thus, IL-12-elicited enhancement of type III IFN-mediated antitumor activity may be due to an indirect effect via the mediators including GM-CSF and IL-15, which are induced by IL-12 in IFN-γ KO mice. In addition, type I IFNs have a biological action to up-regulate expression of the heterodimeric high-affinity receptor for IL-12 composed of β1 and β2 chains [105, 106], which results in enhancement of IL-12 effects. Thus, it was proposed that, like type I IFNs, type III IFNs may enhance the IL-12-mediated biological effects on NK cells and T cells via upregulation of the IL-12 receptor expression, leading to augmentation of the antitumor activity.

Conclusions and Perspectives

Since the discovery of type III IFN and IFN-λR1 (IL-28R) systems in 2002, this novel cytokine family has been demonstrated to have multiple biological effects, which have some similarities with those of type I IFNs. One of the important properties of type III IFNs is the ability to induce antitumor responses. In this chapter, we have reviewed recent studies in vitro and in vivo, describing the potential of type III IFNs in the treatment of cancer. Local production of type III IFN by genetically modified tumor cells elicited a host-mediated antitumor effect, resulting in inhibition of tumor establishment or reduction of tumor growth in vivo. The mechanisms of type III IFN antitumor action are complex. Type III IFNs may utilize effector mechanisms of both innate resistance and adaptive immunity to mediate antitumor resistance, implying that specific tumor antigen recognition may not always be required for the antitumor effects of type III IFNs. Effector cells required for the antitumor effect include polymorphonuclear neutrophils, NK cells, and CD8 T cells. In the MCA205 tumor model, the type III IFN-induced antitumor effect has been displayed to be partially dependent on IFN-γ. IFN-γ-independent antitumor pathways are also demonstrated. The ability of type III IFNs to induce an antigen-specific immunity relies on its capacity to induce cytotoxic T cell responses.

Recent reports investigating the antitumor activity of type III IFNs in *in-vitro* and *in-vivo* tumor models provided clear evidence that type III IFNs have antitumor properties. These studies have revealed the multiple biological activities of type III IFNs that may be relevant for antitumor effects. However, to date much more remains to be elucidated, not only in terms of mechanisms responsible for the antitumor response observed in mouse tumor models but also, if any, in terms of adverse effects. The exploitation of recent findings on the antitumor action of type III IFNs will require more detailed information about the biological activities against various cell types. Especially, the biological actions of type III IFNs against different lymphoid subpopulations, including DCs, have to be fully clarified. In addition, only a few selected points that are specifically important in tumor immunotherapy with type III IFNs, taking into consideration not only the effects on the host immune system but also direct effects on tumor cells, which may cooperate for the generation of long-lasting control of tumor growth, will be emphasized. Furthermore, separate attention should be paid to the role of endogenous type III IFNs in the natural immune control of tumor growth using recently generated IL-28R gene knockout mice [107]. At present, the potential of type III IFNs in a clinical application to cancer therapy is unknown. Further studies will provide a better understanding of whether subtle differences in gene expression induced by type III IFNs relative to type I IFNs may reduce the adverse side effects and increase the efficacy typically seen in type I IFN cancer therapy. Nevertheless, promising data obtained in mouse tumor models of antitumor therapy have raised much hope that type III IFNs could be a powerful therapeutic agent against cancer as already proven for type I IFNs.

References

1. Isaacs, A., and Lindenmann, J. (1957) J Interferon Res 7, 429
2. Weissmann, C., and Weber, H. (1986) Prog Nucleic Acid Res Mol Biol 33, 251
3. Pestka, S., Langer, J. A., Zoon, K. C., and Samuel, C. E. (1987) Annu Rev Biochem 56, 727
4. Pestka, S., Krause, C. D., and Walter, M. R. (2004) Immunol Rev 202, 8
5. Roberts, R. M., Liu, L., Guo, Q., Leaman, D., and Bixby J. (1998) J Interferon Cytokine Res 18, 805
6. LaFleur, D. W., Nardelli, B., Tsareva, T., Mather, D., Feng, P., Semenuk, M., Taylor, K., Buergin, M., Chinchilla, D., Roshke, V., Chen, G., Ruben, S. M., Pitha, P. M., Coleman, T. A., and Moore, P. A. (2001) J Biol Chem 276, 39765
7. Peng, F. W., Duan, Z. J., Zheng, L. S., Xie, Z. P., Gao, H. C., Zhang, H., Li, W. P., and Hou, Y. D. (2007) Protein Expr Purif 53, 356
8. Adolf, G. R. (1990) Virology 175, 410
9. Belardelli, F., Ferrantini, M., Proietti, E., and Kirkwood, J. M. (2002) Cytokine Growth Factor Rev 13, 119
10. Pfeffer, L. M., Dinarello, C. A., Herberman, R. B., Williams, B. R., Borden, E. C., Bordens, R., Walter, M. R., Nagabhushan, T. L., Trotta, P. P., and Pestka, S. (1998) Cancer Res 58, 2489
11. Belardelli, F., and Gresser, I. (1996) Immunol Today 17, 369
12. Kotenko, S. V., Gallagher, G., Baurin, V. V., Lewis-Antes, A., Shen, M., Shah, N. K., Langer, J. A., Sheikh, F., Dickensheets, H., and Donnelly, R. P. (2003) Nat Immunol 4, 69
13. Sheppard, P., Kindsvogel, W., Xu, W., Henderson, K., Schlutsmeyer, S., Whitmore, T. E., Kuestner, R., Garrigues, U., Birks, C., Roraback, J., Ostrander, C., Dong, D., Shin, J., Presnell, S., Fox, B., Haldeman, B., Cooper, E., Taft, D., Gilbert, T., Grant, F. J., Tackett, M., Krivan, W., McKnight, G., Clegg, C., Foster, D., and Klucher, K. M. (2003) Nat Immunol 4, 63
14. Lasfar, A., Lewis-Antes, A., Smirnov, S. V., Anantha, S., Abushahba, W., Tian, B., Reuhl, K., Dickensheets, H., Sheikh, F., Donnelly, R. P., Raveche, E., and Kotenko, S. V. (2006) Cancer Res 66, 4468
15. Onoguchi, K., Yoneyama, M., Takemura, A., Akira, S., Taniguchi, T., Namiki, H., and Fujita, T. (2007) J Biol Chem 282, 7576
16. Ank, N., West, H., Bartholdy, C., Eriksson, K., Thomsen, A. R., and Paludan, S. R. (2006) J Virol 80, 4501
17. Coccia, E. M., Severa, M., Giacomini, E., Monneron, D., Remoli, M. E., Julkunen, I., Cella, M., Lande, R., and Uzé, G. (2004) Eur J Immunol 34, 796
18. Tissari, J., Sirén, J., Meri, S., Julkunen, I., and Matikainen, S. (2005) J Immunol 174, 4289
19. LinksSirén, J., Pirhonen, J., Julkunen, I., and Matikainen, S. (2005) J Immunol 174, 1932
20. Ank, N., Iversen, M. B., Bartholdy, C., Staeheli, P., Hartmann, R., Jensen, U. B., Dagnaes-Hansen, F., Thomsen, A. R., Chen, Z., Haugen, H., Klucher, K., and Paludan, S. R. (2008) J Immunol 180, 2474
21. Langer, J. A., Cutrone, E. C., and Kotenko, S. (2004) Cytokine Growth Factor Rev 15, 33
22. Dumoutier, L., Lejeune, D., Hor, S., Fickenscher, H., and Renauld, J. C. (2003) Biochem J 370, 391
23. Dumoutier, L., Tounsi, A., Michiels, T., Sommereyns, C., Kotenko, S. V., and Renauld, J. C. (2004) J Biol Chem 279, 32269
24. Brand, S., Beigel, F., Olszak, T., Zitzmann, K., Eichhorst, S. T., Otte, J. M., Diebold, J., Diepolder, H., Adler, B., Auernhammer, C. J., Göke, B., and Dambacher, J. (2005) Am J Physiol Gastrointest Liver Physiol 289, G960

25. Zhou, Z., Hamming, O. J., Ank, N., Paludan, S. R., Nielsen, A. L., and Hartmann, R. (2007) J Virol 81, 7749
26. Garbuglia, A. R., Grasso, F., Donà, M. G., Mochi, S., Conti, P., De Lutiis, M. A., Giorgi, C., and Iezzi, T. (2007) Int J Immunopathol Pharmacol 20, 249
27. Spann, K. M., Tran, K. C., Chi, B., Rabin, R. L., Collins, P. L. (2004) J Virol 78(8), 4363
28. Osterlund, P. I., Pietilä, T. E., Veckman, V., Kotenko, S. V., and Julkunen, I. (2007) J Immunol 176, 3434
29. Kotenko, S. V., Krause, C. D., Izotova, L. S., Pollack, B. P., Wu, W., and Pestka, S. (1997) EMBO J., 16, 5894
30. Xie, M. H., Aggarwal, S., Ho, W. H., Foster, J., Zhang, Z., Stinson, J., Wood, W. I., Goddard, A. D., and Gurney, A. L. (2000) J Biol Chem 275, 31335
31. Kotenko, S. V., Izotova, L. S., Mirochnitchenko, O. V., Esterova, E., Dickensheets, H., Donnelly, R. P., and Pestka, S. (2001) J Biol Chem 276, 2725
32. Sheikh, F., Baurin, V. V., Lewis-Antes, A., Shah, N. K., Smirnov, S. V., Anantha, S., Dickensheets, H., Dumoutier, L., Renauld, J. C., Zdanov, A., Donnelly, R. P., Kotenko, S. V. (2004) J Immunol 172, 2006
33. Langer, J. A., Cutrone, E. C., and Kotenko, S. (2004) Cytokine Growth Factor Rev 15, 33
34. Donnelly, R. P., Sheikh, F., Kotenko, S. V., and Dickensheets, H. (2004) J Leukoc Biol 76, 314
35. Yoon, S. I., Logsdon, N. J., Sheikh, F., Donnelly, R. P., and Walter, M. R. (2006) J Biol Chem 281, 35088
36. Wolk, K., and Sabat, R. (2006) Cytokine Growth Factor Rev 17, 367
37. Gibbs, V. C., and Pennica, D. (1997) Gene 186, 97
38. Sommereyns, C., Paul, S., Staeheli, P., and Michiels, T. (2008) PLoS Pathog 4, e1000017
39. Brand, S., Beigel, F., Olszak, T., Zitzmann, K., Eichhorst, S. T., Otte, J. M., Diebold, J., Diepolder, H., Adler, B., Auernhammer, C. J., Göke, B., and Dambacher, J. (2005) Am J Physiol Gastrointest Liver Physiol 289, G960
40. Meager, A., Visvalingam, K., Dilger, P., Bryan, D., and Wadhwa, M. (2005) Cytokine 31, 109
41. Numasaki, M., Tagawa, M., Iwata, F., Suzuki, T., Nakamura, A., Okada, M., Iwakura, Y., Aiba, S., and Yamaya, M. (2007) J Immunol 178, 5086
42. Sato, A., Ohtsuki, M., Hata, M., Kobayashi, E., and Murakami, T. (2006) J Immunol 176, 7686
43. Siebler, J., Wirtz, S., Weigmann, B., Atreya, I., Schmitt, E., Kreft, A., Galle, P. R., and Neurath, M. F. (2007) Gastroenterology 132, 358
44. Pestka, S., Krause, C. D., and Walter, M. R. (2004) Immunol Rev 202, 8
45. Walter, M. R. (2004) Adv Protein Chem 68, 171
46. Brand, S., Zitzmann, K., Dambacher, J., Beigel, F., Olszak, T., Vlotides, G., Eichhorst, S. T., Göke, B., Diepolder, H., and Auernhammer, C. J. (2005) Biochem Biophys Res Commun 331, 543
47. Zitzmann, K., Brand, S., Baehs, S., Göke, B., Meinecke, J., Spöttl, G., Meyer, H., and Auernhammer, C. J. (2006) Biochem Biophys Res Commun 344, 1334
48. Pfeffer, L. M., Dinarello, C. A., Herberman, R. B., Williams, B. R., Borden, E. C., Bordens, R., Walter, M. R., Nagabhushan, T. L., Trotta, P. P., and Pestka, S. (1998) Cancer Res 58, 2489
49. Bracci, L., Proietti, E., and Belardelli, F. (2007) N Y Acad Sci 1112, 256
50. Ferrantini, M., Capone, I., and Belardelli, F. (2007) Biochimie 89, 884
51. Koromilas, A. E., Roy, S., Barber, G. N., Katze, M. G., and Sonenberg, N. (1992) Science 257, 1685
52. Chebath, J., Benech, P., Revel, M., and Vigneron, M. (1987) Nature 330, 587
53. Player, M. R., and Torrence, P. F. (1998) Pharmacol Ther 78, 55
54. Doyle, S. E., Schreckhise, H., Khuu-Duong, K., Henderson, K., Rosler, R., Storey, H., Yao, L., Liu, H., Barahmand-pour, F., Sivakumar, P., Chan, C., Birks, C., Foster, D., Clegg, C. H., Wietzke-Braun, P., Mihm, S., and Klucher, K. M. (2006) Hepatology 44, 896
55. Chin, Y. E., Kitagawa, M., Su, W. C., You, Z. H., Iwamoto, Y., and Fu, X. Y. (1996) Science 272, 719
56. Sangfelt, O., Erickson, S., Einhorn, S., and Grandér, D. (1997) Oncogene 14, 415
57. Sangfelt, O., Erickson, S., Castro, J., Heiden, T., Gustafsson, A., Einhorn, S., and Grandér, D. (1999) Oncogene 18, 2798
58. Iwase, S., Furukawa, Y., Kikuchi, J., Nagai, M., Terui, Y., Nakamura, M., and Yamada, H. (1997) J Biol Chem 272, 12406

59. Kayagaki, N., Yamaguchi, N., Nakayama, M., Eto, H., Okumura, K., and Yagita, H. (1999) J Exp Med 189, 1451
60. Balachandran, S., Kim, C. N., Yeh, W. C., Mak, T. W., Bhalla, K., and Barber, G. N. (1998) EMBO J 17, 6888
61. Chawla-Sarkar, M., Lindner, D. J., Liu, Y. F., Williams, B. R., Sen, G. C., Silverman, R. H., and Borden, E. C. (2003) Apoptosis 8, 237
62. Subramaniam, P. S., Cruz, P. E., Hobeika, A. C., and Johnson, H. M. (1998) Oncogene 16, 1885
63. Sancéau, J., Hiscott, J., Delattre, O., and Wietzerbin, J. (2000) Oncogene 19, 3372
64. Balachandran, S., Roberts, P. C., Kipperman, T., Bhalla, K. N., Compans, R. W., Archer, D. R., and Barber, G. N. (2000) J Virol 74, 1513
65. Ghosh, A., Sarkar, S. N., Rowe, T. M., and Sen, G. C. (2001) J Biol Chem 276, 25447
66. Fidler, I. J. (2000) J Natl Cancer Inst Monogr 28, 10
67. Heyns, A. D., Eldor, A., Vlodavsky, I., Kaiser, N., Fridman, R., and Panet, A. (1985) Exp Cell Res 161, 297
68. Ruszczak, Z., Detmar, M., Imcke, E., and Orfanos, C. E. (1990) J Invest Dermatol 95, 693
69. Hicks, C., Breit, S. N., and Penny, R. (1989) Immunol Cell Biol 67, 271
70. Brouty-Boyé, D., and Zetter, B. R. (1980) Science 208, 516
71. von Marschall, Z., Scholz, A., Cramer, T., Schäfer, G., Schirner, M., Oberg, K., Wiedenmann, B., Höcker, M., and Rosewicz, S. (2003) J Natl Cancer Inst 95, 437
72. Dinney, C. P., Bielenberg, D. R., Perrotte, P., Reich, R., Eve, B. Y., Bucana, C. D., and Fidler, I. J. (1998) Cancer Res 58, 808
73. Singh, R. K., Gutman, M., Llansa, N., and Fidler, I. J. (1996) J Interferon Cytokine Res 16, 577
74. Fabra, A., Nakajima, M., Bucana, C. D., and Fidler, I. J. (1992) Differentiation 52, 101
75. Ezekowitz, R. A., Mulliken, J. B., and Folkman, J. (1992) N Engl J Med 326, 1456
76. Real, F. X., Oettgen, H. F., and Krown, S. E. (1986) J Clin Oncol 4, 544
77. Legha, S. S. (1997) Semin Oncol 24(1 Suppl 4), S39
78. Stadler, W. M., Kuzel, T. M., Raghavan, D., Levine, E., Vogelzang, N. J., Roth, B., Dorr, F. A. (1997) J Cancer 33 Suppl 1, S23
79. Jordan, W. J., Eskdale, J., Boniotto, M., Rodia, M., Kellner, D., and Gallagher, G. (2007) Genes Immun 8, 13
80. Pekarek, V., Srinivas, S., Eskdale, J., and Gallagher, G. (2007) Genes Immun 8, 177
81. Tough, D. F., Borrow, P., and Sprent, J. (1996) Science 272, 1947
82. Marrack, P., Kappler, J., and Mitchell, T. (1999) J Exp Med 189, 521
83. Hung, K., Hayashi, R., Lafond-Walker, A., Lowenstein, C., Pardoll, D., and Levitsky, H. (1998) J Exp Med 188, 2357
84. Segal, B. M., Glass, D. D., and Shevach, E. M. (2002) J Immunol 168, 1
85. Clarke, S. R. (2000) J Leukoc Biol 67, 607
86. Lo, C. H., Lee, S. C., Wu, P. Y., Pan, W. Y., Su, J., Cheng, C. W., Roffler, S. R., Chiang, B. L., Lee, C. N., Wu, C. W., and Tao, M. H. (2003) J Immunol 171, 600
87. Martinotti, A., Stoppacciaro, A., Vagliani, M., Melani, C., Spreafico, F., Wysocka, M., Parmiani, G., Trinchieri, G., and Colombo, M. P. (1995) Eur J Immunol 25, 137
88. Sutmuller, R. P., van Duivenvoorde, L. M., van Elsas, A., Schumacher, T. N., Wildenberg, M. E., Allison, J. P., Toes, R. E., Offringa, R., and Melief, C. J. (2001) J Exp Med 194, 823
89. Mennechet, F. J., and Uzé, G. (2006) Blood 107, 4417
90. Orange, J. S., and Biron, C. A. (1996) J Immunol 156, 4746
91. Biron, C. A., Nguyen, K. B., Pien, G. C., Cousens, L. P., and Salazar-Mather, T. P. (1999) Annu Rev Immunol 17, 189
92. Kasaian, M. T., Whitters, M. J., Carter, L. L., Lowe, L. D., Jussif, J. M., Deng, B., Johnson, K. A., Witek, J. S., Senices, M., Konz, R. F., Wurster, A. L., Donaldson, D. D., Collins, M., Young, D. A., and Grusby, M. J. (2002) Immunity 16, 559
93. Colombo, M. P., Modesti, A., Parmiani, G., and Forni, G. (1992) Cancer Res 52, 4853
94. Stoppacciaro, A., Melani, C., Parenza, M., Mastracchio, A., Bassi, C., Baroni, C., Parmiani, G., and Colombo, M. P. (1993) J Exp Med 178, 151

95. Boehm, U., Klamp, T., Groot, M., and Howard, J. C. (1997) Annu Rev Immunol 15, 749
96. Dighe, A. S., Richards, E., Old, L. J., and Schreiber, R. D. (1994) Immunity 1, 447
97. Angiolillo, A. L., Sgadari, C., Taub, D. D., Liao, F., Farber, J. M., Maheshwari, S., Kleinman, H. K., Reaman, G. H., and Tosato, G. (1995) J Exp Med 182, 155
98. Addison, C. L., Arenberg, D. A., Morris, S. B., Xue, Y. Y., Burdick, M. D., Mulligan, M. S., Iannettoni, M. D., and Strieter, R. M. (2000) Gene Ther 11, 247
99. Cousens, L. P., Orange, J. S., Su, H. C., and Biron, C. A. (1997) Proc Natl Acad Sci USA 94, 634
100. Sareneva, T., Julkunen, I., and Matikainen, S. (2000) J Immunol 165, 1933
101. Wenner, C. A., Güler, M. L., Macatonia, S. E., O'Garra, A., and Murphy, K. M. (1996) J Immunol 156, 1442
102. Mu, J., Zou, J. P., Yamamoto, N., Tsutsui, T., Tai, X. G., Kobayashi, M., Herrmann, S., Fujiwara, H., and Hamaoka, T. (1995) Cancer Res 55, 4404
103. Gri, G., Chiodoni, C., Gallo, E., Stoppacciaro, A., Liew, F. Y., and Colombo, M. P. (2002) Cancer Res 62, 4390
104. Zilocchi, C., Stoppacciaro, A., Chiodoni, C., Parenza, M., Terrazzini, N., and Colombo, M. P. (1998) J Exp Med 188, 133
105. Rogge, L., Barberis-Maino, L., Biffi, M., Passini, N., Presky, D. H., Gubler, U., and Sinigaglia, F. (1997) J Exp Med 185, 825
106. Rogge, L., D'Ambrosio, D., Biffi, M., Penna, G., Minetti, L. J., Presky, D. H., Adorini, L., and Sinigaglia, F. (1998) J Immunol 161, 6567
107. Ank, N., Iversen, M. B., Bartholdy, C., Staeheli, P., Hartmann, R., Jensen, U. B., Dagnaes-Hansen, F., Thomsen, A. R., Chen, Z., Haugen, H., Klucher, K., and Paludan, S. R. (2008) J Immunol 180, 2474

Passive and Active Tumor Homing Cytokine Therapy

Jeffry Cutrera and Shulin Li

Abstract Malignant diseases continue to be one of the deadliest afflictions facing mankind. Research and technology continue to improve the current conventional therapies of surgery, radiation, and chemotherapy, but cancer continues to be a perennial killer mainly due to metastatic tumors as well as residual tumors remaining after treatments. One area of treatment that has the potential to treat all of these tumors is immune modulation with cytokine therapies. Several cytokines have been tested in clinical trials with some being approved as clinical cancer therapies; however, the majority of these therapies fail because of cytokine-induced toxicities. To overcome the toxicity and improve the efficacy of these treatments, several models of tumor-targeted cytokines have been developed. To target the cytokines to the tumor environment, these strategies implement different methods ranging from passive targeting, which exploits the enhanced permeability and retention effect of tumors to active targeting with peptides and antibodies specific for ligands in the tumor environment. This chapter will review the history and progress of tumor-targeted cytokine therapies for the treatment of malignant diseases.

Introduction

In 2008, approximately 565,500 people will die from and more than 2 million people will be diagnosed with cancer in America alone. Although continued progress in conventional therapies such as surgery, radiation, and chemotherapy is being maintained and the 5-year survival of cancer patients is steadily increasing for most types, cancer is still one of the leading causes of death in America, second only to cardiovascular disease [1]. Most cancer deaths are attributed to metastatic disease, which can be distributed throughout the body [2], and residual tumors which

S. Li(✉)
Department of Comparative Biomedical Sciences, School of Veterinary Medicine,
Louisiana State University, Skip Bertman Drive, Baton Rouge, LA 70803, USA
e-mail: sli@vetmed.lsu.edu

J. Lustgarten et al. (eds.), *Targeted Cancer Immune Therapy*,
DOI 10.1007/978-1-4419-0170-5_6,

remain after treatment with conventional therapies [3]. Thus, new cancer treatment strategies must be able to destroy not only the primary tumors but also all of the metastatic or residual tumor cells, which remain after conventional treatments. One of the most promising strategies to accomplish this feat is directly targeting immunostimulatory agents to tumor cells or tumor microenvironments.

The ability of the immune system to attack tumor cells was first hypothesized by Paul Erlich in 1909, but the discovery of cytokines, intracellular signaling proteins produced by immune cells, and their ability to increase the immune response toward cancer really boosted the study of immunomodulation for cancer therapy [4]. Among these cytokines were tumor necrosis factor (TNF)α [5], interleukin (IL)-2 [6], and IL-12 [7]. Interestingly, the biological properties of these cytokines vary tremendously yet all have since shown potential for treating malignancies. For instance, TNFα has direct cytotoxic effects against tumor cells as well as activating antitumor immune responses [8], IL-2 induces proliferation of B, T, and NK cells [9], and IL-12 induces interferon (IFN) γ in T and NK cells [10]. While these and other cytokines are pleiotropic, many have overlapping functions such as the ability of IL-2 and IL-12 to enhance the cytotoxicity of natural killer (NK) and activated T cells [11] and synergistically upregulating the other's receptors via independent signaling pathways [12]. In fact, very quickly after the IL-2 gene was purified in substantial amounts clinical trials in cancer patients began [13, 14].With the continued elucidation of these potential antitumor qualities, several cytokines have been and continue to be clinically evaluated for the treatment of many types of cancer.

Unfortunately, several clinical trials implementing systemic delivery of recombinant cytokines for the treatment of cancer failed to produce positive results and produced severe toxicities. For early IL-2 clinical trials, the only benefits were seen in patient with renal cell carcinoma (RCC) and malignant melanoma. While only a select few patients benefited from the treatments, toxicities ranging from the severe, such as hypotension, vascular leak, and respiratory insufficiencies, to the problematic, like nausea, emesis, diarrhea, etc., limited the levels of cytokines that could be delivered and, therefore, the antitumor effects [4]. Similar results were seen in clinical studies using systemic delivery of recombinant IL-12 and TNFα. So, the succeeding steps to overcome the barriers of systemic cytokine therapies were locoregional delivery of the cytokines and combinational treatment regimens. Unfortunately, the benefits of these treatment strategies have continued to be undermined by the toxicities [4, 8, 10, 12]. Despite the low response rates and high potential for toxicity, IL-2 is clinically approved in the United States, Canada, and the European Union for the treatment of RCC [4].

Nonetheless, the potential benefits of cytokine therapy for the treatment of cancer are present but there are still several obstacles that need to be overcome. With systemic cytokine treatments, the level of cytokine is increased systemically, which leads to most of the toxicities and even death in some cases. Also, the increase in cytokine level was generally not high enough at the target area (i.e., tumor site) to elicit an immune response capable of creating a therapeutic benefit. Another problem with the treatments was the rapid clearance of the cytokine through the body's normal excretory and biotransformation systems. Even with locoregional administrations the minimal level of cytokine concentrations for therapeutic benefits was hard to maintain as well as the fact that most tumors are not available for noninvasive administrations [4, 8, 10, 12]. So, there is a need for treatments that can reach sites distal from the site of administration, reach an immunologically active concentration of the cytokine, and maintain that concentration long enough to induce a therapeutic response.

One such administration technique that could improve the efficacy of cytokine treatments is gene therapy. Local delivery of cytokine-encoding genes is capable of producing therapeutic levels of cytokines at the site of delivery with only slight increases in systemic cytokine levels. Also, the local concentration of cytokines will persist so the immune system can be properly activated. Furthermore, for difficult-to-reach sites of administrations, the frequency of treatment is lower so the therapy is less invasive. Toward this purpose, several types of vectors including multiple viral and nonviral vectors have been tested in animal models as well as clinical trials [2, 4, 15, 16]. There is still much debate about which vector is the best for the treatment of cancer in humans because they all have varying advantages and disadvantages. Several cytokine genes in various vectors have already been investigated via systemic and locoregional administration in preclinical and clinical trials including IL-2, IL-12, TNFα, IFNα, and many more. Another method for local cytokine delivery is adoptive transfer of cells that have been transfected with cytokine producing genes. These cells can be delivered by either intratumoral (i.t.) or peritumoral (p.t.) injection, where they will then produce and secrete the cytokines in the tumor microenvironment [17–20]. Regrettably, most of these cytokine treatment approaches with a few exceptions have yet to successfully overcome enough barriers to meet the requirements necessary to become clinically approved treatments for cancer [4, 15].

A very promising solution to the aforementioned obstacles for cytokine therapy of cancer is targeted delivery of the cytokines to the tumor and tumor microenvironment. For the purpose of this review, targeting entails any method that enhances the delivery, retention, and biological activity of the cytokines at the tumor site. Toward this goal, researchers have developed a wide array of strategies ranging from the passive targeting via the enhanced permeability and retention effect of tumors to the active targeting of tumor and tumor microenvironment antigens. This review will focus on the development, action, progress, and future directions of targeting cytokines to tumor sites for immunomodulatory treatments.

Passive Targeting with Poly-Ethylene Glycol

First described in 1986, tumor environments are characterized by fenestrated vasculature and poor lymphatic drainage [21]. Now termed enhanced permeability and retention (EPR), this tumor-specific trait can be exploited to accumulate high concentrations of systemically delivered treatments. In brief, intravenously delivered agents collect in the tumor tissue by passively transversing large gaps between endothelial cells in the tumor vasculature. Once present in the tumor tissue, these agents remain due to the poor drainage of the lymphatics in the tissue; therefore, the concentration of these agents continues to increase. Most systems that attempt to exploit the EPR effect are nanoparticle colloidal drug carrier systems, which consist of repeating elements conjugated to therapeutic modalities. When these systems are introduced into the blood circulation, they are readily incapacitated by opsonization and then rapidly removed by the mononuclear phagocytic system (MPS) and the reticulo-endothelial system (RES), so the nanoparticles are not present in circulation long enough to utilize the EPR and create an antitumor effect [21, 22].

Several investigators have worked to develop new stealth nanoparticles that can avoid these systems. Several stealth particles were discovered including poly(acrylamide), polysaccharides, and poly(vinyl alcohol). The most widely used and successful technique is the addition of poly(ethylene glycol) (PEG) units onto the surface of particles, which is known as PEGylation. PEG has a structure of $HO–(CH_2CH_2O)_n–CH_2CH_2–OH$. This structure encompasses a chemically inert polyether backbone. Another key component of PEG is the terminal hydroxyl groups, which can be used for conjugation to an extensive list of agents. In vivo, these stealth nanoparticles have longer half-lives in circulation, which leads to an increased invasion of tumor vasculature and accumulation in the tumor site. This stealth characteristic of PEG is determined by several different factors including particle size and surface characteristics. Optimization of these factors has led to the increased efficacy of cytokine-nanoparticle conjugates [23].

IFNα has long been known to be critical in antitumor therapies in addition to its direct antitumor effects [24]. Several clinical trials have shown the potential for IFNα to be used as a treatment for tumors, but the effective dose is hard to reach due to toxicities of systemic treatment. Also, the short half-life ($T_{1/2}$) of IFNα necessitates daily administrations to see any therapeutic effect [25]. PEGylation of IFNα elongates its $T_{1/2}$ in humans from 4 to 16 h for unmodified IFNα to 61–100 h. Likewise, the absorption $T_{1/2}$ increased from 2.3 to approximately 50 h. Several other factors are increased with the PEGylation of IFNα making the treatment of cancer with IFNα more plausible [26].

Indeed, one of the first phase I clinical trials using PEGylated IFNα-2B (one form of IFNα) (PEGIFNα-2B) in patients with chronic myeloid leukemia (CML) showed a dramatic increase in the efficacy of treatments. In this study, the MTD of PEGIFNα-2B was defined as 7.5–9 μg/kg weekly. This dose level given weekly is equivalent to three times the dose level of IFNα-2B in previous CML studies with no increase in toxicities. Furthermore, 53% of patients who were suffering from active disease at the start of the trial showed a therapeutic response. Of the 27 patients in the study who had failed previous IFNα therapy, 13 had a favorable response to this treatment. Also, this study used subcutaneous (s.c.) administrations and the PEGIFNα-2B was readily absorbed with increasing serum concentrations through week 1, but not by week 4. This early clinical study showed the safety, ease of administration, and efficacy of treatment with PEGIFNα-2B [25].

Preclinical and clinical studies with different types of PEGylation conjugated to various cytokines has steadily continued; therefore, the quality of PEG used to modify cytokines has improved. One of the best modifications to PEGylation of cytokines was the creation of poly(methoxypolyethyleneglycol-cyanoacrylate-co-*n*-hexadecyl cyanoacrylate) nanoparticles (PEG-PHDCA). This new formulation is a more rapidly degradable copolymer with higher stealth capabilities. Similar to the original PEG-IFNα studies, PEG-PHDCA conjugated to TNFα increased the T_h of TNFα in the blood circulation. Also, accumulation at the tumor site was increased at 6 h after intravenous injection [27]. So, the PEG-PHDCA increased the length of activity for TNFα, but the characteristics that create this increase were not well understood.

The study of how these characteristics and the formulation of the nanoparticles helped to increase their tumor-targeting capabilities. First, studies to analyze the effects of molecular weight and particle size of surface modifications of PEG-PHDCA conjugated to TNFα resulted in optimized parameters for increased circulation time and tumor accumulation. These studies revealed that nanoparticles with smaller PHDCA particle sizes (~80 nm) and larger molecular weights (5 kDa) decreased serum protein adsorption, which results in decreased phagocytosis, increased circulation time, and higher accumulation in the tumor compared with other tissues. The smaller particle size allows a higher density of MePEG chains, which increases the interaction between the particles and water molecules and prevents the adsorption of serum proteins [23, 28].

Another use of PEG for targeting cytokines to tumors is conjugation to the shell of virus vectors loaded with cytokine-coding genes. Since one of the major limits to viral gene-therapy is the antibody response to the vectors, PEGylation of the vectors can help reduce detection by the humoral immune system. Indeed, intravenous injection of PEGylated adenovirus vectors (PEG-Ad) in mouse models results in reduced CTL production and elongated viral gene expression from 4 to 42 days [29]. Furthermore, PEG-Ad encoding TNFα (PEG-Ad-TNF) has several benefits over unmodified vectors (Ad-TNF). First, the $T_{1/2}$ of PEG-Ad-TNF was 12-fold longer than the unmodified. Second, PEG-Ad-TNF gene expression in the tumor and liver tissue was 35-fold higher and 20-fold lower than Ad-TNF, respectively. The PEG-Ad-TNF also showed increased antitumor activity compared with Ad-TNF. These results show that there is potential for treating tumors with systemic administration of PEG-Ad loaded with cytokine genes [30].

Exploiting the EPR effect for targeting cytokines to tumors can improve the efficacy while reducing the toxicity. This effect is caused by the nature of solid tumors and their effects on the physiologic conditions of the tumor environment. Adding PEG and different variations of PEG can increase the circulation time of cytokines allowing for increased concentrations in the tumor environment and decreased concentrations in toxicity causing tissues such as the liver. Although these effects can be seen in solid tumors, better modalities to exploit more specific tumor-associated characteristics for targeting the cytokines in the tumor environment can further increase the effectiveness and decrease the toxicity of these treatment strategies for tumor therapy.

Active Ligand Targeting with Tumor-Homing Peptides

In addition to the EPR effect, tumors have many other unique attributes, which can be exploited for targeting cytokines. To exploit these traits, several active targeting strategies have been developed such as peptides that home to tumor environments. With the advent of in vivo biopanning with peptide phage display technology, vast amounts of peptides can be expressed on the surface of phage and then analyzed for their ability to bind to ligands in different tissue types [31]. Using this technique, several peptides have been isolated, and new ones continue to be discovered, that preferentially target tumors [32]. Of these tumor-targeting peptides, the most widely studied and most successful peptides do not only target the tumors themselves but also target motifs that are expressed due to unique qualities of the tumor environment. Specifically, these peptides target proteins that are upregulated in tumor vasculature and lymphatic vessels [33].

Peptides that contain the amino acid sequence Arg-Gly-Asp (RGD) were one of the first targeted peptides discovered via biopanning. These peptides target integrins that are upregulated during angiogenesis but bind most specifically to the integrins $\alpha v\beta 3$ and $\alpha v\beta 5$. Along with their ability to bind to these integrins, RGD peptides are also capable of internalizing into the cells, causing cell death, and interrupting the development of more vasculature. There are several different RGD peptide variants, including ACDCRGDCFCG (RGD4C), which have different beneficial abilities [33, 34]. By using knockout mice to isolate the effects of the RGD4C peptide, it was shown that RGD4C has antiangiogenic effects. Using multiple angiogenesis assays in these knockout strains, RGD4C repeatedly demonstrated antiangiogenic capabilities [35]. While these peptides have beneficial properties in addition to their targeting abilities, it is their interactions with integrins that have been used for targeting, imaging, and treating tumors in preclinical models [33–39].

Among these techniques, conjugating RGD sequences to cytokines has shown to increase the therapeutic effect compared with the wild-type (wt) cytokines. RGD-cytokine conjugates can be produced by expression of the fusion protein by recombinant DNA technology or chemical coupling of the purified peptide to purified cytokines. By these methods, several fusions of different RGD peptides with murine and human cytokines have been created, and these fusions have been examined in vitro and in vivo. Most RGD-cytokine conjugates maintain both the binding specificity of the RGD peptide and the biological activity of the conjugated cytokines [36, 37, 39].

One of the most widely studied RGD-cytokine conjugates are those using TNFα. Several different groups have analyzed the RGD binding ability of these conjugates in vitro, and they determined that conjugating RGD peptides does not affect the affinity of the peptide for its receptors [36, 37, 39]. Likewise, the activity of the conjugated TNFα was not lower than the wt cytokine as demonstrated through fibroblast cell viability assays [37, 39]; however, cell viability studies using a cell line that expresses the receptor intregrins specific for RGD showed that the conjugated TNFα does have increased toxicity to these cells. Also, incubating the cells with excess RGD peptide prior to addition of the TNFα and RGD-TNFα decreased the activity of the RGD-TNFα and not wt TNFα. So, the increased activity is due to the binding of the RGD-TNFα to its receptors on the cell surface. Similar results were found by exploiting another attribute of TNFα: ICAM-1 induction. FACS analysis revealed that RGD-TNFα increased the expression of ICAM-1 more than TNFα, and preincubation with free RGD peptide reduced the ICAM-1 expression level to that of the wtTNFα while not reducing the level of ICAM-1 induced by the TNFα [36]. The results from these in vitro studies demonstrate the potential for using RGD-TNFα conjugates in preclinical models.

Indeed, different groups have demonstrated that RGD-TNFα does have increased antitumor activities in vivo. Since TNFα is used to increase the efficacy of chemotherapeutic treatments, one group studied the effect of using RGD4C-TNFα in conjunction with melphalan, a commonly used chemotherapeutic agent. They found that a single treatment of RGD4C-mTNFα (0.3 ng i.p.) when administered in conjunction with one treatment of melphalan (50 ng i.p.) was able to reduce tumor growth in a syngeneic RMA lymphoma model when administration of either agent alone induced no antitumor effects. Although the addition of RGD4C-TNFα to the chemotherapeutic treatment increased antitumor efficacy, there was no corresponding change in animal weight revealing that there is no increase in toxicity with the combinatorial treatments [36]. More recently, another group has shown that treatments of RGD4C conjugated to human TNFα (RGD4C-hTNFα) can improve the antitumor efficacy of hTNFα in a nude mouse model. In these reports, nude mice bearing xenogenic MDA-MB-435 tumors were treated with five consecutive daily i.v. injections of saline, hTNFα, or RGD4C-hTNFα (0.25 mg/kg). Compared with the saline treated group, treatment with hTNFα and RGD4C-hTNFα resulted in tumor volume reductions of 24% and 72%, respectively, by 15 days after treatment. The investigators also monitored animal weight, and there was no difference among the groups throughout the experiment. Additionally, ex vivo staining for CD31 and TUNEL revealed that the RGD4C-hTNFα treatments resulted in selective cytolysis of αvβ3-positive tumor cells and tumor vessels while the saline and hTNFα treatments did not cause any integrin-dependant cytolysis [38]. These in vivo results continue to show the potential for using RGD peptides to increase the antitumor effect of TNFα while reducing the toxicity, which is normally seen in TNFα treatments.

RGD peptides have also been shown to improve the antitumor efficacy of other cytokines. Similar to RGD4C-TNFα in vitro studies, the RGD4C-IL12 conjugate mrIL-12vp binds to the $\alpha_v\beta_3$-positive cell line M21 (human melanoma) and not to the $\alpha_v\beta_3$-negative cell line Saos-2 (human osteosarcoma) while the nontargeted mrIL-12 did not bind to either cell line. Furthermore, in vivo toxicity studies with i.p. injections of 0.025–0.5 μg/d of mrIL-12 resulted in readily observable toxicities such as loss of appetite, weight loss, trouble breathing, and even sudden death after 7 days, and comparable levels of mrIL-12vp did not cause any such toxicity. Also, when NSX2-tumor-bearing mice were treated with PBS, mrIL-12, or mrIL-12vp continuously for 3 weeks (1 μg/day), there was a nearly twofold reduction in tumor volume with the targeted therapy compared with both PBS and nontargeted IL-12 therapies. So, RGD4C can also increase the efficacy of IL-12 for treating tumors while simultaneously decreasing the toxic effects normally seen with IL-12 treatments [35]. All of the aforementioned experiments employing conjugates of RGD peptides and cytokines show that the RGD-integrin interactions can be exploited to enhance the antitumor efficacy and reduce the toxicity of cytokine tumor therapies.

Another set of peptides that target tumor environments are peptides containing the amino acid sequence Asn-Gly-Arg (NGR). Similar to RGD peptides, NGR peptides were first identified via in vivo biopanning [31] and preferentially bind to a ligand, aminopeptidase N (CD13), which is upregulated on tumor vessels during angiogenesis [40]. CD13 is also found in other tissues such as kidney and myeloid cells, but the NGR peptides do not bind to CD13 found in normal tissues [41]. Although there are several different NGR-containing sequences that have been used to target to tumor environments, disulfide-bridged cyclic NGR peptides (CNGRC) show an increased affinity for CD13 and increased antitumor activity, greater than 10-fold higher, when coupled to TNFα compared with a linear NGR peptide (GNGRG) [42]. So, the cyclic-NGR peptides have a lot of potential to be used as tumor targeting vehicles for cytokines.

After the discovery that NGR peptides do indeed target an angiogenesis marker in tumor vasculature, the natural next step was to investigate its ability to facilitate the delivery of antitumor therapies. To this end, NGR was first coupled the murine TNFα (NGR-TNFα) and characterized via in vitro cytotoxicity assays. These experiments using L-M mouse fibroblast cells revealed that coupling the NGR peptides to murine TNFα did not affect the folding, oligomerization, or binding to TNFα receptors. After these proof-of-concept experiments, NGR-TNFα was administered to C57/Bl6 mice bearing syngeneic RMA-T lymphoma tumors. The LD_{50} values of TNFα and NGR-TNFα were 60 and 45 μg, respectively, which are not very different; however, the antitumor effects were drastically different. Impressively, 1 μg of NGR-TNFα delayed tumor growth better than 27 μg of TNFα 14 days after a single i.p. administration 10 days after tumor inoculation. Also, some mice treated with less than the LD_{50} of NGR-TNFα were completely cured of tumors, while no mice treated with any amount of TNFα were completely cured of tumors. The body weights of mice from these experiments were monitored to identify the difference in toxicity from NGR-TNFα when compared with that from TNFα. The efficacy/toxicity ratio of NGR-TNFα was 14 times higher than those of TNFα. Similar experiments were performed using syngeneic B16F1 tumors to analyze the effects of multiple treatments. With treatments at days 11, 17, and 19 after tumor cell inoculation, NGR-TNFα was 12–15 times more effective than the same doses of TNFα while the toxicities were comparable [43]. These studies reveal the increased antitumor activity and decreased toxicity of NGR-TNFα vs. TNFα, which shows the potential for NGR-TNFα in the treatment of tumors.

NGR-TNFα was evaluated also for its ability to enhance the antitumor efficacy of chemotherapeutic agents. Similar to RGD-TNFα, a single administration of subnanogram levels of NGR-TNFα combined with a single dose of melphalan (50 μg) creates a synergistic decrease in tumor volume with no corresponding increase in toxicity as determined by animal weights. Interestingly, only 0.1 ng of NGR-TNFα is needed to see a significant reduction in tumor volume, while no difference is seen in tumor volumes below 0.3 ng of RGD4C-TNFα [36]. More recent studies have shown that pretreatment with NGR-TNFα as opposed to simultaneous treatment greatly increases the efficacy of the chemotherapeutic agents. In several different tumor models and with different chemotherapeutic drugs, a pretreatment with 0.1 μg NGR-TNFα increased the efficacy of the drugs without increasing the toxicity seen with any of the drugs or NGR-TNFα alone. Notably, the increase in efficacy of each drug in combination with NGR-TNFα was different depending on the tumor model used [44, 45]. Interestingly, NGR-TNFα does not increase the cytotoxicity of doxorubicin in in-vitro cytotoxicity assays using the prostate cancer tumor cell line TRAMP-C1, but the in vivo antitumor effect of doxorubicin with NGR-TNFα was significantly increased. This observation demonstrates that NGR-TNFα does not directly increase the cytotoxicity of doxorubicin but instead primes the tumor environment to increase the effect of the doxorubicin on tumor growth [46]. In addition to the direct antitumor activity of NGR-TNFα, it can also synergistically increase the efficacy of chemotherapeutic drugs.

Recent studies have shown that NGR also increases the antitumor efficacy of the human cytokine IFNα2a by targeting to the tumor environment. In vitro studies of EC migration and tube formation using IFNα2a and the NGR-IFNα2a conjugate revealed that the conjugate had consistently increased antiangiogenic effects at all tested concentrations as determined by a reduction of tube formation by HUVEC in matrigel. Similarly, treatment with NGR-IFNα2a to HUVEC induced with bFGF reduced the ability of the cells to migrate through matrigel more than IFNα2a. Also, in two different xyngeneic tumor models in nude mice daily i.p. treatments of NGR-IFNα inhibited tumor growth at levels comparable to those seen with two to fivefold higher doses of IFNα2a. At all treatment doses, no toxicities were observed with either formulation [47]. Further toxicity studies were performed on mice, rats, and monkeys using pharmacologically active doses. Following single doses ranging from 50 to 674 times higher than the clinical dose for adults resulted in no toxicities evidenced by no abnormalities in general signs and animal weights for all species as well as food consumption, urinalysis, hematological examinations, and blood biochemical examinations in monkeys. For repeated-dose studies, rats were administered daily i.m. injections with 1.5×10^6, 4.5×10^6, or 1.25×10^7 U/kg for 90 days and monkeys were given 7.5×10^5, 2.25×10^6, or 6.75×10^6 U/kg for 47 days. In rats, there were no changes in body weights, food intake, or general health and activity. There were some minor changes in some hematological and clinical chemistry parameters, but all levels returned to normal levels after the administrations. The results in the monkey studies were similar with no deaths occurring during the treatments, and most of the clinical and pathology changes returned to normal after the administrations were discontinued [48]. These preclinical efficacy and toxicity data indicate that targeting IFNα2a to tumors using NGR is a very plausible safe and effective treatment for malignant diseases in humans.

Effort continues to be made to discover more peptides that can target tumor environments and to improve the targeting abilities of the peptides. The secret to improving these peptides may not only be based on discovering new peptides [32] but also on improving the current peptide modalities. To such an end, modifying the peptides to increase the amount of ligand interactions they can utilize in the tumor environment would be extremely beneficial. Recently, a shortened version of RGD4C, CDGRC, when fused to murine IFNα and delivered via i.m., i.t., or i.d. injections of plasmid DNA followed by electroporation maintains its ability to anchor in tumor environments and produce antitumor immune responses. This peptide sequence shares homology with NGR peptides as well as RGD peptides so its array of potential ligands is increased to create better homing abilities. Additionally, it has a shorter amino acid sequence than RGD4C, so it is less likely to cause a humoral response to the recombinant fusion protein [49]. Further modifications of these peptides will continue to improve the efficacy of peptide-cytokine treatments for malignancies and possibly propel them into clinical settings.

An alternative method to reduce toxicity and increase efficacy of cytokines is to deliver cytokine genes to tumors. Viral vectors have been studied extensively to deliver genes to various tissue types. Modifying the tropism of the viral vectors to preferentially transduce cells in the tumor or tumor environment would help to sequester the effects of the cytokines and minimize systemic toxicity. To accomplish this goal, viruses armed with cytokine genes are modified to express tumor-targeted peptides on the capsid fibers and home to the tumor vasculature to deliver their payloads. To date, viral vectors have been successfully modified with RGD peptides for the delivery of various genes to the tumor environment with high success [50]. So, it appears to be a potential strategy for the delivery of cytokine genes to the tumor environment.

One of the first viral vectors used to attempt this feat was adenovirus modified to express RGD on the capsid fiber (AdRGD). These vectors were much more efficient at transducing melanoma cells both in vitro and in vivo. Also, i.t. injections of these vectors loaded with TNFα-coding DNA (AdRGD-TNFα) resulted in more hemorrhagic necrosis and inhibition of tumor growth compared with injection of the conventional vector loaded with TNFα genes. However, the TNFα produced from the transduced cells would leak into the circulation resulting in typical TNFα-induced toxicity [51, 52]. Similarly, i.t. injections of AdRGD loaded with IL-12 (AdRGD-IL12) resulted in increased transduction of melanoma cells in vitro, and in a syngeneic melanoma model tumor reduction compared with conventional IL-12 loaded vector at a dose level a magnitude of order less than the nontargeted vector. Different from AdRGD-TNFα, there were no toxic side effects at therapeutic doses, but loss of body weight was seen with doses that were high enough to almost completely reduce tumor volume. Furthermore, combinations of AdRGD-TNFα and AdRGD-IL12 resulted in complete tumor regression in all treated mice, and there were no detectable cytokine levels in the serum [53]. Although these results are exciting for cytokine-loaded-viral vectors to transduce tumor cells, these data do not show any tumor-targeting of the vectors, but further modifications of the vector capsid fibers as well as the cytokine genes will increase the effectiveness of the vectors and allow them to be used for systemic delivery of tumor-targeted cytokine viral vectors.

Active Targeting with Tumor-Targeted Antibodies

By far the most investigated method to target cytokines to tumors is the fusion of antibodies to cytokines to create immunocytokines. Similar to the peptide-cytokine fusions, these immunocytokines actively target antigens on the tumor cells or in the tumor microenvironment and enhance the direct antitumor effects of the cytokines or activate an antitumor immune response against the tumors. Antibodies can be developed to target specific antigens in the tumor environment, whereas most tumor-targeted peptides are derived from in vivo biopanning and so the ligand is not necessarily known. Also, several factors hamper the ability of antibodies to be successfully used to improve therapies. First, they are larger molecules with a full IgG antibody having a molecular weight of approximately 150 kDa. Second, the original antibodies used for therapeutic purposes were created by murine hybridoma technology, so the Fc fragments were not fully compatible with the human immune system. Lastly, because they originated from murine origins, the antibodies elicit an immune response against the antibodies themselves which in turns reduces the therapeutic effect. For these reasons, the antibodies for therapeutics had to be modified to have any potential to be successful in humans [54, 55].

Several different approaches have been used to overcome these initial problems for using antibodies in therapeutic settings, and these approaches differ depending on what the antibody is used for in the therapy. For most cytokine-antibody conjugate therapies, the only region of the antibody that needs to be functioning properly is the variable region. So, removal of the Fc fragment can reduce the size and therefore the immunogenicity of the antibody while maintaining its ability to bind to a specific antigen; however, the resulting fragment is still of murine origin and still immunogenic. Other modifications of antibodies create chimeric antibodies, which are created by combining human portions of antibodies to murine variable regions to reduce the immunogenicity [54, 55]. Regardless of which derivative of an antibody is used, the main goal remains to maintain the specificity of the antibody and the immunomodulatory effects of the cytokine to get the highest antitumor response with the lowest possible toxic side effects. To date, tumor-specific antibodies have been generated for a vast array of tumor environment specific ligands, and these antibodies have been conjugated to a vast array of cytokines.

As in peptide-cytokine therapies, immunocytokines specific for changes specific in tumor vasculature have proven highly successful. One of the first antigens for these immunocytokines utilized the recombinant human single chain antibody L19, which is specific for the domain B isoform of fibronectin. In addition to being found only in tissue undergoing angiogenesis such as tumors and the endometrium, an interesting characteristic of this isoform is that the amino acid sequence is identical in mouse, rat, rabbit, dogs, humans, and several other mammals; therefore, the specificity of L19 is consistent in all these species [56]. L19 conjugated to IL-2 (L19-IL2) was the first L19 immunocytokine used for biodistribution and antitumor studies in mice [57].

These first studies found that the L19-IL2 conjugate did indeed target the tumor neovasculature and increased the antitumor effects of IL-2. Radio-labeled L19-IL2 and the nonspecific conjugate D1.3-IL2 were i.v. administered to nude mice bearing F9 teratocarcinoma tumors. After 24 h, the tumor/blood ratio of the L19-IL2 was 33 whereas the D1.3-IL2 was less than one. Also, microautoradiography showed that the L19-IL2 accumulated around the tumor vasculature in a similar manner to L19 alone proving that the immunocytokine has similar binding affinity for its antigen. They also analyzed the antitumor effects in several tumor cell lines in both syngeneic and xyngeneic models. In all models tested, tumor growth was significantly reduced with treatment of L19-IL2 compared with D1.3-IL2 and saline-treated groups. In addition to a reduction in tumor volume, increases in tumor-infiltrating lymphocytes and necrotic area as well as reduction in the level of mitoses were seen with the L19-IL2 treatments. Also, treatment with a mixture of nonconjugated IL-2 and L19 did not show any significant increases in any of the above-mentioned antitumor immune responses [57]. This first study of an L19-cytokine fusion therapy led the way for several other cytokine conjugates.

L19 was then fused to IL-12 to improve the efficacy and reduce the toxicity of the cytokine treatment for malignancies. In the recombinant L19-IL12 protein, the p35 and p40 subunits were fused with a linker to maintain the proper folding of the heterodimer, which was then attached to the N-terminus of L19. As in L19-IL2, this formulation retained the in vitro bioactivity of the cytokine and the in vivo biodistribution of the antibody. To determine the antitumor activity, two syngeneic tumor models, C51 colon adenocarcinoma and F9 teratocarcinoma, were implanted into Balb/c and 129Sv mice, respectively, and then treated with 2.5 μg of L19-IL12, HyHEL10-IL12 (a nonspecific antibody fusion), or saline every 48 h starting 4 days after tumor implantation. Throughout the treatments tumor volume and animal weights were noted. In both tumor models, tumor growth was drastically reduced with L19-IL12 treatment with at least a fourfold decrease in tumor volume on the last day. Other signs that reveal the increased antitumor effects of L19-IL12 included increased tumor infiltration of immune cells and increased levels of IFNγ in the tumor and serum, which were not seen in either of the control groups. However, in both models there were signs of IL-12 induced hepatotoxicity as well as antibody production against the components of both fusion antibodies. When compared with treatment with IL-12, the L19-IL12 treatments performed better than wt IL-12 even at dose levels as low as 20 times less than the wt cytokine. Also, even when treatments were started as late as 7 days after tumor inoculation, there was an 82% reduction in lung metastases compared with saline-treated groups [56]. These results are very promising for L19-IL12 to be used in clinical settings.

Several other L19-cytokine conjugates have been created and studied including those with IL-15, GM-CSF [58], IFNγ [59], and TNFα [60, 61] further proving the potential for immunocytokines in cancer therapy. In addition, antibodies with different specificities have been created and tested for their ability to target cytokines to tumor environments. Antigens for these cytokines include EGF receptor (ch225) [62, 63], ganglioside GD_2 [62, 64–66], HER2 [67, 68], KSA [9, 69], and many more [54]. However, continual improvement in the design of immunocytokines is needed to develop clinically applicable formulations as evidenced by the IL-12 induced hepatotoxicity described in the L19-IL12 study above. For these reasons, different derivations of immunocytokines have been created and studied.

One subsequent investigation involved the therapeutic potential of two new L19-IL12 derivatives. The first is a disulfuide linked homodimer composed of two L19-IL12 immunocytokines [IL12-SIP(L19)], and the other is a single IL-12 with a single-chain L19 component linked to each subunit of IL-12 (L19-IL12-L19). The biodistribution pattern of IL12-SIP(L19) was very similar to L19-IL12 with tumor uptake of less than 1% of the initial dose, tumor/organ accumulation ratios of approximately 5:1, and high levels of liver uptake; however, L19-IL12-L19 exhibited a much improved pattern with 19% and 9% tumor uptake at 4 and 24 h, respectively, and tumor/organ ratios of approximately 10:1 to 20:1 at 24 h. Also, L19-IL12-L19 performed comparably to wt IL-12 and L19-IL12 in lymphocyte proliferation assays. Single in vivo injections up to 80 μg did not cause any weight loss greater than 5%. Antitumor efficacy studies revealed that indeed the L19-IL12-L19 is the superior agent. Three separate experiments with a single dose of 20 μg, 4 doses every 3 days of 5 μg, or 3 doses every 3 days of 20 μg and 40 μg revealed that IL12-(SIP)L19 retarded tumor growth and extended survival time more than the group treated with saline, and L19-IL12-L19 was even more effective than doses at and half of the IL12 molar equivalent of IL12-(SIP)L19 [70]. These results show that modification of antibodies can increase the performance of immunocytokines for cancer therapies.

Since it has been proved that immunocytokines and modifying the antibody regions of immunocytokines can increase the therapeutic efficacies of cytokines for tumor therapies, further avenues to create stronger therapies are continuing to be examined. One such method is using combinations of immunocytokines to create synergistic therapeutic responses. Several combinatorial cytokine therapies using recombinant wt cytokines have already been proven to be more efficacious than treatments with the individual cytokines such as combinations of IL-12 with several different cytokines [12]. To this end, combinations of immunocytokines as well as versions of immunocytokines wielding two cytokines have been investigated.

One such investigation looked at the benefit of using the L19 antibody conjugated to both IL-12 and TNFα (ILT). In vitro bioactivity studies showed that ILT was able to maintain the function of both cytokines; however, in vivo studies revealed that ILT lacked any significant tumor targeted properties. Experiments to explore the antitumor effects confirmed that ILT showed almost no ability to reduce tumor growth, but coadministrations of L19-IL12 and L19-TNFα were extremely potent for inhibiting tumor growth. In a syngeneic F9 teratocarcinoma model, simultaneous delivery of 2 μg of each immunocytokine completely halted tumor growth while delivery of either agent alone had almost no effect [71]. Another bifunctional immunocytokine was more successful. This human immunocytokine, DCH, consists of two single chain antibodies specific for epithelial cell adhesion molecule (Ep-CAM) with IL-2 and GM-CSF. In vitro assays revealed that both cytokines retain their activities and the antibodies retain their specificities compared with nonfused versions of each [72]. For in vivo experiments, a murine version of DCH (mDCH) was created, which was similar in activity and binding affinity to the original DCH. Treatments with mDCH in syngeneic models did result in some inhibition of tumor growth, but it was not dependent on the tumor targeting ability of the antibody because a nonspecific immunocytokine conferred the same level of tumor inhibition. Also, treatments with the combination of the single cytokine versions of the anti-Ep-CAM immunocytokines resulted in similar levels of tumor inhibition [73]. These results demonstrate that combinations of immunocytokines to exploit the synergistic effects of cytokines can create therapies with high antitumor efficacy, but the combination of cytokines onto the same antibody has yet to show any further benefit. Further exploration and development of immunocytokine combinations and dual-cytokine immunocytokines is needed before any significantly beneficial therapies will emerge.

Summary

Malignant diseases will always be a concern for humanity, and improving treatments will always be needed. The most promising developments for treating these diseases are modulating the immune system to identify the malignant tissue as a disease and implementing a corresponding immune response. To accomplish this goal, cytokines are a valuable resource that can be developed into therapies; however, the innate pleiotropic effects of cytokines makes them a double-edged sword that can cause damage and toxicity as bad as if not worse than the malignancy itself. So, the knowledge to properly wield this sword is paramount to utilizing cytokines as treatments for malignancies. Fortunately, the current technology as well as developing technological advancements is exponentially increasing to allow us to safely and effectively use these cytokines in the near future to treat malignant diseases.

Beginning with the discovery of the EPR effect of the tumor environment, modifications of different cytokines with PEG derivations have allowed targeting to the tumor to reach effective concentrations in the tumor while reducing toxic concentrations in sensitive organs. Also, PEG increased the ability of viruses to specifically deliver cytokine-gene payloads to the tumor environments to achieve reduction in tumor volume while simultaneously reducing toxicity seen with non-PEGylated viruses. Although this passive targeting strategy helped to increase the functionality of cytokine therapies, more active techniques are needed to increase the cytokine therapies to mainstream clinical applications.

Specifically targeting ligands in the tumor environment with tumor environment-specific peptides is one such active method. These peptides have the ability to not only reach the tumor environment but also exhibit antitumor effects such as interrupting angiogenesis. But the true value of these peptides lies in their ability to transfer more destructive agents such as cytokines and viruses loaded with cytokine genes to the tumor environment. The discovery of RGD, NGR, and their derivatives has truly helped to expand the use of cytokines in cancer therapies. These peptides can target various tumor types because they target ligands in the tumor environment and the tumor cells. But these universal targeted peptides may not be beneficial to all patients. The use of in vivo biopanning to discover potential ligands has been shown to identify patient-specific ligands in biopsies [74]. This strategy has the potential to make patient-specific peptide-cytokine conjugates, which will be extremely effective.

Likewise, the use of antibodies as cytokine carriers has proven to be very beneficial for cytokine therapies. These antibodies are very specific for tumor antigens and can be manufactured for any antigen and to be less immunogenic in patients. Also, immunocytokines maintain their specificity for their antigens as well as the bioactivity of the cytokines. These tumor-specific antibodies can also carry cytokine genes loaded in viral vectors to concentrate the cytokine activities in the tumor environment while reducing toxic side effects elsewhere. There is still much room for improvement in these therapies but promising results and preclinical experiments continue to increase the efficacy of these treatments.

Tumor-targeted cytokine treatments are still years away from being a primary treatment for cancer, but continued research into how to modify current treatment strategies will help bring that goal closer every year. Also, the development of new strategies is promising improved treatment strategies. For instance, using mesenchymal stem cells (MSC) to deliver cytokines to the tumor environment are already appearing on the horizon. Several groups have used local delivery of MSC loaded with cytokine genes to decrease tumor volumes, but the successful treatment of tumors with systemic MSC delivery has yet to be realized [17, 19]. Current and future development of these tumor-targeted cytokine therapies is crucial for the continuing improvement of immunomodulatory cancer treatments.

Acknowledgment This study was supported by National Institutes of Health (Bethesda, MD) grant RO1CA120895 and NIH/NIBIB grant R21EB007208

References

1. Society, A. C. (2008) *Cancer Facts & Figures 2008*, American Cancer Society, Atlanta
2. Bazan-Peregrino, M., Seymour, L., and Harris, A. (2007)Cancer Gene Ther 14, 117
3. Haaga, J. R., Exner, A. A., Wang, Y., Stowe, N. T., and Tarcha, P. J. (2005) Radiology 237(3), 911
4. Li, C. Y., Huang, Q., and Kung, H. F. (2005) Cell Mol Immunol 2(2), 81
5. Carswell, E. A., Old, L. J., Kassel, R. L., Green, S., Fiore, N., and Williamson, B. (1975) Proc Natl Acad Sci USA 72(9), 3666
6. Morgan, D. A., Ruscetti, F. W., and Gallo, R. (1976) Science 193(4257), 1007
7. Kobayashi, M., Fitz, L., Ryan, M., Hewick, R. M., Clark, S. C., Chan, S., Loudon, R., Sherman, F., Perussia, B., and Trinchieri, G. (1989) J Exp Med 170(3), 827
8. Jiang, Y. Y., Liu, C., Hong, M. H., Zhu, S. J., and Pei, Y. Y. (2007) Bioconjugate Chem 18(1), 41
9. Xiang, R., Lode, H. N., Dolman, C. S., Dreier, T., Varki, N. M., Qian, X., Lo, K. M., Lan, Y., Super, M., Gillies, S. D., and Reisfeld, R. A. (1997) Cancer Res 57(21), 4948
10. Del Vecchio, M., Bajetta, E., Canova, S., Lotze, M. T., Wesa, A., Parmiani, G., and Anichini, A. (2007) Clin Cancer Res 13(16), 4677
11. Soiffer, R. J., Robertson, M. J., Murray, C., Cochran, K., and Ritz, J. (1993) Blood 82(9), 2790
12. Weiss, J. M., Subleski, J. J., Wigginton, J. M., and Wiltrout, R. H. (2007) Expert Opin Biol Ther 7(11), 1705

13. Rosenberg, S. A., Lotze, M. T., Yang, J. C., Aebersold, P. M., Linehan, W. M., Seipp, C. A., and White, D. E. (1989) Ann Surg 210(4), 474
14. Atkins, M. B., Sparano, J., Fisher, R. I., Weiss, G. R., Margolin, K. A., Fink, K. I., Rubinstein, L., Louie, A., Mier, J. W., Gucalp, R., et al. (1993) J Clin Oncol 11(4), 661
15. Loisel-Meyer, S., Foley, R., and Medin, J. A. (2008) Front Biosci 13, 3202
16. Schatzlein, A. G. (2003) J Biomed Biotechnol 2003(2), 149
17. Hamada, H., Kobune, M., Nakamura, K., Kawano, Y., Kato, K., Honmou, O., Houkin, K., Matsunaga, T., and Niitsu, Y. (2005) Cancer Sci 96(3), 149
18. Nakamura, K., Ito, Y., Kawano, Y., Kurozumi, K., Kobune, M., Tsuda, H., Bizen, A., Honmou, O., Niitsu, Y., and Hamada, H. (2004) Gene Ther 11(14), 1155
19. Reiser, J., Zhang, X. Y., Hemenway, C. S., Mondal, D., Pradhan, L., and La Russa, V. F. (2005) Expert Opin Biol Ther 5(12), 1571
20. Stagg, J., Lejeune, L., Paquin, A., and Galipeau, J. (2004) Hum Gene Ther 15(6), 597
21. Matsumura, Y., and Maeda, H. (1986) Cancer Res 46(12_Part_1), 6387
22. Maeda, H., Wu, J., Sawa, T., Matsumura, Y., and Hori, K. (2000) J Contr Release 65(1–2), 271
23. van Vlerken, L. E., Vyas, T. K., and Amiji, M. M. (2007) Pharm Res 24(8), 1405
24. Brassard, D. L., Grace, M. J., and Bordens, R. W. (2002) J Leukoc Biol 71(4), 565
25. Talpaz, M., O'Brien, S., Rose, E., Gupta, S., Shan, J., Cortes, J., Giles, F. J., Faderl, S., and Kantarjian, H. M. (2001) Blood 98(6), 1708
26. Matthews, S. J. and McCoy, C. (2004) Clin Ther 26(7), 991
27. Li, Y. P., Pei, Y. Y., Zhou, Z. H., Zhang, X. Y., Gu, Z. H., Ding, J., Zhou, J. J., Gao, X. J., and Zhu, J. H. (2001) Biol Pharm Bull 24(6), 662
28. Fang, C., Shi, B., Pei, Y.-Y., Hong, M.-H., Wu, J., and Chen, H.-Z. (2006) Eur J Pharmaceut Sci 27, 27
29. Croyle, M. A., Chirmule, N., Zhang, Y., and Wilson, J. M. (2001) J Virol 75(10), 4792
30. Gao, J.-Q., Eto, Y., Yoshioka, Y., Sekiguchi, F., Kurachi, S., Morishige, T., Yao, X., Watanabe, H., Asavatanabodee, R., Sakurai, F., Mizuguchi, H., Okada, Y., Mukai, Y., Tsutsumi, Y., Mayumi, T., Okada, N., and Nakagawa, S. (2007) J Contr Release 122(1), 102
31. Pasqualini, R., and Ruoslahti, E. (1996) Nature 380(6572), 364
32. Craig, R., and Li, S. (2006) Mini Rev Med Chem 6, 109
33. Enback, J., and Laakkonen, P. (2007) Biochem Soc Trans 35(Pt 4), 780
34. Maubant, S., Saint-Dizier, D., Boutillon, M., Perron-Sierra, F., Casara, P. J., Hickman, J. A., Tucker, G. C., and Van Obberghen-Schilling, E. (2006) Am Soc Hematol 108(9), 3035
35. Dickerson, E. B., Akhtar, N., Steinberg, H., Wang, Z.-Y., Lindstrom, M. J., Padilla, M. L., Auerbach, R., and Helfand, S. C. (2004) Mol Cancer Res 2(12), 663
36. Curnis, F., Gasparri, A., Sacchi, A., Longhi, R., and Corti, A. (2004) Cancer Res 64(2), 565
37. Ma, D., Chen, Y., Fang, L., Jin, G., Zhou, B., Cao, L., Ye, J., and Hua, Z. (2007) J Chromatogr B Analyt Technol Biomed Life Sci 857(2), 231
38. Wang, H., Chen, K., Cai, W., Li, Z., He, L., Kashefi, A., and Chen, X. (2008) Mol Cancer Ther 7(5), 1044
39. Wang, H., Yan, Z., Shi, J., Han, W., and Zhang, Y. (2006) Protein Expr Purif 45(1), 60
40. Pasqualini, R., Koivunen, E., Kain, R., Lahdenranta, J., Sakamoto, M., Stryhn, A., Ashmun, R. A., Shapiro, L. H., Arap, W., and Ruoslahti, E. (2000) Cancer Res 60(3), 722
41. Curnis, F., Arrigoni, G., Sacchi, A., Fischetti, L., Arap, W., Pasqualini, R., and Corti, A. (2002) Cancer Res 62, 867
42. Colombo, G., Curnis, F., De Mori, G. M., Gasparri, A., Longoni, C., Sacchi, A., Longhi, R., and Corti, A. (2002) J Biol Chem 277(49), 47891
43. Curnis, F., Sacchi, A., Borgna, L., Magni, F., Gasparri, A., and Corti, A. (2000) Nat Biotech 18(11), 1185
44. Curnis, F., Sacchi, A., and Corti, A. (2002) J Clin Invest 110(4), 475
45. Sacchi, A., Gasparri, A., Gallo-Stampino, C., Toma, S., Curnis, F., and Corti, A. (2006) Clin Cancer Res 12(1), 175

46. Bertilaccio, M. T., Grioni, M., Sutherland, B. W., Degl'Innocenti, E., Freschi, M., Jachetti, E., Greenberg, N. M., Corti, A., and Bellone, M. (2008) Prostate 68(10), 1105
47. Meng, J., Yan, Z., Wu, J., Li, L., Xue, X., Li, M., Li, W., Hao, Q., Wan, Y., Qin, X., Zhang, C., You, Y., Han, W., and Zhang, Y. (2007) Cytotherapy 9(1), 60
48. Meng, J., Yan, Z., Wu, Y., Gao, M., Li, W., Gao, F., Wang, H., Han, W., and Zhang, Y. (2008) Regul Toxicol Pharmacol 50(3), 294
49. Craig, R., Cutrera, J., Zhu, S., Xia, X., Lee, Y. H., and Li, S. (2008) Mol Ther 16(5), 901
50. Temming, K., Schiffelers, R. M., Molema, G., and Kok, R. J. (2005) Drug Resistance Updates 8(6), 381
51. Okada, Y., Okada, N., Mizuguchi, H., Hayakawa, T., Mayumi, T., and Mizuno, N. (2003) Gene Ther 10(8), 700
52. Okada, Y., Okada, N., Nakagawa, S., Mizuguchi, H., Takahashi, K., Mizuno, N., Fujita, T., Yamamoto, A., Hayakawa, T., and Mayumi, T. (2002) Jpn J Cancer Res 93(4), 436
53.Okada, Y., Okada, N., Mizuguchi, H., Takahashi, K., Hayakawa, T., Mayumi, T., and Mizuno, N. (2004) Biochim Biophys Acta General Subj 1670(3), 172
54. Ortiz-Sanchez, E., Helguera, G., Daniels, T. R., and Penichet, M. L. (2008) Informa Helthcare 8(5), 609
55. Schrama, D., Reisfeld, R. A., and Becker, J. C. (2006) Nat Rev 5, 147
56. Halin, C., Rondini, S., Nilsson, F., Berndt, A., Kosmehl, H., Zardi, L., and Neri, D. (2002) Nat Biotechnol 20(3), 264
57. Carnemolla, B., Borsi, L., Balza, E., Castellani, P., Meazza, R., Berndt, A., Ferrini, S., Kosmehl, H., Neri, D., and Zardi, L. (2002) Blood 99(5), 1659
58. Kaspar, M., Trachsel, E., and Meri, D. (2007) Cancer Res 67(10), 4940
59. Ebbinghaus, C., Ronca, R., Kaspar, M., Grabulovski, D., Berndt, A., Kosmehl, H., Zardi, L., and Neri, D. (2005) Int J Cancer 116, 304
60. Balza, E., Mortara, L., Sassi, F., Monteghirfo, S., Carnemolla, B., Castellani, P., Neri, D., Accolla, R. S., Zardi, L., and Borsi, L. (2006) Clin Cancer Res 8, 2575
61. Borsi, L., Balza, E., Carnemolla, B., Sassi, F., Castellani, P., Berndt, A., Kosmehl, H., Biro, A., Siri, A., Orecchia, P., Grassi, J., Neri, D., and Zardi, L. (2003) Blood 102(13), 4384
62. Becker, J. C., Pancook, J. D., Gillies, S. D., Mendelsohn, J., and Reisfeld, R. A. (1996) Proc Natl Acad Sci USA 93(7), 2702
63. Reisfeld, R. A., Gillies, S. D., Mendelsohn, J., Varki, N. M., and Becker, J. C. (1996) Cancer Res 56, 1707
64. King, D. M., Albertini, M. R., Schalch, H., Hank, J. A., Gan, J., Surfus, J., Mahvi, D., Schiller, J. H., Warner, T., Kim, K., Eickhoff, J., Kendra, K., Reisfeld, R. A., Gillies, S. D., and Sondel, P. (2004) J Clin Oncol 22(22), 4463
65. Metelitsa, L. S., Gillies, S. D., Super, M., Shimada, H., Renolds, C. P., and Seeger, R. C. (2002) Blood 99(11), 4166
66. Schrama, D., Straten, P.t., Fischer, W. H., McLellan, A. D., Brocker, E.-B., Reisfeld, R. A., and Becker, J. C. (2001) Immunity 14, 111
67. Dela Cruz, J. S., Trinh, K. R., Morrison, S. L., and Penichet, M. L. (2000) J Immunol 165(9), 5112
68. Peng, L. S., Penichet, M. L., and Morrison, S. L. (1999) J Immunol 163, 250
69. Ko, Y. J., Bubley, G. J., Weber, R., Redfern, C., Gold, D. P., Finke, L., Kovar, A., Dahl, T., and Gillies, S. D. (2004) J Immunother 27(3), 232
70. Gafner, V., Trachsel, E., and Neri, D. (2006) Int J Cancer 119, 2205
71. Halin, C., Gafner, V., Villani, M. E., Borsi, L., Berndt, A., Kosmehl, H., Zardi, L., and Neri, D. (2003) Cancer Res 63, 3202
72. Schanzer, J. M., Baeuerle, P. A., Dreier, T., and Kufer, P. (2006) Cancer Immun 6, 4
73. Schanzer, J. M., Fichtner, I., Baeuerle, P. A., and Kufer, P. (2006) J Immunother 29(5), 477
74. Krag, D. N., Shukla, G. S., Shen, G. P., Pero, S., Ashikaga, T., Fuller, S., Weaver, D. L., Burdette-Radoux, S., and Thomas, C. (2006) Cancer Res 66(15), 7724

Part II
Cell-based Immune Therapy

New Strategies to Improve Tumor Cell Vaccine Therapy

Jian Qiao and Haidong Dong

Abstract The advantage of using a tumor cell vaccine is that it is rich in multiple tumor-associated antigens. The immune responses to those antigens are elicited by most of current tumor cell vaccines that are transduced with immunostimulatory cytokines or costimulatory molecules. However, the lack of long-lasting and objective tumor regression in clinical trials prompted reevaluation of the immunogenicity of tumor cell vaccines and the molecular basis of the immune responses they induced. New vectors for the genetic modification of tumor cell vaccines to improve immunogenicity have been developed. The identification of negative regulators during vaccination has lead to the discovery of new reagents to specifically target regulatory cells or molecules to improve the efficacy of these vaccines. On the basis of their enhancing effects during the cross-priming of CD8 T cells, toll-like receptor ligands have been used in the modification of tumor cells to improve their immunogenicity. Therefore, the endeavors in developing new tumor cell vaccines not only extend our knowledge about the tumor-reactive immunity but also promise an effective treatment regimen in human cancers.

Introduction

Tumor cell vaccine therapy has been defined as a promising treatment regimen for decades because they are the richest source of rejection antigens. In combination with a nonspecific immune stimulatory adjuvant, a tumor cell vaccine is used to stimulate tumor-specific immune responses for the prevention of tumor metastasis or reoccurrence, or even to reject progressive tumors. Although this concept has been validated in numerous experimental therapeutic studies in laboratory animals, clinical trials indicate that we are still far from developing a reliable and consistent

H. Dong (✉)
Departments of Urology and Immunology, College of Medicine, Mayo Clinic, Rochester, MN 55905, USA
e-mail: dong.haidong@mayo.edu

J. Lustgarten et al. (eds.), *Targeted Cancer Immune Therapy*,
DOI 10.1007/978-1-4419-0170-5_7,

vaccine to achieve significant tumor regression in many human cancers. Recent advancements in understanding how the immune system responds to tumor antigens and in manipulating the immune response have suggested the redesign and improvement of current protocols using tumor cell vaccines in the treatment of human cancer. The strategy is to enhance the immune responses to tumor cells through transduction of cytokines and costimulatory molecules, and depletion of negative regulator cells or molecules. To improve the efficacy of tumor cells as a vaccine, we should consider breaking the self-tolerance in immune responses to tumor antigens.

Increasing the Immunogenicity of Tumor Cell Vaccines

The Immunogenicity of Tumor Cell Vaccines

Immunogenicity is the ability of an antigen to elicit an immune response or the degree to which it provokes a response. Immunogenicity is influenced by multiple characteristics of an antigen, such as foreignness, molecular size, protein structure, and epitope density. Immunization, also referred to as vaccination, is the deliberate induction of an immune response to develop protective immunity. The natural specificity and the inducibility of the immune system determines the efficacy of immunizations [1]. The concept of cancer immunoediting extends our understanding of the interaction between tumor cells and the immune system, and provides the foundation to address the immunogenicity of tumor cell vaccines [2]. Cancer immunoediting is a three-phase process: (1) elimination (cancer immunosurveillance, in which immunity functions as an extrinsic tumor suppressor in naïve hosts); (2) equilibrium (expansion of transformed cells held in check by immunity); and (3) escape (tumor cell variants with dampened immunogenicity or the capacity to attenuate immune responses grow into clinically apparent cancers) [3]. As a result, the immune system will either protect the host against tumor development or facilitate tumor outgrowth. Therefore, how to maintain or increase immunogenicity has become a critical issue in designing tumor cell vaccines.

Many tumors show some antigenicity, and can be recognized by the adaptive immune system, because of the presence of known tumor-associated antigens (TAAs), which include nonmutated, overexpressed, or inappropriately expressed tissue differentiation antigens [4]. The antigenicity of tumor cells provides the foundation for adaptive immunity in tumor control, especially in the equilibrium phase [3]. Particularly, the identification of unique tumor antigens in human tumors further validated the antigenicity of tumor cells [5]. These unique tumor antigens are largely the result of somatic point mutations occurring in many different proteins expressed by tumor cells [6]. Clinical vaccine trials for patients with malignant melanoma have demonstrated that vaccination against a single antigen can induce tumor-specific cytotoxic T lymphocytes (CTLs), but carry the risk of promoting tumor antigen escape variants [7]. A better clinical response has correlated with the generation of CTLs that are primed by tumor vaccines containing three or more tumor antigens [8]. However, for many tumors, few, if any, antigenic epitopes are known. To circumvent this limitation, whole tumor cells containing a spectrum of known and unknown unique tumor antigens may be more immunogenic and promote a better antitumor immune response.

It would be highly desirable that antitumor immune responses include multiple T cell clones against multiple tumor antigens. Tumor cell vaccines have several advantages in generating tumor-specific immunity. They can be modified to present major histocompatibility complex (MHC) class I and class II epitopes to prime diverse immune responses including a broader repertoire of $CD8^+$ and $CD4^+$ T cells. In turn, primed T cells are able to recruit other effectors such as macrophages and eosinophils into the tumor sites to suppress tumor growth [9]. The additional presence of epitopes for T helper lymphocytes could be beneficial because MHC class II-restricted activation of T helper lymphocytes plays a pivotal role in the physiological immune response to pathogens; therefore, this may be considerably important in the tumor rejection process [10]. The T cell help is a critical determinant in the recall response of memory $CD8^+$ T cell in response to secondary antigen exposure [11]; they provide critical interleukin (IL)-2 during memory $CD8^+$ T cell priming [12]. An important feature of tumor cell vaccines is to generate protective memory T cell responses because the presence of tumor-reactive memory $CD8^+$ T cells is significantly correlated to an improved prognosis in many human cancers [13]; therefore, the immunogenicity of a tumor cell vaccine warrants good quality of tumor-reactive $CD8^+$ T cells.

Transduction of Costimulatory Molecules in the Tumor Cell Vaccine

Lymphocyte activation and the development of adaptive immunity require specific antigen recognition by lymphocytes (signal 1) and additional costimulatory signals (signal 2). This two-signal concept explains why adaptive immunity is elicited by infection and not by self-antigens. The first members of the costimulatory family to be described are B7–1 and B7–2, which bind to CD28 or CTLA-4. B7–1 and B7–2 promote IL-2 production and the development of effector T cells by signaling through CD28 [14]. The expression of B7–1 in some tumor cells increases their immunogenicity and leads to tumor regression [15]. The fundamental importance and therapeutic potential of costimulatory signals for T cell activation prompted efforts in designing tumor cell vaccines. Equally important, the blockage of negative regulators provides additional tools in manipulating the immune response in tumor vaccine therapy [14]. One of the B7/CD28 family molecules, CTLA-4, has been intensively investigated in combination with tumor cell vaccines for breaking T cell tolerance to self/tumor antigens.

Several in vitro studies have demonstrated that B7–1-modified human tumor cells can induce primary CTL activity from autologous, human lymphocyte antigen (HLA) class I-matched allogeneic peripheral lymphocytes and purified $CD8^+$ T cells [16, 17].

CTLs generated by B7–1 costimulation are tumor specific and HLA class I restricted, and $CD8^+$ T cells are primarily responsible for this specific cytotoxicity. Furthermore, CTLs generated from HLA class I-matched $CD8^+$ T cells by B7–1 are cytolytic to tumor cells autologous to the stimulated T cells, suggesting that B7–1-modified tumor cells can be used as a potent tumor vaccine for autologous and HLA class I-matched allogeneic patients.

Phase I and II trials of B7–1-transduced autologous tumor cell vaccine has been conducted [18, 19]. The vaccine is postulated to costimulate the tumor-reactive T cells that will be subsequently expanded by IL-2. The B7 gene-modified autologous tumor (renal cell carcinoma) vaccine is safe and can be combined with the systemic use of IL-2 with acceptable toxicity. More than half of the enrolled patients have stabilized diseases with 3% and 5% having pathologically complete and partial responses. Interestingly, most of the patients experienced delayed-type hypersensitivity (DTH) after treatment, and some patient DTH tissue sites contained significant lymphocytic infiltration that correlated with prolonged patient survival [18]. Many tumor cells are poor antigen presenting cells because of their low level expression of MHC class I or II molecules, the use of costimulatory molecules on tumor cells to direct prime T cells will be a limitation in cancer therapy. Therefore, additional approaches are necessary to increase tumor antigen presentation in vivo.

Transduction of GM-CSF in Tumor Cell Vaccines

Tumor cell vaccine induced-tumor immunity is a multistep process. A successful antitumoral T cell response will include the (1) priming and differentiation of multifunctional tumor antigen-reactive T cells, and (2) homing of effector T cells to the tumor site where reactivation by tumor antigens leads to tumor elimination. Therefore, an appropriate presentation of tumor antigens carried by a tumor cell vaccine will be a critical step in determining the immunogenicity of a vaccine.

Granulocyte-macrophage colony-stimulating factor (GM-CSF) induces the differentiation of myeloid dendritic cells (DCs) that promote the development of T cell responses. Tumor cells engineered to secrete GM-CSF are particularly effective as antitumor vaccines, and the addition of GM-CSF to standard vaccines may increase their effectiveness by recruiting DCs to the vaccine site [20]. This approach is applied to increase the immunogenicity of autologous tumor cell vaccines. An autologous tumor cell vaccine is prepared by tumor cells from the patient undergoing subsequent treatments. The merit of this vaccine is that tumor cells may carry tumor antigens unique to the patient. Autologous tumor cells genetically modified to secrete GM-CSF have been used in several human cancers. Evidence of vaccine-induced immune activation was demonstrated. For example, tumor vaccines composed of autologous tumor cells genetically modified to secrete GM-CSF (GVAX™) have demonstrated clinical activity in advanced-stage nonsmall-cell lung cancer (NSCLC) [21]. In addition, retrovirally GM-CSF-transduced autologous renal tumor cell vaccines (GVAX™) from patients with stage IV renal cell cancer (RCC) show substantially enhanced antitumor cellular and humoral immune responses [22]. However, a significant limitation in the use of GM-CSF as an immunostimulatory agent is that objective antitumor responses are infrequent and not often long-lasting. Effective and persistent antitumor immunity will likely require novel methods to eliminate negative regulatory immune responses that limit the activation and expansion of CTLs. This approach requires additional manipulation of immune responses to improve efficacy.

Using Allogeneic Tumor Cell Vaccine to Improve the Immunogenicity

A limitation of autologous tumor cell vaccine is the number of cells that can be recovered from the resected tumor to produce a vaccine. Alternatively, an allogeneic tumor cell vaccine is considered. Allogeneic tumor cell vaccines are prepared by using tumor cells of a particular cancer type originally derived from someone other than the vaccine recipient. Allogeneic tumor cell vaccines are usually generated with established stable tumor cell lines derived from tumor patients. The rationale for the use of these vaccines is that there are shared tumor antigens among patients. The current approach, based on the use of allogeneic tumor cell lines to induce responses against shared tumor antigens, presents numerous advantages: (1) these relatively well-characterized antigen sources allow a more accurate clinical assessment of antigen-specific responses than less-defined autologous tumor cell vaccines [23]; (2) their applicability to patients regardless of HLA type because the professional antigen-presenting cells (APCs) of the host, rather than the vaccinating tumor cells, are responsible for generation of tumor-specific $CD8^+$ T cells through cross-priming mechanisms [24]; and (3) the activation and generation of tumor-specific $CD4^+$ responses that are crucial in tumor immunity of some animal models [25]. Additionally, the allogeneic features of this type of vaccine can provide a strong natural adjuvant that is released from the dead cells [26].

Allogeneic tumor vaccines in an MHC-mismatched animal host have been shown to prevent tumor establishment upon challenge by immunization of a cell vaccine [27]. A clinical trial with a GM-CSF-transduced allogeneic tumor cell vaccine demonstrated that this approach is safe with the potential to trigger systemic antitumor immunity in pancreatic cancer patients [28]. For example, irradiated allogeneic cells in Canvaxin™, a polyvalent vaccine containing more than 20 tumor antigens, was used to treat melanoma and colon cancer. The Canvaxin™ vaccine induces polyvalent humoral and cell-mediated immune responses to a wide variety of protein and ganglioside melanoma antigens. Furthermore, vaccine-induced immune responses have been correlated with survival after the resection of local, regional, and distant melanoma [29].

Genetic Approaches to Increase the Immunogenicity of Tumor Cell Vaccines Using Viral Vectors

Given the potential immunostimulatory role of costimulatory molecules and cytokines that are transduced into tumor cells during vaccine preparation, there are still limitations in the transduction efficiency of primary tumor cells because they are often difficult to expand in vitro. Several viral vectors, including the vaccinia virus, adenoviruses, alphaviruses, newcastle disease virus (NDV), herpes simplex virus (HSV), and retroviruses have been used to genetically modify tumor cells. The development of modified tumor cell vaccines through engineered viruses designed to express immune modulators (e.g., cytokine or costimulatory molecules) or TAAs has been aimed to induce effective active immunization against tumors. Within the last 5–10 years, vectors for the gene delivery into tumor cells have improved greatly. A number of genetically modified autologous or allogeneic tumor cell vaccines have been tested in clinical trials [28, 30, 31]. This chapter focuses primarily on viral vectors that have been widely tested in preclinical or clinical trials.

Vaccinia virus-based vectors are particularly attractive for gene delivery because of their high efficacy in infecting target-cells and favorable safety profiles in humans. The vaccinia virus replicates in the cytoplasm without integrating into the host cellular genome. Vaccinia-based viral vectors are easily genetically manipulated with a large insertion capacity (up to 25 kb). Several vectors engineered to express immunostimulatory molecules (e.g., GM-CSF) or tumor antigens including human papilloma virus (HPV) proteins and carcinoembryonic antigen genes have been tested in clinical trials for cancer treatment [32, 33].

Adenoviruses are 30–35 kb, double-stranded DNA viruses. They have been widely used for cancer treatment including replicating defective or competent adenoviruses. Conditionally replicating adenoviruses (CRADs) have been developed as a promising new treatment for cancer, which specifically replicate in and kill tumor cells while sparing normal cells. Within a solid tumor mass, progeny viruses newly released from infected tumor cells allow neighboring tumor or immune cells to be infected, amplifying engineered immunostimulatory molecules, or TAA gene expression [34]. Additionally, recombinant adenoviruses have several advantages for the development of tumor cell vaccines; for example, therapeutic genes can be easily inserted into the viral genome and high-titer viruses can be produced.

Alphaviruses including Semliki Forest Virus (SFV), Sindbis Virus (SIN), and Venezuelan Equine Encephalitis Virus (VEE) are positive-strand RNA viruses that have broad tropisms with high levels of infection efficiency and foreign gene expression in various types of tumor cells. In contrast to retroviruses, alphaviral vectors do not integrate into the host cellular genome following viral infection and the use of SFV encoding HPV E6 and E7 genes has shown long-lasting cellular immunity against cervical cancer in a preclinical model [35]. In addition, alphaviral vectors expressing cytokines including IL-12 [36], IL15 [37], or GM-CSF [38] and vectors expressing a tumor antigen such as rat *neu* [39] have been generated and used to enhance the immune responses against cancer in murine tumor models.

The obstacle to the clinical evaluation of viral vectors is the development of viral producer cells for large-scale vector production.

NDV is an enveloped virus, containing a single-stranded, negative-sense, non-segmented RNA genome. An NDV-infected autologous tumor cell vaccine has been used to immunize patients with advanced head and neck squamous cell carcinomas. Encouragingly, the specific cellular immune response against cancer was still observed 5 years after the first vaccination [40]. With the availability of the reverse genetics system for NDV, it is now possible to engineer the NDV genome by inserting additional immunostimulatory molecules or TAA genes to enhance the efficacy of NDV-modified tumor cell vaccines [41, 42].

HSV is a double-stranded DNA virus approximately 150 kb in genome length. Tumor cell destruction by replicating HSV oncolytic viruses has induced antitumor responses against tumor antigens released from the lysed tumor cells in several murine tumor models. This biologic functionality of HSV coupled with its readily manipulated viral genome has promoted the development of HSV vectors for gene transfer and offers more potent tumor cell vaccines. Replicating oncolytic HSV vectors expressing cytokines including IL-12 [43] or GM-CSF[44] and viruses expressing melanoma antigens gp100 and MART-1, or the tyrosinase gene, have been generated and used for in vivo tumor cell infection, leading to the inhibition of local and distant metastatic tumors in animal models. Recently, HSV encoding GM-CSF has been used in clinical trials to treat several solid tumors such as melanoma, breast, head and neck, and pancreatic cancer. Alternatively, the HSV-1 amplicon, a plasmid-based gene transfer vector, has been developed with a high efficiency of gene transfer into a broad range of cells. The great advantage of the HSV amplicon is its insertion capacity; the amplicon vector contains approximately 1% of the 152-kb HSV-1 genome [45], which enables them to introduce several foreign genes into target tumor cells.

Recombinant Moloney murine leukemia virus (Mo-MuLV)-based retroviral vectors have been extensively developed for gene transfer. The specific targeting of dividing cells with murine leukemia virus (MLV) vectors provides an excellent opportunity for tumor cell transfer because it integrates into the host cellular genome, stably expressing the genes introduced, and prolonging cytokine production or tumor antigen persistence in the tumor cells. The irradiated autologous tumor cells transduced by retroviral vectors expressing GM-CSF have been tested in patients with advanced prostate cancer and metastatic malignant melanoma [30, 46]. The extensive inflammatory infiltration in biopsied tumors from 11 of 16 patients was observed. A number of other genetically modified autologous and allogeneic tumor cell vaccines with retroviruses expressing IL-2, IL-4, B7–1, and a-(1,3) galactosyltransferase also have been tested in clinical trials [19, 47]. Recently, semi or fully replication competent MLV vectors have been developed to achieve a high efficiency of gene transfer [48, 49]. In contrast to replicating competent oncolytic viruses, replication competent retroviruses can replicate in tumor cells without immediate cell lysis. Furthermore, due to its low immunogenicity, MLV is unlikely to cause a stronger immune response against its viral antigens than the weaker tumor antigens that it expresses.

In summary, the optimal delivery vectors to introduce cytokines, immunostimulatory molecules, or tumor antigens into tumor cells have different properties. The ideal vectors for the development of tumor cell vaccines are required to efficiently transfer genes of interest into tumor cells to induce a specific, effective, and long-lasting immune response against cancer cells while having no toxicity in host.

Improving the Immunological Response of Tumor Cell Vaccines

Because most cancer vaccine strategies are examined as a therapy for existing tumors, rather than as a prophylaxis, the consequences of antigen-specific T cell interaction with tumors is a critical parameter in their efficacy. The lack of clinical effectiveness, despite the ability to generate antitumor T cells in vivo, has been the subject of considerable immunologic investigation. Even after prolonged immunization with a tumor antigen vaccine, there was little effect of the T cells on the incidence of recurrent tumors expressing high levels of target antigens used in the vaccine [27].

Cancer vaccines are designed to initiate a tumor-specific immune response; however, the outcome of these responses is controlled by the regulatory constraints on immune responses. Antigenicity is only at one end of the tumor vaccine immunogenicity equation [1, 2]. The other end of this equation is determined by regulators that control the immune response. The quantity and quality of tumor-reactive T cells that are primed by tumor cell vaccine have a critical role in the final outcome of therapy. The mechanism by which tumor cell vaccines prime T cell responses remains a controversial issue. Two primary possibilities can be presented: (1) tumor cells directly present antigen through endogenous MHC/peptide complexes to prime naïve T cells, and (2) tumor antigens are processed by APCs such as DCs to prime T cells, a mechanism known as "cross-priming" [24]. Because many human tumor cells lose their MHC molecules or downregulate their expression, the priming of T cell responses is mainly dependent on the cross-presentation process in vivo. Actually, cross-priming has been identified as a crucial process for tumor cell vaccines to induce in vivo antitumor immunity [25]. However, it is still not clear which signals determine the cross-presentation that leads to T cell activation (cross-priming), or T cell inactivation (cross-tolerance), because they are based on the cross-presentation mediated by the same $CD8\alpha^+$ DCs in vivo [50, 51].

In the tumor host, the expansion of tumor-induced regulatory T (T_{reg}) cells, alterations in T cells signaling transduction, and tumor-induction of T cell apoptosis [52, 53] all contribute to the failure of most clinical trials using tumor cell vaccines. We will briefly review how tumor cell antigens could be efficiently presented and what the negative regulatory mechanisms are, and evaluate potential approaches to circumvent these barriers to improve the efficacy of tumor cell vaccines.

Improving the Cross-Priming of $CD8^+$ T Cells

The effectiveness of tumor cell vaccine relays on how well the tumor antigens are presented to T cells, either directly by the modified tumors or more likely through the crossing-priming of tumor cell-associated antigens to CD8$^+$ T cells via professional APCs, such as denritic cells (DCs) [50]. In fact, the function of GM-CSF in tumor vaccine setting is to promote DC differential and maturation resulting in enhanced tumor antigen presentation. Recent studies demonstrated that professional APCs and DCs express high level of toll-like receptors (TLRs) and thus immune stimulatory function can be further augmented in their efficacy in cross-priming and T cell activation [54–58]. Applying this approach to design a tumor cell vaccine, McBride et al. showed that only cell-associated, insoluble, dsRNA enhances tumor-specific T cell induction that results in an antitumor effect in vivo [59]. Therefore, the incorporation of dsRNA into tumor cell vaccines represents a feasible approach to applying antitumor CD8$^+$ T cell immunity. This approach would deliver dsRNA to DCs in an optimal manner because, after phagocytosis of the tumor vaccine, the dsRNA becomes available in endosomes that express the cognate receptor (e.g., TLR3 for poly I:C). A preclinical study indicated that a therapeutic protocol is able to enhance the survival of tumor-bearing mice that lack CD4$^+$ helper T cells. Thus, introduction of TLR3 signals in tumor cell vaccines has promise in improving their efficacy through the generation of protective immunity against tumors.

Several clinical observations have supported the concept that cross-priming is a key process in mediating the therapeutic effects of tumor cell vaccines. Vaccination with GM-CSF-transduced pancreatic cancer lines demonstrated DTH responses to autologous tumor after vaccination in 3 out of 14 treated patients [60]. A consistent induction of CD8$^+$ T cell responses to multiple HLA-A2, A3, and A24-restricted tumor-specific epitopes was observed exclusively in those three patients with vaccine-induced DTH responses. Importantly, neither of the vaccinating pancreatic cancer cell lines expressed HLA-A2, A3, or A24. These results provide the first direct evidence that CD8$^+$ T cell responses can be generated through cross-presentation by an immunotherapy approach designed to recruit APCs to the vaccination site. Additionally, Eguchi et al. found that IL-4-transfected tumor cells activate tumor-infiltrating DCs and, adoptively transferring of these DCs confers protection on a tumor-challenged recipient [61]. These results suggest that DCs can uptake tumor antigens and cross-present these antigen to prime a protective CD8$^+$ T cell response, which has been confirmed in a vaccine against melanoma antigens [62]. Therefore, enhacing the cross-priming process will be one of the key steps in increasing the immunologic responses to tumor vaccines.

Blockade of Coinhibitory Signals in Immunization

Full activation of naïve T cells not only requires an antigen-specific signal provided by TCR engagement with the appropriate MHC/peptide complexes, but also requires secondary "costimulatory signals" that are delivered by the APCs. In addition, cytokine growth factors such as IL-2 and IL-15 are considered as tertiary signals during activated T cell expansion. T cell receptor engagement in the absence of a costimulatory signal results in T cells that fail to develop full effector function and are rendered anergic [63]. As previously discussed, several studies have enhanced the generation of functional antitumor T cells through the vaccination of B7-1-transduced tumor cells [15, 64]. Nevertheless, this strategy of improving the efficacy of tumor vaccines is limited in several cases. Tumor cells such as B cell lymphomas express high levels of MHC class I and class II, have inducible expression of B7-1, and can process and present antigen to T cells in vitro [65, 66]. However, lymphoma is often a highly aggressive cancer that progresses in the very compartment where tumor-specific T cell responses are normally generated. One explanation for these findings is that B7-1 or B7-2 expressed by lymphoma cells favorably binds to the CTLA-4 coinhibitory receptor on activated T cells [67].

The blockage of CTLA-4 by employing GM-CSF transduced cells improves tumor cell vaccines. Periodic infusions of anti-CTLA-4 antibody, after vaccination with autologous tumor cells transduced to produce GM-CSF (GVAX™), generate objective responses of metastatic melanoma with minimal toxicities [68]. This clinical trial indicates the importance of cancer patient management after vaccination to maintain an efficient antitumor immune response against progressing tumor cells. CTLA-4 is a second T cell receptor for B7-1 and B7-2 that plays an inhibitory role in the regulation of T cell responses. Several studies have demonstrated that an antibody blocking CTLA-4 can enhance the T cell response, whereas cross-linking CTLA-4 results in diminished cytokine production and decreased proliferation [69, 70]. Improving tumor cell vaccine therapy by blocking CTLA-4 seems to occur at the host-derived APC level [71], emphasizing the importance of approaches that enhance T cell priming at the host level. The blocking CTLA-4 and administration of GM-CSF-tumor cell vaccines reject tumors shortly after tumor inoculation [72], during the early priming stage. The tumor free mice establish long-term protection from the same tumors upon future challenges, suggesting enhanced priming is a tumor-specific T cell response not only required for the rejection of established tumors, but also for generating antitumor memory responses.

The timing involved in blocking negative regulatory signals is also important in tumor vaccine therapy. Gregor et al. observed that the blockage of CTLA-4, when used during secondary/booster vaccinations, induced stronger antitumor immunity [73]. There are a few reasons why blocking CTLA-4 is only effective when administering with the second or third vaccine. First, after each immunization, the number of antigen-specific T cells increases, which are activated by the blockage of the negative CTLA-4 signal. Second, it is possible that the expression of CTLA-4 is upregulated on functional effector T cells that are enriched after several rounds of immunization. It is also possible that higher avidity T cells are generated after repeated immunization, and these cells are more sensitive to CTLA-4-mediated suppression [74]. Finally, the suppressive function of T_{reg} cells generated after a priming immunization may be partially inhibited by the anti-CTLA-4 antibody because of the high CTLA-4 expression on T_{reg} cells. Therefore, blocking inhibitory signals at the priming stage of T cell activation is required in designing effective tumor vaccines.

Enhancing the Recall Responses of Tumor-Reactive Memory T Cells

An important requirement of a tumor vaccine is the generation of protective T cell memory. The ability of memory T cells to rapidly respond to antigens makes them key players in protective immunity against cancers and infections. The presence of tumor-specific memory $CD8^+$ T cells has been noted in several human cancer patients [75–77]. Tumor infiltration by these effector memory $CD8^+$ T cells in colon and breast cancers, as well as in other tumors, such as colorectal carcinoma, has been associated with a better prognosis [13]. Developing a method of using tumor cell vaccines to recall these tumor-reactive memory T cells in cancer patients is challenging.

Chronic exposure to tumor antigens, negative regulators and suppression by T_{reg} cells suppress protective T cell memory in a tumor host [78]. As indicated by Klebanoff et al. [78], the mere generation of T cell memory may not guarantee the efficacy of tumor vaccine. Tumor vaccines may fail if they fail to effectively rescue the suppressed memory T cells. In an animal renal cell carcinoma (RENCA), we identified tumor-specific functional memory $CD8^+$ T cells in the bone marrow of tumor mice [79], but not in the tumor draining lymph nodes or spleen. Our study suggested that immunization with an irradiated tumor cell vaccine could recall the antitumor responses of these tumor-specific memory $CD8^+$ T cells, which could not reject the established tumors. Further studies indicate that antitumor function of these memory $CD8^+$ T cells is restrained by the presence of T_{reg} cells and the negative costimulatory signals of B7-H1, a negative costimulatory molecule on tumor cells [79].

Regulatory T cells have been found to inhibit the proliferation and function of memory $CD8^+$ T cells in vivo [80, 81]. Therefore, depletion of T_{reg} cells is critical in enhancing the recall responses of memory $CD8^+$ T cells. This depletion of T_{reg} cells is based on the removal of $CD25^+$ cells, a surrogate T_{reg} cell surface marker [82]. Nanni et al. reported that the depletion of T_{reg} cells by the injection of anti-CD25 significantly enhanced the therapeutic effects of an allogeneic tumor cell vaccine [83]. We have observed that an increased accumulation of T_{reg} cells in the draining lymph nodes of mice with progressive renal cell carcinoma (RENCA) and cotransfer of T_{reg} cells dramatically inhibit the antitumor function of memory $CD8^+$ T cells [79]. These increased T_{reg} cells show the effector marker CD103 on their surface. Irradiated whole RENCA cells are immunogenic in preventing tumorigenesis upon challenge after the immunization of naïve mice [79]. However, this tumor cell vaccine alone could not reject established tumors therapeutically. In combination with the depletion of T_{reg} cells using an anti-CD4 antibody and blockage of B7-H1, we found that the RENCA cell vaccine induced completed rejection of established RENCA tumors. This dramatic therapeutic effect was attributed to the strong recall responses of preexisting tumor-reactive memory $CD8^+$ T cells in tumor host [79].

Although the original role of T_{reg} cells is to control self-reactive immunity, increasing experimental and clinical evidence indicates that T_{reg} cells have a detrimental impact on the T cell response to tumors [84]. Several animal models show that tumor-specific immunity is augmented when $CD4^+$ $CD25^+T_{reg}$ cells are depleted [85–87]. Given the nature of priming immune responses by a tumor vaccine, it would not be a surprised to observe that the vaccination of a tumor-bearing host coincides with the expansion of tumor-induced T_{reg} cells and effector cells [88]. However, the suppressive function of T_{reg} cells is dominant and suppresses the expansion of naïve tumor-specific T cells. These vaccine-induced T_{reg} cells also block the execution of effector cells in vivo and in vitro, suggesting the possibility that a therapeutic vaccination could worsen host tolerance to tumor antigens. For that reason, strategies that inactivate or deplete T_{reg} cells should be included in treatment paradigms that aim to generate functional tumor-specific T cells.

Summary

The efficacy of T cell immunity is determined by the quality, rather than the quantity of tumor-reactive T cells, induced by tumor cell vaccines. High avidity and affinity T cells are needed to fight progressive tumors. Many efforts have been invested to increase the priming of T cells by improving the immunogenicity of tumor cell vaccines through the transduction of costimulatory molecules or cytokines. However, the overall low responsive rate and temporal regression of tumors after vaccination suggests that multiple approaches in improving the immunostimulatory efficacy of tumor cell vaccines and alleviating immunosuppressive components may be required. The blockade of negative regulators and depletion of T_{reg} cells provide additional promise in increasing the efficacy of tumor cell vaccines. New knowledge of the molecular mechanisms that regulate immunological responses to vaccines is warranted in the design and application of effective tumor cell vaccines for prevention and treatment.

References

1. Boon, T., Van Pel, A., and De Plaen, E. (1989) Cancer Cells 1, 25
2. Dunn, G. P., Bruce, A. T., Ikeda, H., Old, L. J., and Schreiber, R. D. (2002) Nat Immunol 3, 991
3. Koebel, C. M., Vermi, W., Swann, J. B., Zerafa, N., Rodig, S. J., Old, L. J., Smyth, M. J., and Schreiber, R. D. (2007) Nature 450, 903
4. Gilboa, E. (1999) Immunity 11, 263
5. Lewis, J. J. (2004) Proc Natl Acad Sci USA 101 Suppl 2, 14653
6. Parmiani, G., De Filippo, A., Novellino, L., and Castelli, C. (2007) J Immunol 178, 1975
7. Thurner, B., Haendle, I., Roder, C., Dieckmann, D., Keikavoussi, P., Jonuleit, H., Bender, A., Maczek, C., Schreiner, D., von den Driesch, P., Brocker, E. B., Steinman, R. M., Enk, A., Kampgen, E., and Schuler, G. (1999) J Exp Med 190, 1669
8. Banchereau, J., Palucka, A. K., Dhodapkar, M., Burkeholder, S., Taquet, N., Rolland, A., Taquet, S., Coquery, S., Wittkowski, K. M., Bhardwaj, N., Pineiro, L., Steinman, R., and Fay, J. (2001) Cancer Res 61, 6451

9. Hung, K., Hayashi, R., Lafond-Walker, A., Lowenstein, C., Pardoll, D., and Levitsky, H. (1998) J Exp Med 188, 2357
10. Bennett, S. R., Carbone, F. R., Karamalis, F., Miller, J. F., and Heath, W. R. (1997) J Exp Med 186, 65
11. Hamilton, S. E., Wolkers, M. C., Schoenberger, S. P., and Jameson, S. C. (2006) Nat Immunol 7, 475
12. Williams, M. A., Tyznik, A. J., and Bevan, M. J. (2006) Nature 441, 890
13. Pages, F., Berger, A., Camus, M., Sanchez-Cabo, F., Costes, A., Molidor, R., Mlecnik, B., Kirilovsky, A., Nilsson, M., Damotte, D., Meatchi, T., Bruneval, P., Cugnenc, P. H., Trajanoski, Z., Fridman, W. H., and Galon, J. (2005) N Engl J Med 353, 2654
14. Zang, X., and Allison, J. P. (2007) Clin Cancer Res 13, 5271
15. Chen, L., Ashe, S., Brady, W. A., Hellstrom, I., Hellstrom, K. E., Ledbetter, J. A., McGowan, P., and Linsley, P. S. (1992) Cell 71, 1093
16. Yang, S., Darrow, T. L., and Seigler, H. F. (1997) Cancer Res 57, 1561
17. Mazzocchi, A., Melani, C., Rivoltini, L., Castelli, C., Del Vecchio, M., Lombardo, C., Colombo, M. P., and Parmiani, G. (2001) Cancer Immunol Immunother 50, 199
18. Fishman, M., Hunter, T. B., Soliman, H., Thompson, P., Dunn, M., Smilee, R., Farmelo, M. J., Noyes, D. R., Mahany, J. J., Lee, J. H., Cantor, A., Messina, J., Seigne, J., Pow-Sang, J., Janssen, W., and Antonia, S. J. (2008) J Immunother 31, 72
19. Antonia, S. J., Seigne, J., Diaz, J., Muro-Cacho, C., Extermann, M., Farmelo, M. J., Friberg, M., Alsarraj, M., Mahany, J. J., Pow-Sang, J., Cantor, A., and Janssen, W. (2002) J Urol 167, 1995
20. Hege, K. M., Jooss, K., and Pardoll, D. (2006) Int Rev Immunol 25, 321
21. Nemunaitis, J., Jahan, T., Ross, H., Sterman, D., Richards, D., Fox, B., Jablons, D., Aimi, J., Lin, A., and Hege, K. (2006) Cancer Gene Ther 13, 555
22. Tani, K., Azuma, M., Nakazaki, Y., Oyaizu, N., Hase, H., Ohata, J., Takahashi, K., OiwaMonna, M., Hanazawa, K., Wakumoto, Y., Kawai, K., Noguchi, M., Soda, Y., Kunisaki, R., Watari, K., Takahashi, S., Machida, U., Satoh, N., Tojo, A., Maekawa, T., Eriguchi, M., Tomikawa, S., Tahara, H., Inoue, Y., Yoshikawa, H., Yamada, Y., Iwamoto, A., Hamada, H., Yamashita, N., Okumura, K., Kakizoe, T., Akaza, H., Fujime, M., Clift, S., Ando, D., Mulligan, R., and Asano, S. (2004) Mol Ther 10, 799
23. Boon, T., and van der Bruggen, P. (1996) J Exp Med 183, 725
24. Huang, A. Y., Golumbek, P., Ahmadzadeh, M., Jaffee, E., Pardoll, D., and Levitsky, H. (1994) Science 264, 961
25. Pardoll, D. M. (1998) Nat Med 4, 525
26. Kono, H., and Rock, K. L. (2008) Nat Rev Immunol 8, 279
27. Rosenberg, S. A., Sherry, R. M., Morton, K. E., Scharfman, W. J., Yang, J. C., Topalian, S. L., Royal, R. E., Kammula, U., Restifo, N. P., Hughes, M. S., Schwartzentruber, D., Berman, D. M., Schwarz, S. L., Ngo, L. T., Mavroukakis, S. A., White, D. E., and Steinberg, S. M. (2005) J Immunol 175, 6169
28. Jaffee, E. M., Hruban, R. H., Biedrzycki, B., Laheru, D., Schepers, K., Sauter, P. R., Goemann, M., Coleman, J., Grochow, L., Donehower, R. C., Lillemoe, K. D., O'Reilly, S., Abrams, R. A., Pardoll, D. M., Cameron, J. L., and Yeo, C. J. (2001) J Clin Oncol 19, 145
29. Morton, D. L. (2004) Dev Biol (Basel) 116, 209
30. Soiffer, R., Lynch, T., Mihm, M., Jung, K., Rhuda, C., Schmollinger, J. C., Hodi, F. S., Liebster, L., Lam, P., Mentzer, S., Singer, S., Tanabe, K. K., Cosimi, A. B., Duda, R., Sober, A., Bhan, A., Daley, J., Neuberg, D., Parry, G., Rokovich, J., Richards, L., Drayer, J., Berns, A., Clift, S., Cohen, L. K., Mulligan, R. C., and Dranoff, G. (1998) Proc Natl Acad Sci USA 95, 13141
31. Salgia, R., Lynch, T., Skarin, A., Lucca, J., Lynch, C., Jung, K., Hodi, F. S., Jaklitsch, M., Mentzer, S., Swanson, S., Lukanich, J., Bueno, R., Wain, J., Mathisen, D., Wright, C., Fidias, P., Donahue, D., Clift, S., Hardy, S., Neuberg, D., Mulligan, R., Webb, I., Sugarbaker, D., Mihm, M., and Dranoff, G. (2003) J Clin Oncol 21, 624.
32. Borysiewicz, L. K., Fiander, A., Nimako, M., Man, S., Wilkinson, G. W., Westmoreland, D., Evans, A. S., Adams, M., Stacey, S. N., Boursnell, M. E., Rutherford, E., Hickling, J. K., and Inglis, S. C. (1996) Lancet 347, 1523

33. McAneny, D., Ryan, C. A., Beazley, R. M., and Kaufman, H. L. (1996) Ann Surg Oncol 3, 495
34. Mathis, J. M., Stoff-Khalili, M. A., and Curiel, D. T. (2005) Oncogene 24, 7775
35. Daemen, T., Regts, J., Holtrop, M., and Wilschut, J. (2002) Gene Ther 9, 85
36. Asselin-Paturel, C., Lassau, N., Guinebretiere, J. M., Zhang, J., Gay, F., Bex, F., Hallez, S., Leclere, J., Peronneau, P., Mami-Chouaib, F., and Chouaib, S. (1999) Gene Ther 6, 606
37. Tseng, J. C., Hurtado, A., Yee, H., Levin, B., Boivin, C., Benet, M., Blank, S. V., Pellicer, A., and Meruelo, D. (2004) Cancer Res 64, 6684
38. Klimp, A. H., van der Vaart, E., Lansink, P. O., Withoff, S., de Vries, E. G., Scherphof, G. L., Wilschut, J., and Daemen, T. (2001) Gene Ther 8, 300
39. Nelson, E. L., Prieto, D., Alexander, T. G., Pushko, P., Lofts, L. A., Rayner, J. O., Kamrud, K. I., Fralish, B., and Smith, J. F. (2003) Breast Cancer Res Treat 82, 169
40. Karcher, J., Dyckhoff, G., Beckhove, P., Reisser, C., Brysch, M., Ziouta, Y., Helmke, B. H., Weidauer, H., Schirrmacher, V., and Herold-Mende, C. (2004) Cancer Res 64, 8057
41. Krishnamurthy, S., Huang, Z., and Samal, S. K. (2000) Virology 278, 168
42. Huang, Z., Krishnamurthy, S., Panda, A., and Samal, S. K. (2001) J Gen Virol 82, 1729
43. Toda, M., Martuza, R. L., Kojima, H., and Rabkin, S. D. (1998) J Immunol 160 4457
44. Parkinson, R. J., Mian, S., Bishop, M. C., Gray, T., Li, G., McArdle, S. E., Ali, S., and Rees, R. C. (2003) Prostate 56, 65
45. Saeki, Y., Ichikawa, T., Saeki, A., Chiocca, E. A., Tobler, K., Ackermann, M., Breakefield, X. O., and Fraefel, C. (1998) Hum Gene Ther 9, 2787
46. Simons, J. W., Mikhak, B., Chang, J. F., DeMarzo, A. M., Carducci, M. A., Lim, M., Weber, C. E., Baccala, A. A., Goemann, M. A., Clift, S. M., Ando, D. G., Levitsky, H. I., Cohen, L. K., Sanda, M. G., Mulligan, R. C., Partin, A. W., Carter, H. B., Piantadosi, S., Marshall, F. F., and Nelson, W. G. (1999) Cancer Res 59, 5160
47. Maio, M., Fonsatti, E., Lamaj, E., Altomonte, M., Cattarossi, I., Santantonio, C., Melani, C., Belli, F., Arienti, F., Colombo, M. P., and Parmiani, G. (2002) Cancer Immunol Immunother 51, 9
48. Qiao, J., Moreno, J., Sanchez-Perez, L., Kottke, T., Thompson, J., Caruso, M., Diaz, R. M., and Vile, R. (2006) Gene Ther 13, 1457
49. Logg, C. R., Tai, C. K., Logg, A., Anderson, W. F., and Kasahara, N. (2001) Hum Gene Ther 12, 921
50. den Haan, J. M., Lehar, S. M., and Bevan, M. J. (2000) J Exp Med 192, 1685
51. Belz, G. T., Behrens, G. M., Smith, C. M., Miller, J. F., Jones, C., Lejon, K., Fathman, C. G., Mueller, S. N., Shortman, K., Carbone, F. R., and Heath, W. R. (2002) J Exp Med 196, 1099
52. Hahne, M., Rimoldi, D., Schroter, M., Romero, P., Schreier, M., French, L. E., Schneider, P., Bornand, T., Fontana, A., Lienard, D., Cerottini, J., and Tschopp, J. (1996) Science 274, 1363
53. Dong, H., Strome, S. E., Salomao, D. R., Tamura, H., Hirano, F., Flies, D. B., Roche, P. C., Lu, J., Zhu, G., Tamada, K., Lennon, V. A., Celis, E., and Chen, L. (2002) Nat Med 8, 793
54. Le Bon, A., Etchart, N., Rossmann, C., Ashton, M., Hou, S., Gewert, D., Borrow, P., and Tough, D. F. (2003) Nat Immunol 4, 1009
55. Tough, D. F., Borrow, P., and Sprent, J. (1996) Science 272, 1947
56. Datta, S. K., Redecke, V., Prilliman, K. R., Takabayashi, K., Corr, M., Tallant, T., DiDonato, J., Dziarski, R., Akira, S., Schoenberger, S. P., and Raz, E. (2003) J Immunol 170, 4102
57. Schulz, O., Diebold, S. S., Chen, M., Naslund, T. I., Nolte, M. A., Alexopoulou, L., Azuma, Y. T., Flavell, R. A., Liljestrom, P., and Reis e Sousa, C. (2005) Nature 433, 887
58. Kolumam, G. A., Thomas, S., Thompson, L. J., Sprent, J., and Murali-Krishna, K. (2005) J Exp Med 202, 637
59. McBride, S., Hoebe, K., Georgel, P., and Janssen, E. (2006) J Immunol 177, 6122
60. Thomas, A. M., Santarsiero, L. M., Lutz, E. R., Armstrong, T. D., Chen, Y. C., Huang, L. Q., Laheru, D. A., Goggins, M., Hruban, R. H., and Jaffee, E. M. (2004) J Exp Med 200, 297
61. Eguchi, J., Kuwashima, N., Hatano, M., Nishimura, F., Dusak, J. E., Storkus, W. J., and Okada, H. (2005) J Immunol 174, 7194
62. Berard, F., Blanco, P., Davoust, J., Neidhart-Berard, E. M., Nouri-Shirazi, M., Taquet, N., Rimoldi, D., Cerottini, J. C., Banchereau, J., and Palucka, A. K. (2000) J Exp Med 192, 1535

63. Kang, S. M., Beverly, B., Tran, A. C., Brorson, K., Schwartz, R. H., and Lenardo, M. J. (1992) Science 257, 1134
64. Townsend, S. E., and Allison, J. P. (1993) Science 259, 368
65. Ashwell, J. D., DeFranco, A. L., Paul, W. E., and Schwartz, R. H. (1984) J Exp Med 159, 881
66. Schultze, J. L., Cardoso, A. A., Freeman, G. J., Seamon, M. J., Daley, J., Pinkus, G. S., Gribben, J. G., and Nadler, L. M. (1995) Proc Natl Acad Sci USA 92, 8200
67. Leach, D. R., Krummel, M. F., and Allison, J. P. (1996) Science 271, 1734
68. Hodi, F. S., Butler, M., Oble, D. A., Seiden, M. V., Haluska, F. G., Kruse, A., Macrae, S., Nelson, M., Canning, C., Lowy, I., Korman, A., Lautz, D., Russell, S., Jaklitsch, M. T., Ramaiya, N., Chen, T. C., Neuberg, D., Allison, J. P., Mihm, M. C., and Dranoff, G. (2008) Proc Natl Acad Sci USA 105, 3005
69. Krummel, M. F., and Allison, J. P. (1996) J Exp Med 183, 2533
70. Walunas, T. L., Bakker, C. Y., and Bluestone, J. A. (1996) J Exp Med 183, 2541
71. Hurwitz, A. A., Yu, T. F., Leach, D. R., and Allison, J. P. (1998) Proc Natl Acad Sci USA 95, 10067
72. van Elsas, A., Hurwitz, A. A., and Allison, J. P. (1999) J Exp Med 190, 355
73. Gregor, P. D., Wolchok, J. D., Ferrone, C. R., Buchinshky, H., Guevara-Patino, J. A., Perales, M. A., Mortazavi, F., Bacich, D., Heston, W., Latouche, J. B., Sadelain, M., Allison, J. P., Scher, H. I., and Houghton, A. N. (2004) Vaccine 22, 1700
74. Egen, J. G., and Allison, J. P. (2002) Immunity 16, 23
75. D'Souza, S., Rimoldi, D., Lienard, D., Lejeune, F., Cerottini, J. C., and Romero, P. (1998) Int J Cancer 78, 699.
76. Choi, C., Witzens, M., Bucur, M., Feuerer, M., Sommerfeldt, N., Trojan, A., Ho, A., Schirrmacher, V., Goldschmidt, H., and Beckhove, P. (2005) Blood, 105, 2132
77. Feuerer, M., Beckhove, P., Bai, L., Solomayer, E. F., Bastert, G., Diel, I. J., Pedain, C., Oberniedermayr, M., Schirrmacher, V., and Umansky, V. (2001) Nat Med 7, 452
78. Klebanoff, C. A., Gattinoni, L., and Restifo, N. P. (2006) Immunol Rev 211, 214
79. Webster, W. S., Thompson, R. H., Harris, K. J., Frigola, X., Kuntz, S., Inman, B. A., and Dong, H. (2007) J Immunol 179, 2860
80. Kursar, M., Bonhagen, K., Fensterle, J., Kohler, A., Hurwitz, R., Kamradt, T., Kaufmann, S. H., and Mittrucker, H. W. (2002) J Exp Med 196, 1585
81. Murakami, M., Sakamoto, A., Bender, J., Kappler, J., and Marrack, P. (2002) Proc Natl Acad Sci USA 99, 8832
82. Sakaguchi, S. (2005) Nat Immunol 6, 345
83. Nanni, P., Nicoletti, G., Palladini, A., Croci, S., Murgo, A., Antognoli, A., Landuzzi, L., Fabbi, M., Ferrini, S., Musiani, P., Iezzi, M., De Giovanni, C., and Lollini, P. L. (2007) Cancer Res 67, 11037
84. Zou, W. (2005) Nat Rev Cancer 5, 263
85. Shimizu, J., Yamazaki, S., and Sakaguchi, S. (1999) J Immunol 163, 5211
86. Turk, M. J., Guevara-Patino, J. A., Rizzuto, G. A., Engelhorn, M. E., Sakaguchi, S., and Houghton, A. N. (2004) J Exp Med 200, 771
87. Curiel, T. J., Coukos, G., Zou, L., Alvarez, X., Cheng, P., Mottram, P., Evdemon-Hogan, M., J. R., C.-G., Zhang, L., Burow, M., Zhu, Y., Wei, S., Kryczek, I., Daniel, B., Gordon, A., Myers, L., Lackner, A., Disis, M. L., Knutson, K. L., Chen, L., and Zou, W. (2004) Nat Med 10, 942
88. Zhou, G., Drake, C. G., and Levitsky, H. I. (2006) Blood 107, 628

Modification of Dendritic Cells to Enhance Cancer Vaccine Potency

Archana Monie, Chien-Fu Hung, and T.-C. Wu

Abstract Antigen-specific immunotherapy has emerged as an attractive approach for the treatment of cancers because it has the potency to specifically eradicate systemic tumors and control metastases without damaging normal cells. It is now clear that professional antigen-presenting cells (APCs), such as dendritic cells (DCs) play a central role in the generation of antigen-specific immune responses induced by cancer vaccines. Therefore, strategies to enhance the potency of cancer vaccines should focus on the modification of the properties of DCs either in vivo or ex vivo. These strategies include (1) increasing the number of antigen-expressing DCs; (2) improving antigen expression, processing, and presentation in DCs; (3) promoting DC activation and function; and (4) enhancing DC and T cell interaction to augment vaccine-elicited T cell immune responses. Because many of these strategies modify the properties of DCs to enhance cancer vaccine potency through different mechanisms, they could potentially be combined to generate highly potent cancer vaccines. The encouraging results from preclinical studies employing these strategies have led to several clinical trials. Continued exploration of innovative strategies to enhance cancer vaccine potency through the modification of DC properties may lead to the generation of more effective vaccines for the control of cancer.

Introduction

Immunotherapy has Emerged as an Alternative Treatment for Cancer

Cancer remains as one of the deadliest diseases of our time. Current strategies for the treatment of advanced stage cancers involve conventional therapies such as radiation and chemotherapy. However, advanced stage cancers are difficult to control using

---

T.-C. Wu (✉)
Department of Pathology, Johns Hopkins School of Medicine, Cancer Research Building II Room 309, 1550 Orleans St, Baltimore, MD 21231, USA
e-mail: wutc@jhmi.edu

J. Lustgarten et al. (eds.), *Targeted Cancer Immune Therapy*,
DOI 10.1007/978-1-4419-0170-5_8,

these conventional therapies alone. Therefore, there is an urgent need to develop novel therapies that may be used in conjunction with these conventional therapies in order to further improve the treatment of advanced stage cancers. Antigen-specific immunotherapy has emerged as a potential approach to the treatment of cancers because it has the potency to specifically eradicate systemic tumors and control metastases without damaging normal cells. Antigen-specific immunotherapy has the advantage of being more specific to the tumor and a high degree of safety. It is less likely to generate nonspecific autoimmunity and has the potential to correlate the clinical outcome to a specific immune response [1]. The development of effective antigen-specific immunotherapy should consider targeting the antigen to key antigen-presenting cells (APCs), such as dendritic cells (DCs).

Importance of DCs for Cancer Immunotherapy

DCs are professional APCs and play a key role in the initiation of the adaptive immune response and in the generation of antigen-specific antiviral and antitumor T cell immune responses. It has been established that the generation of cell-mediated immunity is essential in controlling viral infections and malignant tumors. $CD8^+$ T cells are involved in the direct killing of viral-infected cells or tumors, while $CD4^+$ T helper cells augment the $CD8^+$ immune responses as well as antibody-mediated immunity. DCs are responsible for the presentation of antigen to naïve $CD4^+$ and $CD8^+$ T cells, thus promoting the differentiation of effector $CD4^+$ and $CD8^+$ T cells. In peripheral tissues, immature DCs efficiently uptake antigens and process them into antigenic peptides. These peptides are then loaded onto major histocompatibility (MHC) class I and class II molecules and presented on the surface of the DCs. These immature DCs possess several surface receptors, including toll-like receptors (TLRs), cytokine receptors, FcR, tumor necrosis factor (TNF)-receptor family molecules, and sensors for cell death, that enable them to respond to danger signals, such as bacterial or viral components, or inflammatory cytokines, indicating the presence of an infection. In response to a danger signal, the DCs undergo a maturation process, and upregulate adhesion and costimulatory molecules. This converts them into efficient APCs that migrate to the lymphoid organs and activate antigen-specific T cells [2–4]. The understanding of DC biology and the importance of DCs in T cell activation has led to innovative strategies to enhance cancer vaccine potency through modification of DCs.

Modification of the Properties of DCs

Several innovative strategies have been developed in the past decade to modify the properties of DCs for enhancing cancer vaccine potency (Fig. 1). In general, DCs

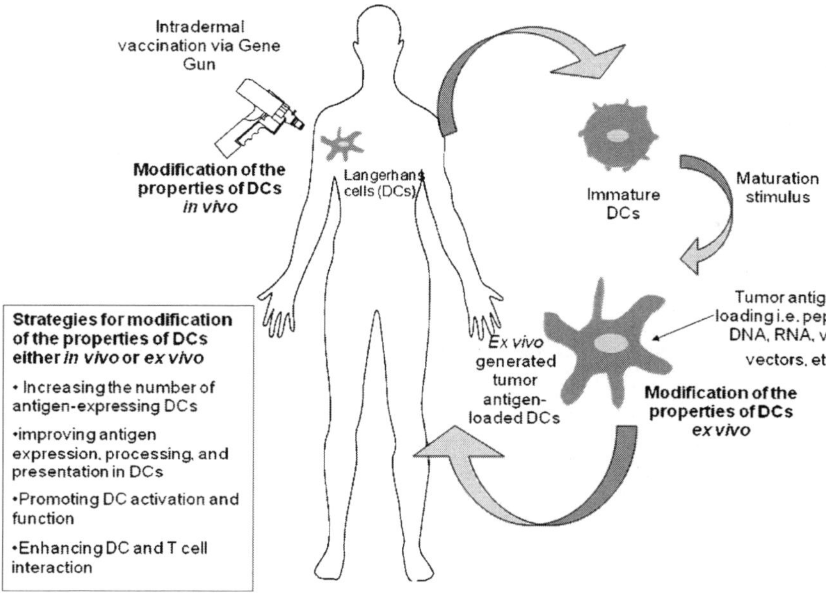

Fig. 1 Modification of the properties of dendritic cells to enhance cancer vaccine potency. One approach of cancer vaccination is to immunize patients with autologous, patient-derived DCs loaded with tumor antigens ex vivo. DCs generated ex vivo are induced to mature, loaded with tumor antigen, and are then injected into the host to generate $CD4^{+}$ and $CD8^{+}$ T cell responses in the cancer patient. Alternatively, cancer vaccines have been developed using strategies for targeting antigen to DCs in vivo, for example intradermal administration of DNA vaccines via gene gun. We and others have used the gene gun delivery system to develop several strategies to enhance DNA vaccine potency in vivo by modifying the properties of DCs, including (1) increasing the number of antigen-expressing DCs; (2) improving antigen expression, processing, and presentation in DCs; (3) promoting DC activation and function; and (4) enhancing DC and T cell interaction to augment vaccine-elicited T cell immune responses. In addition, these strategies have also been used for the modification of the properties of ex vivo generated DCs to further enhance cancer vaccine potency

can be isolated and expanded from patients and modified ex vivo to serve as a DC-based vaccine. Numerous reviews are available on ex vivo-modified DC-based cancer vaccines [5–10]. Alternatively, strategies have been developed for targeting antigen to DCs that involve direct modification of the properties of DCs in vivo. In vivo and ex vivo modification strategies have their advantages and disadvantages. For example, first, in vivo-targeted DCs can be generated in large amounts at lower costs, whereas ex vivo-generated DCs need to be customized and involve labor-intensive and expensive procedures. Second, in vivo targeting can target the antigen to multiple subsets of DCs at multiple sites in the body, while the ex vivo strategy is limited to the DC subsets that can be easily isolated and cultured in sufficient quantities. Another important aspect is the specificity of the each approach.

Table 1 Advantages and disadvantages of in vivo and ex vivo modification of DCs

	In vivo modification of DCs	Ex vivo modification of DCs
Production	Low-cost of production, simple and single procedure	Labor-intensive and high cost of production, multiple procedures
Accessibility	Accessible to large number of patients	Accessible to a limited number of patients
DC subsets and in vivo distribution	Can be targeted to multiple DC subsets and at multiple sites	Limited to DC subsets that can be isolated and cultured in vitro in sufficient numbers
Specificity	Limited specificity	High specificity as only the ex vivo cultured DCs are injected
Maturation and activation	Poor control as DCs are matured and activated in vivo	High control as DCs are stimulated and matured ex vivo before administration

The ex vivo cultured DCs are highly specific to a particular antigen compared with in vivo-targeted DCs. Furthermore, the ex vivo-generated DCs are at a highly controlled maturation and activation state compared with those targeted in vivo. Additional factors such as the duration of antigen presentation and stability of the vaccine after administration may also contribute to the efficacy of the in vivo and ex vivo targeting strategies. A summary of the advantages and disadvantages of in vivo and ex vivo targeting strategies is illustrated in Table 1.

In the current review, we mainly focus on strategies to modify the properties of DCs in vivo. We particularly focus on our experience in the modification of DCs to increase the potency of DNA vaccines. These vaccines have become an attractive and potentially effective strategy for antigen-specific immunotherapy because of their safety, stability, and cost-effectiveness [11–13]. Among the previously explored routes of DNA administration, intradermal vaccination using a gene gun represents one of the most efficient methods for delivering DNA directly into DCs. The gene gun can deliver DNA-coated gold particles into intradermal Langerhans cells in vivo [14]; these cells mature and migrate to the lymphoid organs for T cell priming [15]. The gene gun administration system allows us to test several strategies to modify the properties of DCs in vivo. We and others have used the gene gun delivery system to develop several strategies to enhance DNA vaccine potency by modifying the properties of DCs including (1) increasing the number of antigen-expressing DCs; (2) improving antigen expression, processing, and presentation in DCs; (3) promoting DC activation and function; and (4) enhancing DC and T cell interaction to augment vaccine-elicited T cell immune responses. In addition, we will also provide a brief summary of some of the strategies to enhance cancer vaccine potency by the modification of the properties of ex vivo generated DCs. Table 2 summarizes several of the strategies that have been employed to enhance cancer vaccine potency by the modification of DCs either in vivo or ex vivo.

Table 2 Strategies to enhance cancer vaccine potency by modification of DCs

	Modification of DCs in vivo		Modification of DCs ex vivo	
Increasing the number of antigen-expressing DCs	Efficient routes for delivery	[16–27, 29]	Generation of DCs ex vivo	[114, 118–122]
	Linkage of antigen to molecules capable of binding to DCs	[28–33]	Antigen-loading (e.g., peptides, proteins, DNA, RNA, viral vectors)	[9, 124–139]
	Intercellular antigen spreading	[34–45]	Efficient routes for delivery	[144, 145, 149, 150]
	Employment of chemotherapy-induced apoptosis	[46, 47]		
Enhancing antigen expression, processing, and presentation in DCs	Codon optimization	[48–50]	Employment of intracellular targeting strategies to enhance MHC class I and II antigen presentation in DCs	[127, 128, 136–138, 147, 151, 185, 186]
	Employment of intracellular targeting strategies to enhance MHC class I and II antigen presentation in DCs	[51–60, 63–66, 130]		
	Circumventing antigen processing	[68, 69]		
Promoting DC activation and function	Employment of TLR ligands and adjuvants	[73–79, 81–93, 97]	Employment of TLR ligands and adjuvants	[152–156]
	Inhibition of immunosuppressive factors	[98, 100]	Inhibiting negative regulatory pathways (SOCS-1, GILZ, etc.)	[112, 157–160]
Enhancing DC and T cell interaction	Employment of cytokines and co-stimulatory molecules	[15]	Induction of CD4⁺ T cell help	[127, 128]
	Prolong DC survival	[103, 104]	Inhibition of immunosuppressive regulatory T cells	[162–164, 167]
	Induction of CD4⁺ T cell help	[66, 105–108]		
	Inhibition of immunosuppressive regulatory T cells	[111, 113, 184]		
	Promote in vivo DC expansion	[28, 114–116]		

DC Dendritic cell, *MHC* major histocompatibility complex, *TLR* toll-like receptor

Strategies to Enhance Vaccine Potency by Modifying the Properties of Dendritic Cells In Vivo

Increasing the Number of Antigen-Expressing DCs

One approach for increasing the number of antigen-expressing DCs is by an effective route of vaccine delivery directly into DCs in vivo. For example, DNA vaccines have been most commonly administered by the intramuscular or intradermal route [12]. Among the previously explored routes of administration, intradermal vaccination using a gene gun has been shown to be one of the most efficient methods for delivering DNA directly into DCs. The gene gun can deliver DNA-coated gold particles into intradermal Langerhans cells in vivo [14]; these cells then mature and migrate to the lymphoid organs for T cell priming [15]. In addition, gene gun immunization is significantly more dose-efficient than intramuscular or subcutaneous injection [12, 13].

Another important method for the direct delivery of vaccines to DCs is by intranodal injection. Direct lymph nodal injection of canary pox viral vector-based vaccines expressing the melanoma antigen, gp100, has been shown to enhance the tumor-specific immunity in patients [16]. Several groups have also shown that intralymphatic delivery of vaccines into the lymph nodes or spleen can also significantly enhance the vaccine immunogenicity [17–20]. By targeting the vaccines encoding antigen to DC-rich areas such as the secondary lymphoid tissues, intralymphatic immunization may increase the likelihood of transfecting large numbers of local APCs resulting in strong $CD8^+$ T cell immune responses [18].

Electroporation has also emerged as an efficient method for improving cellular uptake to increase the number of antigen-expressing DCs. The employment of electroporation, a technique widely used to improve in vitro gene transfection, can potentially facilitate the uptake and expression of DNA by target cells in vivo and lead to an increase in the number of antigen-expressing DCs, augmenting vaccine-elicited immune responses. Several studies have employed electroporation to improve the antigen expression and thus enhance vaccine-elicited antigen-specific immune responses in vivo [21–27]. Thus, electroporation may represent a feasible option to tackle the limited transfection efficiency of vaccines.

Another strategy to increase the number of antigen-expressing or antigen-loaded DCs is the linkage of antigen to molecules that target the antigen to the surface of DCs in the context of DNA vaccines. For example, linkage of antigen to Fms-like tyrosine kinase 3-ligand can also target antigen to DCs; a chimeric *Flt-3L-E7* fusion gene was shown to significantly improve cytotoxic T lymphocyte (CTL) responses in mice compared with that of vaccination with wild-type E7 DNA [28]. Furthermore, linkage of antigen to a secreted form of heat shock protein 70, which bind to scavenger receptors on the surface of DCs such as CD91, may represent an effective method for targeting linked antigen to DCs and enhancing antigen-specific immunity [29–31]. Antigen may also be linked to cytotoxic lymphocyte antigen 4 (CTLA-4), which binds to B7-expressing cells such as DCs, to direct antigen to sites of immune induction and enhance the vaccine-generated immune response [32]. In addition, linkage of antigen to the Fc portion of immunoglobulin G (IgG) can target antigen to Fc receptors on the surface of DCs, promote receptor-mediated internalization of the antigen-Fc complexes by DCs and result in enhanced vaccine potency [33]. Several receptors expressed on DCs have also been used to target antigen to DCs, including mannose receptor, CD205, CD40, and the Fcγ receptors [10]. Thus, it would be important to further explore if antigens linked to these molecules would be capable of targeting antigen to DCs as well as augmenting vaccine-elicited immune responses from multiple arms of the adaptive immunity.

This strategy mainly applies to DNA vaccines because their potency is limited by their inability to naturally amplify and spread among DCs in vivo. The antigen encoded in the DNA vaccine can be spread in vivo by linkage of the antigen to proteins capable of intercellular transport. This has been demonstrated using the herpes simplex virus type 1 (HSV-1) tegument protein VP22, which is capable of antigen spreading. The linkage of this protein to the antigen of interest has been shown to significantly increase the number of antigen-expressing DCs in the lymph nodes in several studies [34–39]. Specifically, the linkage of VP22 to E7 antigen led to the enhancement of E7-specific long-term memory $CD8^+$ T cell immune responses and antitumor effects against E7-expressing tumor cells [40, 41]. In addition, two other proteins with some homology to VP22, bovine herpesvirus VP22 (BVP22) and Marek's disease virus VP22 (MVP22), have also been shown to be capable of intercellular spreading and transport and have been used in several preclinical studies [42–45].

Coadministration of cancer vaccines with chemotherapeutic agents can promote the release of antigen from apoptotic tumor cells. This can potentially facilitate antigen uptake by local DCs, resulting in enhancement of vaccine potency. A recent study by Kang et al. showed that the chemotherapeutic agent epigallocatechin-3-gallate (EGCG), a chemical derived from green tea, could induce tumor apoptosis and enhance the tumor antigen-specific T cell immune responses elicited by DNA vaccination [46]. Another study demonstrated that pretreatment with cisplatin enhanced the antigen-specific antitumor immunity induced by DNA vaccination [47]. Thus, it may be of interest to explore whether other chemotherapeutic agents could exhibit similar synergistic effects when combined with cancer vaccination.

Enhancing Antigen Expression, Processing, and Presentation in DCs

Codon optimization involves the modification of antigenic gene sequences by replacement of codons that are rarely recognized by cellular protein synthesis machinery with more commonly recognized codons. This has emerged as a promising approach to enhance the expression of encoded antigen in DCs. For example, studies have shown that immunization of mice with either codon-optimized human papillomavirus type 16 (HPV-16) E6 DNA [48] or codon-optimized HPV-16 E7 DNA [49] was shown to generate greater immune responses than vaccination of mice with wild-type E6 or E7 DNA, respectively. Codon-optimization has also been effectively employed in adenovirus-based vaccines. For example, intranasal administration of a recombinant replication-deficient adenovirus-based vaccine expressing the soluble core domain of G glycoprotein of respiratory syncytial virus (RSV) engineered by codon optimization was shown to effectively generate protective immunity against RSV infection [50].

Targeting the intracellular processing and presentation pathways may serve to enhance antigen presentation in DCs. Thus, strategies to enhance MHC class I processing and presentation in DCs may increase the activation of CD8$^+$ T cells, leading to stronger antitumor or antiviral immunity. The linkage of antigen to proteins that target the antigen for proteasomal degradation or entry into the endoplasmic reticulum (ER) has been shown to facilitate MHC class I presentation of linked antigen in DCs. For example, linkage of antigen to calreticulin (CRT) [51], *Mycobacterium tuberculosis* heat shock protein 70 (hsp70) [52], γ-tubulin [53], the translocation domain of *Pseudomonas aeruginosa* exotoxin A (ETA(dII)) [54], or ER insertion signal sequences [55] can significantly improve MHC class I presentation of nuclear or cytosolic antigens. In a comparison of HPV-16 E7 DNA vaccines employing intracellular targeting strategies, Kim et al. found that a DNA vaccine encoding E7 linked to CRT generated the greatest E7-specific CTL responses and antitumor effects against E7-expressing tumors in a preclinical model [56]. MHC class II presentation of antigen encoded by DNA vaccines can also be enhanced to increase vaccine potency. CD4$^+$ helper T cells are known to play a major role in the priming of CD8$^+$ T cells and generation of memory T cells [57]. For example, the sorting signal of lysosomal-associated membrane protein type 1 (LAMP-1) fused to the HPV-16 E7 antigen has been shown to target the E7 antigen to cellular endosomal/lysosomal compartments, facilitating class II presentation of E7 and leading to increased numbers of E7-specific CD4$^+$ T cells and E7-specific CTL activity [58, 59]. Furthermore, vaccination with LAMP-1 linked to the human immunodeficiency virus-1 (HIV-1) Gag antigen in a DNA vaccine demonstrated enhanced CD4$^+$ and CD8$^+$ T cell memory responses compared with vaccination with wild-type Gag alone [60]. The MHC class II-associated invariant chain (Ii) can also be potentially used for improving class II presentation of antigen in DCs. The class II-associated peptide (CLIP) region of Ii in the ER can be substituted with a desired epitope, which can be efficiently presented through the MHC class II pathway in DCs for the stimulation of peptide-specific CD4$^+$ T cells [61, 62]. Studies have shown that the transfection of MHC class II-positive cells with DNA encoding an Ii chain in which CLIP is replaced with a CD4$^+$ T cell epitope of an antigen of interest can lead to presentation of the CD4$^+$ T cell epitope through the MHC class II pathway [63–65]. More recently, Hung et al. have demonstrated that a DNA vaccine encoding Ii with the CLIP region replaced with the pan HLA-DR binding epitope (PADRE) could elicit potent PADRE-specific CD4$^+$ T cell responses in vaccinated mice [66]. Furthermore, coadministration of the Ii-PADRE vaccine with DNA encoding HPV-16 E7 generated significantly greater CD8$^+$ T cell immune responses relative to a coadministration of DNA encoding HPV-16 E7 with DNA encoding unmodified Ii [66].

Recent studies have demonstrated the possibility of circumventing antigen processing through the generation of stable MHC class I presentation. The employment of MHC class I single-chain trimer (SCT) technology involves linkage of the gene encoding an antigenic peptide to β2-microglobulin and a MHC class I heavy chain, producing a single-chain construct encoding the peptide antigen fused to an MHC class I molecule [67]. The expression of this construct within DCs may allow stable presentation of the antigenic peptide through MHC class I molecules on the cell surface. For example, a DNA vaccine encoding a SCT encoding a HPV-16 E6 CTL epitope, β2-microglobulin, and H-$2K^b$ MHC class I heavy chain has been shown to generate enhanced E6 peptide-specific $CD8^+$ T cell responses in vaccinated mice relative to immunization with DNA encoding wild-type HPV-16 E6 [68]. In addition, a DNA vaccine employing an SCT of human leukocyte antigen (HLA)-A2 linked to a peptide of the tumor-associated antigen mesothelin was recently shown to generate strong human mesothelin peptide-specific $CD8^+$ T cell responses and prevent the growth of mesothelin-expressing tumors in HLA-A2 transgenic mice [69].

Promoting DC Activation and Function

It is now clear that TLRs on DCs play a crucial role in innate and adaptive immune responses [70–72]. DCs are stimulated by signals including TLR ligands or inflammatory cytokines to mature and differentiate into potent activators of antigen-specific T cells [4]. Thus, vaccine potency may be enhanced by providing these signals to facilitate DC activation. For example, the TLR-9 ligand, CpG motifs, which are bacterial-derived immunostimulatory gene sequences, have been shown to enhance vaccine potency by promoting the growth and activation of transfected DC [73–75]. In addition, modification of the CpG content of a DNA plasmid backbone has also been shown to affect the immunogenicity of the plasmid [76, 77], thus enhancing the potency of vaccines administered with them [78]. TLR-4 ligands such as monophosphoryl lipid A (MPL), a detoxified derivative of the lipopolysaccharide (LPS) of *Salmonella minnesota* R595 [79] have also been shown to enhance DNA vaccine potency [80]. Administration of MPL in conjunction with DNA vaccines has been shown to enhance antibody- and CTL-mediated immunity induced by DNA vaccination against HIV-1 viral-encoded antigens in mice [81].

Other agents that modify TLR-mediated signal transduction pathways may also be useful for enhancing vaccine potency through their actions on TLRs on the surface of DCs. Therefore, vaccines administered in conjunction with these agents may lead to DC activation and result in enhanced vaccine-elicited immune responses. Imiquimod and its analog resiquimod are two immune response modifiers that have been shown to bind to and activate TLR-7 and TLR-8 on DCs [82, 83]. They have been used as adjuvants to increase the number and maturation status of DCs in lymphoid organs [84] and enhance tumor-specific [85] and viral antigen-specific [86, 87] immune responses in vaccinated mice.

DNA encoding TLR adaptor molecules may also be useful as genetic adjuvants for augmenting vaccine-elicited immune responses and improving the potency of cancer vaccines. Vaccination in conjunction with DNA encoding the TLR adaptor molecules myeloid differentiation factor 88 (MyD88) and Toll-interleukin (IL)-1 receptor domain-containing adaptor-inducing IFN-β (TRIF) have been shown to enhance the antigen-specific immune responses generated by DNA vaccines [88].

The employment of cationic lipid–DNA complexes (CLDCs) consisting of liposomes complexed to plasmid DNA has also been used to activate DCs [89], which shown to induce the release of significant levels of T helper type 1 (Th1)-biasing cytokines such as IL-12 by DCs, leading to enhanced antigen-specific immune responses [90]. In addition, CLDCs were selectively taken up by splenic DCs, and thus CLDCs may represent a method for the efficient transfection of DCs in vivo as well as for the activation of DCs [89, 90].

Other immunostimulatory adjuvants for vaccination strategies that may be related to DC activation include cholera toxin (CT) [91] and *Escherichia coli* heat-labile enterotoxin (LT) [92, 93], two closely related molecules capable of inducing maturation in DCs and eliciting robust immune responses when administered through the mucosal and parenteral routes [94–96]. It has been shown that intradermal administration of DNA vaccines in conjunction with CT and LT plasmid vectors could significantly enhance Th1 and Th2 cytokine responses against viral antigens and induce strong protective immunity [97]. Thus, these and other bacterial toxin-based adjuvants may represent effective means of promoting the activation of DCs to enhance DNA vaccine potency.

A new strategy for promoting DC activation is the inhibition of natural immune attenuators, such as suppressor of cytokine signaling 1 (SOCS-1), in DCs. SOCS-1 participates in the negative regulation of the JAK-STAT pathway and suppresses DC activation [98, 99]. Coadministration of HIV-1 DNA vaccines with DNA encoding small interfering RNA (siRNA) targeting SOCS-1 has been shown to significantly improve DNA vaccine-elicited HIV-1 envelope-specific $CD8^+$ and $CD4^+$ T cell immune responses, presumably by enhanced production of inflammatory cytokines such as interleukin (IL)-12 by DCs [100]. These studies suggest that the inhibition of other immunosuppressive factors in DCs may represent effective strategies for enhancing cancer vaccine potency in the future.

Enhancing DC and T Cell Interaction

It is important to optimize the interaction between T cells and the immune system's central players, DCs, to enhance vaccine potency. Employing cytokines and costimulatory molecules represents one strategy for more efficient T cell activation. Priming naïve T cells to proliferate and differentiate into effector cells requires two distinct sets of extracellular signals. One signal comes from T cell receptors binding to the appropriate peptide–MHC complex on the surface of DCs. The second required signal is provided by costimulatory molecules on the DC surface that function together with antigens to stimulate T cells. Since cytokines may augment or serve as the secondary costimulatory signal, employing cytokines and costimulatory molecules with cancer vaccines can lead to enhanced T cell activation and cancer vaccine potency.

Several studies have shown the success of this strategy applied to DNA vaccines. For example, coadministration of DNA vaccines with DNA encoding costimulatory molecules such as B7 may lead to more efficient activation of antigen-specific T cells [15]. Coadministration of DNA vaccines with DNA encoding cytokines fused to Fc domains of IgG has been shown to further enhance DNA vaccine potency. Codelivery of vaccines with DNA encoding various cytokines such as IL-2, IL-12, IL-18, or granulocyte-macrophage colony stimulating factor (GMCSF) can enhance vaccine-elicited immune responses [12, 101, 102].

Another important strategy to enhance the interaction between T cells and DCs is to prolong the life of DCs, which can improve the number of antigen-expressing DCs, enhance their long-term ability to prime T cells, and augment T cell responses and enhance cancer vaccine potency. Because DCs become susceptible to T cell-mediated apoptosis after T cell priming, one strategy to prolong DC survival would be to use DNA encoding antiapoptotic factors such as Bcl-xL, Bcl-2, X-linked inhibitor of apoptosis protein (XIAP), and dominant negative mutants (dn) of caspases (e.g., dn caspase-9 and dn caspase-8). It has been shown that codelivery of DNA encoding E7 with DNA encoding antiapoptotic factors enhanced E7-specific $CD8^+$ T cell responses in mice and elicited antitumor effects against E7-expressing tumors [103]. However, the introduction of DNA encoding antiapoptotic proteins into cells is complicated by issues of oncogenicity. An alternative approach, such as inhibition of proapoptotic proteins using RNA interference (RNAi), may alleviate these concerns of cellular malignant transformation. It has been shown that coadministration of DNA vaccines encoding E7 with short interfering RNA (siRNA) targeting the key proapoptotic proteins *Bak* and *Bax* was able to effectively improve DC resistance to apoptosis and enhance antitumor $CD8^+$ T cell responses in mice [104]. It would be of interest to further explore coadministration of cancer vaccines with siRNA targeting other key proapoptotic proteins, such as caspase-8, caspase-9 and/or caspase-3, to enhance cancer vaccine potency.

$CD4^+$ T helper cells play a major role in stimulating and augmenting $CD8^+$ T cell levels, activating macrophages and other effector molecules to supplement $CD8^+$ T cell immune responses. Therefore, recruiting $CD4^+$ T helper cells at sites of $CD8^+$ T cell priming can potentially enhance CTL immune responses. This strategy has been utilized in several cancer vaccines. Hung et al. demonstrated that coadministration of DNA vaccines with DNA encoding an Ii chain with the CLIP region replaced with pan HLA-DR binding epitope (PADRE) could lead to significant enhancement in antigen-specific $CD8^+$ immune responses [66]. An agent that has been shown to be useful in recruiting $CD4^+$ T cell help is fragment C (FrC) of tetanus toxin, which contains universally immunogenic T helper cell epitopes that can bind to many different types of MHC class II molecules [105]. Some DNA vaccines encoding FrC of tetanus toxin have been shown to significantly enhance antigen-specific $CD8^+$ T cell immune responses [106–108]. $CD4^+$ T cell-mediated augmentation of

$CD8^+$ T cell priming represents a plausibly effective vaccine strategy for potentiating cancer vaccines.

Natural regulatory T cells (T_{reg} cells) are important for the maintenance of host homeostasis and can limit the level of effector immune responses against infection and malignancies. Natural T_{reg} cells constitutively express CD25 and the T cell inhibitory receptor CTLA-4 and directly and indirectly inhibit $CD8^+$ T cell and DC interaction [109, 110]. T_{reg} cell depletion is a potential strategy for enhancing the potency of cancer vaccines. Several agents have been used to deplete T_{reg} cells in vivo, such as cyclophosphamide, fludarabine, IL-2 immunotoxin, and COX-2 inhibitors [110]. Administration of cancer vaccines in conjunction with agents to deplete T_{reg} cells has been shown to result in enhancement in antigen-specific $CD8^+$ T cell responses [111, 112]. High level expression of transcription factor Forkhead box p3 (Foxp3) is a distinctive marker for T_{reg} cells. It has recently been demonstrated that vaccination of mice with Foxp3-transfected DCs could generate Foxp3-specific CTL, depletion of $T_{reg,}$ and enhance tumor immunity [113]. T_{reg} cell depletion represents a conceivable strategy for eliminating negative immunoregulation, enhancing T cell activation and function, and improving the interaction between T cells and DCs.

Another approach to improve DC and T cell interaction is the use of cytokines involved in DC expansion. One effective DC growth factor is Fms-like tyrosine kinase 3-ligand (Flt-3L). For example, a DNA vaccine encoding a fusion protein comprising the tumor antigen MUC-1 and human Flt-3L was shown to elicit MUC-1-specific CTL responses and potent tumor regression in mice [114]. Additionally, codelivery of a DNA vaccine encoding antigen with DNA encoding Flt-3L recruited large numbers of DCs and generated significant antigen-specific immune responses in mice [115]. Furthermore, as previously mentioned, the linkage of antigen to Flt-3L may also target antigen to DCs, resulting in improved T cell activation and augmented cytotoxic T lymphocyte (CTL) responses in mice [28].

To further enhance cancer vaccine potency, strategies to expand DCs in vivo can be paired with strategies to attract DCs to sites of vaccination. Codelivery of plasmids encoding the chemokine macrophage inflammatory protein-1alpha (MIP-1alpha) and Flt-3L with a DNA vaccine was shown to result in enhanced recruitment, expansion, and activation of DCs at the site of DNA vaccination and lead to augmented antigen-specific cellular and humoral immune responses [116].

Strategies to Enhance Vaccine Potency by Modifying the Properties of Dendritic Cells Ex Vivo

One approach of cancer vaccination is to immunize patients with autologous, patient-derived DCs loaded with tumor antigens ex vivo. DCs generated ex vivo are modified away from the immunosuppressive effects of certain tumor-secreted factors such as interleukin-10 (IL-10), transforming growth factor-β (TGF-β), and vascular endothelial growth factor (VEGF) that inhibit DC development and function [117].

These DCs are injected into the host to stimulate robust and enduring $CD4^+$ and $CD8^+$ T cell responses in the cancer patient. The efficiency and control provided by ex vivo manipulation of DCs aims to generate an optimally activated antigen-presenting cell. However, ex vivo-generated DCs are still unable to fully mimic the development of immature DCs, particularly the process of DC activation, to increase numbers of mature DCs and accordingly increase the magnitude of immune response. There is a need to improve the efficacy of vaccines using ex vivo DCs.

Several strategies can be used to modify the properties of DCs ex vivo to further enhance the potency of these cancer vaccines by (1) increasing the number of antigen-expressing DCs; (2) improving antigen expression, processing, and presentation in DCs; (3) promoting DC activation and function; and (4) enhancing DC and T cell interaction to augment vaccine-elicited T cell immune responses.

Increasing the Number of Antigen-Expressing DCs

Multiple strategies have been developed to generate large number of DCs ex vivo. DCs can be generated from monocytes in peripheral blood cultured with IL-4 and granulocyte macrophage colony stimulating factor (GM-CSF) [118]. They may also be generated ex vivo by the differentiation of $CD34^+$ precursor cells present in the peripheral blood, cord blood, or bone marrow by incubating them with various cytokine combinations in vitro [119–122]. Another strategy is to treat patients with Flt-3 ligand (Flt-3L), which activates the Flt-3 receptor, and serves as a growth and differentiation factor for hematopoietic progenitors, leading to the expansion of DCs in vivo [114]. These types of ex vivo generated DCs are, however, mainly immature DCs and have a low capacity to activate T cells. However, these DCs can be induced to develop into mature DCs, which are more immunogenic and express higher levels of MHC and costimulatory molecules [123].

The potency of cancer vaccines may be significantly enhanced by maximizing the number of ex vivo antigen-loaded DCs. One of the most important design considerations in cancer vaccines is the form of antigen used to load DCs. The form of antigen has a big impact on its ability to access MHC class I and II presentation pathways and induce $CD8^+$ and $CD4^+$ T cells responses. There are several methods that have been employed to load DCs with tumor antigen ex vivo. The antigen can be presented by the DCs exogenously, as peptides [124], whole protein, tumor lysate, or complexed with antibody [125]. DCs can also be engineered to synthesize antigen(s) endogenously by transfection with mRNA [126] or tumor-derived RNA [127, 128]. Additionally, they could be loaded by viral vectors [9, 129], killed tumor cells [130, 131], and DC-derived exosomes [7, 132].

The most common strategy to load antigen has been the use of MHC class I and MHC class II peptides derived from defined antigens [133, 134]. These peptides are advantageous in that they are chemically defined, relatively stable, and simple to prepare and store. However, the limitation to using peptides is the need to determine the human leukocyte antigen (HLA) type of the patient. However, due to the highly polymorphic nature of these HLA molecules, it is necessary to identify specific immunogenic epitopes of antigens before a vaccine can be developed. It may be difficult to produce a vaccine that is effective in a variety of patients with different HLA haplotypes, making it impractical for large-scale vaccination treatments. There is also limited persistence of peptide–MHC complexes on DCs. Using whole antigen is preferred because it is likely to contain peptides that can be effectively presented by most MHC molecules. An approach that can possibly address the limitations of proteins and peptides is the use of overlapping long (20–25 aa) peptides that cover most, but not necessarily all, of the coding sequence of the tumor antigen [135]. This approach should provide MHC class I and II epitopes and does not require knowledge of an individual's MHC haplotype. Furthermore, mRNA transfection of DCs also permits efficient loading of MHC class I by the endogenous route, and mRNA-transfected DCs have been shown to elicit enhanced antigen-specific T cell responses in vitro [128]. In fact, several phase I clinical trials in patients with immunized with antigen-specific antigen mRNA-transfected DCs demonstrated that the majority of patients exhibited a significant antigen-specific T cell response [136–138]. Thus, immunization with mRNA-transfected DCs is a promising strategy to stimulate potent antitumor immunity. Another strategy to improve antigen loading and presentation to DCs can be focused on antigen preparation and formulation. For example, Shi et al. demonstrated that tumor hyperthermia led to enhanced cross-priming of melanoma-specific CTLs [139]. Heat treatment of tumor cells upregulated levels of hsp70 and increased tumor antigen expression, resulting in generation of antigen-specific CTL responses, improved DC activation and improved cross-priming. The emphasis on enhancing antigen loading of DCs can overshadow the fact that persistence of antigen presentation in the ex vivo-loaded DC may be a more critical issue in determining DC immunogenicity. It takes several hours for the injected DCs to reach the lymph nodes and continued antigen presentation to induce an effective antitumor response [140, 141].

It is of interest to explore the optimal routes of delivery to increase the number of antigen-expressing DCs. Several routes of administration were explored for ex vivo-generated DCs, including intradermal, intranodal, intralymphatic, and intratumoral injections [142, 143]. Intradermal is the most commonly used for ex vivo DC vaccination. Generally, only a small fraction (less than 5%) of intradermally administered mature DCs reaches the draining lymph nodes due to inefficient homing [144, 145]. Direct intralymphatic injection may circumvent the skin migration problem [144]. However, DC migration was shown to improve when the injection site was conditioned with TNF [146]. Studies have also employed intramuscular administration of transfected DCs and demonstrated significant tumor-specific immune responses [147]. Recent studies also demonstrated that intranodal injection may result in the trapping of the DCs in the fat tissue surrounding the lymph node [148]. However, it is not clear if overloading the lymph node with large numbers of DCs would enhance vaccine potency [149]. A pilot clinical trial conducted on patients with metastatic prostate cancer immunized with Ag-pulsed DC by intravenous, intradermal, or intralymphatic injection demonstrated that all the patients developed Ag-specific T cell immune responses following immunization, regardless of the route of administration.

However, induction of IFN-γ production was seen only with intralymphatic and intradermal routes of administration. This suggests that the route of administration of the modified DCs plays an important role in the generation of significant antigen-specific immune responses in vaccinated hosts [150].

Enhancing Antigen Expression, Processing, and Presentation in DCs

The pathways by which DCs capture antigen and deliver it into distinct intracellular DC compartments determine subsequent processing and presentation. Some of the strategies that have been employed to enhance MHC class I and II processing and presentation in DCs in vivo have also been tested using ex vivo generated DCs. These strategies include linkage of antigen to proteins that target the antigen for proteasomal degradation or entry into the ER (such as CRT), hsp70, ER insertion signal sequences, or peptide translocation domains [151]. Fusing a lysosomal targeting signal to the antigen can direct cytoplasmic antigens to the MHC class II presentation pathway [58]. For example, a recent study by Kang et al. demonstrated the employment of an intracellular targeting approach that routed the HPV-16 E7 antigen into the endosomal and lysosomal compartments by linking with the sorting signal of lysosome-associated membrane protein 1 (LAMP-1) to enhance the presentation of antigen to MHC class I-restricted $CD8^+$ T cells and MHC class II-restricted $CD4^+$ T cells. The authors demonstrated that DCs retrovirally transduced with the E7 antigen linked to LAMP-1 dramatically increased in vitro activation and expansion of E7-specific $CD4^+$ and $CD8^+$ T cells and generated greater antitumor immunity compared with DCs transduced with E7 alone [147]. Another study also demonstrated that DCs transfected with RNA encoding antigen linked to LAMP-1 lysosomal targeting signal, which can target the antigen to cellular endosomal/lysosomal compartments and facilitate class II presentation, could significantly enhance the induction of antigen-specific $CD4^+$ T cells [127].

Strategies to Promote DC Activation and Function

Cotransduction of DCs with a TLR gene or immunostimulatory cytokine genes such as IL-12 or CD40-ligand is one strategy to enhance DC function [152]. TLRs are the main agents through which DCs mature in response to the presence of pathogens. Hence, culturing DCs with TLR ligands or their analogs (e.g., TLR4 ligand LPS, TLR3 ligand polyinosinic-polycytidylic acid [polyI/C], TLR9 ligand oligodeoxynucleotide containing one or more unmethylated CpG dinucleotides [CpG ODN] and TLR7/8 ligands R848 and imiquimod) can induce the functional maturation of DCs. This maturation may be augmented by using certain combinations of TLR agonists [153]. Recent studies demonstrated that the costimulation of DCs with several TLR ligands, including TLR7 and TLR3 ligands induced activation of bone marrow-derived DCs with increased secretion of proinflammatory cytokines and costimulatory molecules. Furthermore, ex vivo injection of peptide-loaded bone marrow derived DCs stimulated by the combinations of TLR7 and TLR3 ligands led to a significant increase in the CTL effector functions in vaccinated mice [153]. Additionally, there have been studies demonstrating phagosome maturation, which permits antigen presentation on MHC class II and is regulated by TLR signals associated with phagocytosis of apoptotic cells [154, 155].

Still, optimal DC maturation ex vivo may require a combination of TLR ligands and cytokines. Costimulatory molecules such as OX40 and 4-1BB are cross-linked by ligands, expressed on activated DCs, and help provide survival signals to activate T cells. Transfection of genes encoding the corresponding ligands into antigen-loaded DCs represents another approach to enhancing DC activation. For example, transfection of mRNA encoding OX40 into DCs has been shown to potentiate the ability of mouse DCs to induce antitumor immunity and enhance the DCs activation in vitro [156]. Thus, TLR ligands have been shown to enhance the potency of DC-based vaccines.

An approach to promote DC activation and function is to inhibit regulatory pathways that lower levels of DC maturation. It has been shown that the stimulatory capacity of DCs and the magnitude of the adaptive immune response are negatively regulated by SOCS1 in DCs [157]. Shen et al. demonstrated that siRNA inhibition of SOCS1 in DCs potentiates DC immunogenicity and strongly enhances antigen-specific antitumor immunity [158]. Another attractive target is glucocorticoid-induced leucine zipper (GILZ), which is the common effector of suppressive signals mediated by glucocorticoids IL-10 and TGF-ß [112].

Recently, there has been evidence that the receptor tyrosine kinase Mer (MerTK) plays a key role in mediating apoptotic cell-induced inhibition of DC activation and maturation [159]. It has been also previously demonstrated that apoptotic cells immunoregulate DCs by selective inhibition of the NF-κβ pathway, which regulates expression of several genes involved in DC activation and maturation, through signals mediated by MerTK [160]. Incubation of DCs prepared ex vivo from nonobese diabetic mice with apoptotic cells was shown to block secretion of proinflammatory cytokines, upregulation of costimulatory molecules, and T cell activation, leading to inhibition of DC activation and function. The inhibition of the suppressive factor MerTK in DCs may potentially be explored in the context of ex vivo DC-based vaccines. Therefore, inhibition of immunoregulatory pathways in DCs represents a plausible strategy to improve DC function, thus further enhancing cancer vaccine potency.

Enhancing DC and T Cell Interaction

As previously mentioned, $CD4^+$ T helper cells play a critical role in the induction of $CD8^+$ T cell immune responses [161]. Therefore, recruiting $CD4^+$ T helper cells at sites of $CD8^+$ T cell priming can potentially enhance CTL immune responses. This strategy has been utilized in several cancer vaccines in vivo in ex vivo. For example, a study by Nair et al. demonstrated the induction of $CD4^+$ T cells improved DC and T cell interaction by transfecting DCs with RNA encoding defined tumor antigens or tumor-derived RNA to introduce multiple tumor antigen epitopes into DCs. The authors demonstrated that DCs transfected with carcinoembryonic antigen (CEA) mRNA generated a potent CEA-specific $CD8^+$ cytotoxic T lymphocyte (CTL) response in vitro. They also found that DCs transfected with RNA encoding a chimeric CEA/LAMP-1 lysosomal targeting signal enhanced the induction of CEA-specific $CD4^+$ T cells, providing a strategy to induce T cell assistance [127, 128].

Another strategy to enhance the interaction between DCs and T cells is by eliminating the immunosuppressive T_{reg} cells and improving T cell priming. DCs loaded with antigen have been shown to efficiently expand T_{reg} cells in vitro [162]. This has been demonstrated in clinical studies wherein the injection of immature antigen-loaded DCs led to the specific inhibition of antigen-specific $CD8^+$ T cell effector function in freshly isolated T cells because of the presence of IL-10 secreting antigen-specific T_{reg} cells [163]. This indicates that the injection of antigen-loaded immature DCs ex vivo leads to the induction of antigen-specific regulatory $CD8^+$ T cells [164]. Thus, it is important to develop strategies to limit the generation of T_{reg} cells or inhibit the suppressive function of T_{reg} cells to enhance DC and T cell interaction [6, 165, 166]. A recent clinical trial showed that depletion of T_{reg} cells could significantly improve the tumor-specific T cell responses in cancer patients vaccinated with ex vivo generated DC-based vaccines [167].

Clinical Trials with Ex Vivo Generated DC-Based Vaccines

Several clinical trials have been conducted using ex vivo generated DC-based vaccines and generated mixed results [5, 6]. Many of these strategies employ different methods of generating the DCs and loading the antigens [168]. However, from the results of these trials, it is not clear if these DC-based vaccines represent an efficient strategy to induce protective and therapeutic immunity in cancer patients. A phase III trial in melanoma patients failed to demonstrate that DC-based vaccination provided a significant improvement in the therapeutic efficacy compared with conventional treatments. Nevertheless, several clinical studies using ex vivo generated DC-based vaccines have also shown promising results in enhancing the tumor-specific immune responses in cancer patients [137, 138, 167, 169]. Specifically, in a phase I study in patients with metastatic prostate cancer, autologous DCs transfected with mRNA encoding prostate-specific antigen (PSA) were shown to stimulate potent T cell-mediated antitumor immune responses in vitro [169]. Another study employing renal tumor RNA-transfected DCs demonstrated significant immunological and clinical responses in metastatic renal cancer patients [138]. Therefore, it is important to consider multiple factors while interpreting the results from clinical trials using DC-based vaccines.

Summary

It is important to continue to elucidate the biological functions of DCs. A better understanding of DC biology would create the opportunity for the development of innovative strategies to manipulate DCs in vivo or ex vivo to enhance cancer vaccine potency. Because many of these strategies to modify DCs may act by different mechanisms, it is conceivable that the future of cancer vaccine development likely requires the combination of various strategies for further enhancing cancer vaccine potency. For example, we have shown that the potency of a DNA vaccine combining an intracellular targeting strategy as well as a strategy to prolong the life of DCs can be further enhanced by addition of DNA that is capable of increasing $CD4^+$ T cell help [170]. Thus, the combination of several strategies represents a promising approach to enhance cancer vaccine potency.

As mentioned earlier, several clinical trials conducted using ex vivo-generated DC-based vaccines have generated mixed results. There are many explanations for the inconsistent outcomes. For example, there may be variations in the disease states of patients, formulation techniques for DCs, antigens loaded, route of administration of DCs, and the regimen for DC administration. All these factors may influence the efficacy of the DC-based vaccines. Among these factors, the effectiveness of antigen loading, processing and presentation, maturation of the DCs, and the homing and targeting of DCs to the appropriate microenvironment for T cell priming may prove to be the most crucial. Thus, it is important to consider these factors for the future development of ex vivo-generated DC-based vaccines.

Cancer vaccines employing strategies for in vivo targeting of DCs allow the antigen to be efficiently targeted to multiple DC subsets in the natural environment and at multiple sites. Furthermore, in vivo targeting of DCs involves an easier and cost-effective production that can be applied to a large number of patients. On the basis of these advantages, it is conceivable that future endeavors should also focus on the development of cancer vaccines employing in vivo targeting strategies for future clinical translation.

The therapeutic effects of vaccination may be further enhanced by their combination by blocking the factors that inhibit T cell activation, such as CTLA-4 and PD-1. These molecules are negative coregulators in the T cell costimulatory pathway. The antibody-mediated blockade of CTLA-4 and PD-1 can potentially be used to prolong antitumoral T cell responses [171, 172]. The combination of cancer vaccines with agents that influence the tumor microenvironment may also potentially be used to generate enhanced therapeutic effects against various cancers. It is clear that several factors present in the tumor microenvironment may potentially hinder immunotherapy. These factors include the expression of B7-H1 [173], STAT3 [174], and MIC-A and B [175], indoleamine 2,3-dioxygenase (IDO) enzyme [176], and galectin-1 [177] on tumor cells, immunosuppressive cytokines such as IL-10 [178] and TGF-β [179], T regulatory cells [180], and myeloid-derived suppressor cells [181]. It is conceivable that agents capable of blocking these molecules may be used to enhance cancer vaccine potency.

Treatment of established and advanced cancers would most likely require multimodality treatments that combine conventional cancer therapies including chemotherapy, radiation, or other biotherapeutic agents with antigen-specific immunotherapy to generate significant therapeutic effects. Furthermore, some chemotherapeutic agents and radiotherapy can lead to apoptosis or lysis of tumor cells, which can potentially boost the immune responses generated by therapeutic cancer vaccines. For example, pretreatment with the chemotherapeutic drug, cisplatin has been shown to enhance antigen-specific $CD8^+$ T cell-mediated antitumor immunity induced by DNA vaccination [47]. Studies combining therapeutic vaccines with anticancer agents have been shown to be effective in the treatment of several cancers [182, 183].

Acknowledgments We gratefully acknowledge Ms. Barbara Ma for assistance in preparation of the review. This review is not intended to be an encyclopedic one, and the authors apologize to those not cited. This work is supported by the NCI SPORE in Cervical Cancer P50 CA098252, NCI 1RO1 CA114425–01 and 1RO1 CA118790 and American Cancer Society (ACS).

References

1. Sznol, M., and Holmlund, J. (1997) Semin Oncol 24, 173
2. Steinman, R. M. (1991) Annu Rev Immunol 9, 271
3. Banchereau, J., Briere, F., Caux, C., Davoust, J., Lebecque, S., Liu, Y.J., Pulendran, B., and Palucka, K. (2000) Annu Rev Immunol 18, 767
4. Guermonprez, P., Valladeau, J., Zitvogel, L., Thery, C., and Amigorena, S. (2002) Annu Rev Immunol 20, 621
5. Gilboa, E. (2007) J Clin Investig 117, 1195
6. Palucka, A. K., Ueno, H., Fay, J. W., and Banchereau, J. (2007) Immunol Rev 220, 129
7. Markiewicz, M. A., and Kast, W. M. (2004) Cancer Invest 22, 417
8. Ribas, A. (2005) Curr Gene Ther 5, 619
9. Ribas, A., Butterfield, L. H., Glaspy, J. A., and Economou, J. S. (2002) Curr Gene Ther 2, 57
10. Tacken, P. J., de Vries, I. J., Torensma, R., and Figdor, C. G. (2007) Nat Rev 7, 790
11. Donnelly, J. J., Ulmer, J. B., Shiver, J. W., and Liu, M. A. (1997) Annu Rev Immunol 15, 617
12. Gurunathan, S., Klinman, D. M., and Seder, R. A. (2000) Annu Rev Immunol 18, 927
13. Payne, L. G., Fuller, D. H., and Haynes, J. R. (2002) Curr Opin Mol Ther 4, 459
14. Condon, C., Watkins, S. C., Celluzzi, C. M., Thompson, K., and Falo, L. D., Jr. (1996) Nat Med 2, 1122
15. Porgador, A., Irvine, K. R., Iwasaki, A., Barber, B. H., Restifo, N. P., and Germain, R. N. (1998) J Exp Med 188, 1075
16. Spaner, D. E., Astsaturov, I., Vogel, T., Petrella, T., Elias, I., Burdett-Radoux, S., Verma, S., Iscoe, N., Hamilton, P., and Berinstein, N. L. (2006) Cancer 106, 890
17. Jeglum, K. A., Mangan, C., and Wheeler, J. E. (1985) Cancer Drug Deliv 2, 127.
18. Maloy, K. J., Erdmann, I., Basch, V., Sierro, S., Kramps, T. A., Zinkernagel, R. M., Oehen, S., and Kundig, T. M. (2001) Proc Natl Acad Sci USA 98, 3299
19. Tagawa, S. T., Lee, P., Snively, J., Boswell, W., Ounpraseuth, S., Lee, S., Hickingbottom, B., Smith, J., Johnson, D., and Weber, J. S. (2003) Cancer 98, 144
20. Munoz-Montesino, C., Andrews, E., Rivers, R., Gonzalez-Smith, A., Moraga-Cid, G., Folch, H., Cespedes, S., and Onate, A. A. (2004) Infect Immun 72, 2081
21. Widera, G., Austin, M., Rabussay, D., Goldbeck, C., Barnett, S. W., Chen, M., Leung, L., Otten, G. R., Thudium, K., Selby, M. J., and Ulmer, J. B. (2000) J Immunol 164, 4635

22. Paster, W., Zehetner, M., Kalat, M., Schuller, S., and Schweighoffer, T. (2003) Gene Ther 10, 717
23. Kalat, M., Kupcu, Z., Schuller, S., Zalusky, D., Zehetner, M., Paster, W., and Schweighoffer, T. (2002) Cancer Res 62, 5489
24. Otten, G., Schaefer, M., Doe, B., Liu, H., Srivastava, I., zur Megede, J., O'Hagan, D., Donnelly, J., Widera, G., Rabussay, D., Lewis, M. G., Barnett, S., and Ulmer, J. B. (2004) Vaccine 22, 2489
25. Babiuk, S., Baca-Estrada, M. E., Foldvari, M., Storms, M., Rabussay, D., Widera, G., and Babiuk, L. A. (2002) Vaccine 20, 3399
26. Scheerlinck, J. P., Karlis, J., Tjelle, T. E., Presidente, P. J., Mathiesen, I., and Newton, S. E. (2004) Vaccine 22, 1820
27. Zhang, X., Divangahi, M., Ngai, P., Santosuosso, M., Millar, J., Zganiacz, A., Wang, J., Bramson, J., and Xing, Z. (2007) Vaccine 25, 1342
28. Hung, C. F., Hsu, K. F., Cheng, W. F., Chai, C. Y., He, L., Ling, M., and Wu, T. C. (2001) Cancer Res 61, 1080
29. Trimble, C., Lin, C. T., Hung, C. F., Pai, S., Juang, J., He, L., Gillison, M., Pardoll, D., Wu, L., and Wu, T. C. (2003) Vaccine 21, 4036
30. Hauser, H., and Chen, S. Y. (2003) Methods 31, 225
31. Hauser, H., Shen, L., Gu, Q. L., Krueger, S., and Chen, S. Y. (2004) Gene Ther 11, 924
32. Boyle, J. S., Brady, J. L., and Lew, A. M. (1998) Nature 392, 408
33. You, Z., Huang, X., Hester, J., Toh, H. C., and Chen, S. Y. (2001) Cancer Res 61, 3704
34. Elliott, G., and O'Hare, P. (1997) Cell 88, 223
35. Phelan, A., Elliott, G., and O'Hare, P. (1998) Nat Biotechnol 16, 440
36. Dilber, M. S., Phelan, A., Aints, A., Mohamed, A. J., Elliott, G., Smith, C. I., and O'Hare, P. (1999) Gene Ther 6, 12
37. Wybranietz, W. A., Gross, C. D., Phelan, A., O'Hare, P., Spiegel, M., Graepler, F., Bitzer, M., Stahler, P., Gregor, M., and Lauer, U. M. (2001) Gene Ther 8, 1654
38. Peng, S., Trimble, C., Ji, H., He, L., Tsai, Y.C., Macaes, B., Hung, C. F., and Wu, T. C. (2005) J Biomed Sci 12, 689
39. Saha, S., Yoshida, S., Ohba, K., Matsui, K., Matsuda, T., Takeshita, F., Umeda, K., Tamura, Y., Okuda, K., Klinman, D., Xin, K. Q., and Okuda, K. (2006) Virology 354, 48
40. Hung, C. F., Cheng, W. F., Chai, C. Y., Hsu, K. F., He, L., Ling, M., and Wu, T. C. (2001) J Immunol 166, 5733
41. Kim, T. W., Hung, C. F., Kim, J. W., Juang, J., Chen, P. J., He, L., Boyd, D. A., and Wu, T. C. (2004) Hum Gene Ther 15, 167
42. Harms, J. S., Ren, X., Oliveira, S. C., and Splitter, G. A. (2000) J Virol 74, 3301
43. Koptidesova, D., Kopacek, J., Zelnik, V., Ross, N. L., Pastorekova, S., and Pastorek, J. (1995) Arch Virol 140, 355
44. Dorange, F., El Mehdaoui, S., Pichon, C., Coursaget, P., and Vautherot, J. F. (2000) J Gen Virol 81, 2219
45. Mwangi, W., Brown, W. C., Splitter, G. A., Zhuang, Y., Kegerreis, K., and Palmer, G. H. (2005) J Leukoc Biol 78, 401
46. Kang, T. H., Lee, J. H., Song, C. K., Han, H. D., Shin, B. C., Pai, S. I., Hung, C. F., Trimble, C., Lim, J. S., Kim, T. W., and Wu, T. C. (2007) Cancer Res 67, 802
47. Tseng, C. W., Hung, C. F., Alvarez, R. D., Trimble, C., Huh, W. K., Kim, D., Chuang, C. M., Lin, C. T., Tsai, Y. C., He, L., Monie, A., and Wu, T. C. (2008) Clin Cancer Res 14, 3185
48. Lin, C. T., Tsai, Y. C., He, L., Calizo, R., Chou, H. H., Chang, T. C., Soong, Y. K., Hung, C. F., and Lai, C. H. (2006) J Biomed Sci 13, 481
49. Liu, W. J., Gao, F., Zhao, K. N., Zhao, W., Fernando, G. J., Thomas, R., and Frazer, I. H. (2002) Virology 301, 43
50. Yu, J. R., Kim, S., Lee, J. B., and Chang, J. (2008), J Virol 82, 2350
51. Cheng, W. F., Hung, C. F., Chai, C. Y., Hsu, K. F., He, L., Ling, M., and Wu, T. C. (2001) J Clin Investig 108, 669
52. Chen, C. H., Wang, T. L., Hung, C. F., Yang, Y., Young, R. A., Pardoll, D. M., and Wu, T. C. (2000) Cancer Res 60, 1035

53. Hung, C. F., Cheng, W. F., He, L., Ling, M., Juang, J., Lin, C. T., and Wu, T. C. (2003) Cancer Res 63, 2393
54. Hung, C. F., Cheng, W. F., Hsu, K. F., Chai, C. Y., He, L., Ling, M., and Wu, T. C. (2001) Cancer Res 61, 3698
55. Ciernik, I. F., Berzofsky, J. A., and Carbone, D. P. (1996) J Immunol 156, 2369
56. Kim, J. W., Hung, C. F., Juang, J., He, L., Kim, T. W., Armstrong, D. K., Pai, S. I., Chen, P. J., Lin, C. T., Boyd, D. A., and Wu, T. C. (2004) Gene Ther 11, 1011
57. Castellino, F., and Germain, R. N. (2006) Annu Rev Immunol 24, 519
58. Wu, T.-C., Guarnieri, F. G., Staveley-O'Carroll, K. F., Viscidi, R. P., Levitsky, H. I., Hedrick, L., Cho, K. R., August, T., and Pardoll, D. M. (1995) Proc Natl Acad Sci 92, 11671
59. Ji, H., Wang, T.-L., Chen, C.-H., Hung, C.-F., Pai, S., Lin, K.-Y., Kurman, R. J., Pardoll, D. M., and Wu, T.-C. T (1999) Hum Gene Ther 10, 2727
60. de Arruda, L. B., Chikhlikar, P. R., August, J. T., and Marques, E. T. (2004) Immunology 112, 126
61. Cresswell, P. (1994) Annu Rev Immunol 12, 259
62. Trombetta, E. S., and Mellman, I. (2005) Annu Rev Immunol 23, 975
63. Fujii, S., Senju, S., Chen, Y. Z., Ando, M., Matsushita, S., and Nishimura, Y. (1998) Hum Immunol 59, 607
64. Malcherek, G., Wirblich, C., Willcox, N., Rammensee, H. G., Trowsdale, J., and Melms, A. (1998) Eur J Immunol 28, 1524
65. Nagata, T., Higashi, T., Aoshi, T., Suzuki, M., Uchijima, M., and Koide, Y. (2001) Vaccine 20, 105
66. Hung, C. F., Tsai, Y. C., He, L., and Wu, T. C. (2007) Mol Ther 15, 1211
67. Primeau, T., Myers, N. B., Yu, Y. Y., Lybarger, L., Wang, X., Truscott, S. M., Hansen, T. H., and Connolly, J. M. (2005) Immunol Res 32, 109
68. Huang, C. H., Peng, S., He, L., Tsai, Y. C., Boyd, D. A., Hansen, T. H., Wu, T. C., and Hung, C. F. (2005) Gene Ther 12, 1180
69. Hung, C. F., Calizo, R., Tsai, Y. C., He, L., and Wu, T. C. (2007) Vaccine 25, 127
70. Iwasaki, A., and Medzhitov, R. (2004) Nat Immunol 5, 987
71. Aderem, A., and Ulevitch, R. J. T (2000) Nature 406, 782.
72. Akira, S., and Takeda, K. (2004) Nat Rev 4, 499
73. Hemmi, H., Takeuchi, O., Kawai, T., Kaisho, T., Sato, S., Sanjo, H., Matsumoto, M., Hoshino, K., Wagner, H., Takeda, K., and Akira, S. (2000) Nature 408, 740
74. Hartmann, G., Weiner, G. J., and Krieg, A. M. (1999) Proc Natl Acad Sci USA 96, 9305
75. Klinman, D. M., Yamshchikov, G., and Ishigatsubo, Y. (1997) J Immunol 158, 3635
76. Coban, C., Ishii, K. J., Gursel, M., Klinman, D. M., and Kumar, N. (2005) J Leukoc Biol 78, 647
77. Zhang, A., Jin, H., Zhang, F., Ma, Z., Tu, Y., Ren, Z., Zhang, X., Zhu, K., and Wang, B. (2005) DNA Cell Biol 24, 292
78. Kojima, Y., Xin, K. Q., Ooki, T., Hamajima, K., Oikawa, T., Shinoda, K., Ozaki, T., Hoshino, Y., Jounai, N., Nakazawa, M., Klinman, D., and Okuda, K. (2002) Vaccine 20, 2857
79. Ulrich, J. T., and Myers, K. R. (1995) Pharm Biotechnol 6, 495
80. Baldridge, J. R., McGowan, P., Evans, J. T., Cluff, C., Mossman, S., Johnson, D., and Persing, D. (2004) Expert Opin Biol Ther 4, 1129
81. Sasaki, S., Tsuji, T., Hamajima, K., Fukushima, J., Ishii, N., Kaneko, T., Xin, K. Q., Mohri, H., Aoki, I., Okubo, T., Nishioka, K., and Okuda, K. (1997) Infect Immun 65, 3520
82. Hemmi, H., Kaisho, T., Takeuchi, O., Sato, S., Sanjo, H., Hoshino, K., Horiuchi, T., Tomizawa, H., Takeda, K., and Akira, S. (2002) Nat Immunol 3, 196
83. Schon, M. P., and Schon, M. (2004) Apoptosis 9, 291
84. Thomsen, L. L., Topley, P., Daly, M. G., Brett, S. J., and Tite, J. P. (2004) Vaccine 22, 1799
85. Smorlesi, A., Papalini, F., Orlando, F., Donnini, A., Re, F., and Provinciali, M. (2005) Gene Ther 12, 1324
86. Zuber, A. K., Brave, A., Engstrom, G., Zuber, B., Ljungberg, K., Fredriksson, M., Benthin, R., Isaguliants, M. G., Sandstrom, E., Hinkula, J., and Wahren, B. (2004) Vaccine 22, 1791

87. Otero, M., Calarota, S. A., Felber, B., Laddy, D., Pavlakis, G., Boyer, J. D., and Weiner, D. B. (2004) Vaccine 22, 1782
88. Takeshita, F., Tanaka, T., Matsuda, T., Tozuka, M., Kobiyama, K., Saha, S., Matsui, K., Ishii, K. J., Coban, C., Akira, S., Ishii, N., Suzuki, K., Klinman, D. M., Okuda, K., and Sasaki, S. (2006) J Virol 80, 6218
89. Dow, S. W., Fradkin, L. G., Liggitt, D. H., Willson, A. P., Heath, T. D., and Potter, T. A. (1999) J Immunol 163, 1552
90. U'Ren, L., Kedl, R., and Dow, S. (2006) Cancer Gene Ther 13, 1033
91. Gagliardi, M. C., Sallusto, F., Marinaro, M., Langenkamp, A., and Lanzavecchia, A. (2000) Eur J Immunol 30, 2394
92. Martin, M., Sharpe, A., Clements, J. D., and Michalek, S. M. (2002) J Immunol 169, 1744
93. Bagley, K. C., Abdelwahab, S. F., Tuskan, R. G., Fouts, T. R., and Lewis, G. K. (2002) Infect Immun 70, 5533
94. Rappuoli, R., Pizza, M., Douce, G., and Dougan, G. (1999) Immunol Today 20, 493
95. Williams, N. A., Hirst, T. R., and Nashar, T. O. (1999) Immunol Today 20, 95
96. Holmgren, J., Adamsson, J., Anjuere, F., Clemens, J., Czerkinsky, C., Eriksson, K., Flach, C. F., George-Chandy, A., Harandi, A. M., Lebens, M., Lehner, T., Lindblad, M., Nygren, E., Raghavan, S., Sanchez, J., Stanford, M., Sun, J. B., Svennerholm, A. M., and Tengvall, S. (2005) Immunol Lett 97, 181
97. Arrington, J., Braun, R. P., Dong, L., Fuller, D. H., Macklin, M. D., Umlauf, S. W., Wagner, S. J., Wu, M. S., Payne, L. G., and Haynes, J. R. (2002) J Virol 76, 4536
98. Endo, T. A., Masuhara, M., Yokouchi, M., Suzuki, R., Sakamoto, H., Mitsui, K., Matsumoto, A., Tanimura, S., Ohtsubo, M., Misawa, H., Miyazaki, T., Leonor, N., Taniguchi, T., Fujita, T., Kanakura, Y., Komiya, S., and Yoshimura, A. (1997) Nature 387, 921
99. Alexander, W. S. (2002) Nat Rev 2, 410
100. Song, X. T., Evel-Kabler, K., Rollins, L., Aldrich, M., Gao, F., Huang, X. F., and Chen, S. Y. (2006) PLoS Med 3, 11
101. Lori, F., Weiner, D. B., Calarota, S. A., Kelly, L. M., and Lisziewicz, J. (2006) Springer Semin Immunopathol 28, 231
102. Laddy, D. J., and Weiner, D. B. (2006) Int Rev Immunol 25, 99
103. Kim, T. W., Hung, C. F., Ling, M., Juang, J., He, L., Hardwick, J. M., Kumar, S., and Wu, T. C. (2003) J Clin Investig 112, 109
104. Kim, T. W., Lee, J. H., He, L., Boyd, D. A., Hardwick, J. M., Hung, C. F., and Wu, T. C. (2005) Cancer Res 65, 309
105. Panina-Bordignon, P., Tan, A., Termijtelen, A., Demotz, S., Corradin, G., and Lanzavecchia, A. (1989) Eur J Immunol 19, 2237
106. Rice, J., Elliott, T., Buchan, S., and Stevenson, F. K. (2001) J Immunol 167, 1558
107. Rice, J., Buchan, S., and Stevenson, F. K. (2002) J Immunol 169, 3908
108. Rice, J., Buchan, S., Dewchand, H., Simpson, E., and Stevenson, F. K. (2004) J Immunol 173, 4492
109. Belkaid, Y., and Rouse, B. T. (2005) Nat Immunol 6, 353
110. Beyer, M., and Schultze, J. L. (2006) Blood 108, 804
111. Toka, F. N., Suvas, S., and Rouse, B. T. (2004) J Virol 78, 13082
112. Cohen, N., Mouly, E., Hamdi, H., Maillot, M. C., Pallardy, M., Godot, V., Capel, F., Balian, A., Naveau, S., Galanaud, P., Lemoine, F. M., and Emilie, D. (2006) Blood 107, 2037
113. Nair, S., Boczkowski, D., Fassnacht, M., Pisetsky, D., and Gilboa, E. (2007) Cancer Res 67, 371
114. Fong, C. L., Mok, C. L., and Hui, K. M. (2006) Gene Ther 13, 245
115. Nayak, B. P., Sailaja, G., and Jabbar, A. M. (2006) Virology 348, 277
116. Sumida, S. M., McKay, P. F., Truitt, D. M., Kishko, M. G., Arthur, J. C., Seaman, M. S., Jackson, S. S., Gorgone, D. A., Lifton, M. A., Letvin, N. L., and Barouch, D. H. (2004) J Clin Investig 114, 1334
117. Rabinovich, G. A., Gabrilovich, D., and Sotomayor, E. M. (2007) Annu Rev Immunol 25, 267
118. Sallusto, F., and Lanzavecchia, A. (1994) J Exp Med 179, 1109

119. Romani, N., Gruner, S., Brang, D., Kampgen, E., Lenz, A., Trockenbacher, B., Konwalinka, G., Fritsch, P. O., Steinman, R. M., and Schuler, G. (1994) J Exp Med 180, 83
120. Caux, C., Dezutter-Dambuyant, C., Schmitt, D., and Banchereau, J. (1992) Nature, 360, 258
121. Strunk, D., Rappersberger, K., Egger, C., Strobl, H., Kromer, E., Elbe, A., Maurer, D., and Stingl, G. (1996) Blood, 87, 1292
122. Szabolcs, P., Moore, M. A., and Young, J. W. E. (1995) J Immunol 154, 5851
123. Steinman, R. M., and Dhodapkar, M. (2001) Int J Cancer 94, 459
124. Zwaveling, S., Ferreira Mota, S. C., Nouta, J., Johnson, M., Lipford, G. B., Offringa, R., van der Burg, S. H., and Melief, C. J. (2002) J Immunol 169, 350
125. Regnault, A., Lankar, D., Lacabanne, V., Rodriguez, A., Thery, C., Rescigno, M., Saito, T., Verbeek, S., Bonnerot, C., Ricciardi-Castagnoli, P., and Amigorena, S. (1999) J Exp Med 189, 371
126. Boczkowski, D., Nair, S. K., Snyder, D., and Gilboa, E. (1996) J Exp Med 184, 465
127. Nair, S. K., Boczkowski, D., Morse, M., Cumming, R. I., Lyerly, H. K., and Gilboa, E. (1998) Nat Biotechnol 16, 364
128. Nair, S. K., Hull, S., Coleman, D., Gilboa, E., Lyerly, H. K., and Morse, M. A. (1999) Int J Cancer 82, 121
129. Brown, K., Gao, W., Alber, S., Trichel, A., Murphey-Corb, M., Watkins, S. C., Gambotto, A., and Barratt-Boyes, S. M. (2003) J Immunol 171, 6875
130. Berard, F., Blanco, P., Davoust, J., Neidhart-Berard, E. M., Nouri-Shirazi, M., Taquet, N., Rimoldi, D., Cerottini, J. C., Banchereau, J., and Palucka, A. K. (2000) J Exp Med 192, 1535
131. Albert, M. L., Sauter, B., and Bhardwaj, N. (1998) Nature 392, 86
132. Ferrone, C. R., Perales, M. A., Goldberg, S. M., Somberg, C. J., Hirschhorn-Cymerman, D., Gregor, P. D., Turk, M. J., Ramirez-Montagut, T., Gold, J. S., Houghton, A. N., and Wolchok, J. D. (2006) Clin Cancer Res 12, 5511
133. Gilboa, E. (1999) Immunity 11, 263
134. Wang, R. F., and Rosenberg, S. A. (1999) Immunol Rev 170, 85
135. Vambutas, A., DeVoti, J., Nouri, M., Drijfhout, J. W., Lipford, G. B., Bonagura, V. R., van der Burg, S. H., and Melief, C. J. (2005) Vaccine 23, 5271
136. Gilboa, E., and Vieweg, J. (2004) Immunol Rev 199, 251
137. Su, Z., Dannull, J., Yang, B. K., Dahm, P., Coleman, D., Yancey, D., Sichi, S., Niedzwiecki, D., Boczkowski, D., Gilboa, E., and Vieweg, J. (2005) J Immunol 174, 3798
138. Su, Z., Dannull, J., Heiser, A., Yancey, D., Pruitt, S., Madden, J., Coleman, D., Niedzwiecki, D., Gilboa, E., and Vieweg, J. (2003) Cancer Res 63, 2127
139. Shi, H., Cao, T., Connolly, J. E., Monnet, L., Bennett, L., Chapel, S., Bagnis, C., Mannoni, P., Davoust, J., Palucka, A. K., and Banchereau, J. (2006) J Immunol 176, 2134
140. Busch, D. H., Kerksiek, K. M., and Pamer, E. G. (2000) J Immunol 164, 4063
141. Bachmann, M. F., Beerli, R. R., Agnellini, P., Wolint, P., Schwarz, K., and Oxenius, A. (2006) Eur J Immunol 36, 842
142. Figdor, C. G., de Vries, I. J., Lesterhuis, W. J., and Melief, C. J. (2004) Nat Med 10, 475
143. Verdijk, P., Aarntzen, E. H., Punt, C. J., de Vries, I. J., and Figdor, C. G. (2008) Expert Opin Biol Ther 8, 865
144. De Vries, I. J., Krooshoop, D. J., Scharenborg, N. M., Lesterhuis, W. J., Diepstra, J. H., Van Muijen, G. N., Strijk, S. P., Ruers, T. J., Boerman, O. C., Oyen, W. J., Adema, G. J., Punt, C. J., and Figdor, C. G. (2003) Cancer Res 63, 12
145. Morse, M. A., Coleman, R. E., Akabani, G., Niehaus, N., Coleman, D., and Lyerly, H. K. (1999) Cancer Res 59, 56
146. MartIn-Fontecha, A., Sebastiani, S., Hopken, U. E., Uguccioni, M., Lipp, M., Lanzavecchia, A., and Sallusto, F. (2003) J Exp Med 198, 615
147. Kang, T. H., Lee, J. H., Bae, H. C., Noh, K. H., Kim, J. H., Song, C. K., Shin, B. C., Hung, C. F., Wu, T. C., Park, J. S., and Kim, T. W. (2006) Immunol Lett 106, 126
148. Figdor, C. (2008) Cancer Immunology, Immunotherapy, 57 (suppl 1), S5

149. Lesimple, T., Neidhard, E. M., Vignard, V., Lefeuvre, C., Adamski, H., Labarriere, N., Carsin, A., Monnier, D., Collet, B., Clapisson, G., Birebent, B., Philip, I., Toujas, L., Chokri, M., and Quillien, V. (2006) Clin Cancer Res 12, 7380
150. Fong, L., Brockstedt, D., Benike, C., Wu, L., and Engleman, E. G. (2001) J Immunol 166, 4254
151. Leifert, J. A., Rodriguez-Carreno, M. P., Rodriguez, F., and Whitton, J. L. (2004) Immunol Rev 199, 40
152. Reis e Sousa, C. (2004) Curr Opin Immunol 16, 21
153. Warger, T., Osterloh, P., Rechtsteiner, G., Fassbender, M., Heib, V., Schmid, B., Schmitt, E., Schild, H., and Radsak, M. P. (2006) Blood 108, 544
154. Blander, J. M., and Medzhitov, R. (2004) Science 304, 1014
155. Blander, J. M., and Medzhitov, R. (2006) Nat Immunol 7, 1029
156. Dannull, J., Nair, S., Su, Z., Boczkowski, D., DeBeck, C., Yang, B., Gilboa, E., and Vieweg, J. (2005) Blood 105, 3206
157. Gilboa, E. (2004) Nat Biotechnol 22, 1521
158. Shen, L., Evel-Kabler, K., Strube, R., and Chen, S. Y. (2004) Nat Biotechnol 22, 1546
159. Wallet, M. A., Sen, P., Flores, R. R., Wang, Y., Yi, Z., Huang, Y., Mathews, C. E., Earp, H. S., Matsushima, G., Wang, B., and Tisch, R. (2008) J Exp Med 205, 219
160. Sen, P., Wallet, M. A., Yi, Z., Huang, Y., Henderson, M., Mathews, C. E., Earp, H. S., Matsushima, G., Baldwin, A. S., Jr., and Tisch, R. M. (2007) Blood 109, 653
161. Porgador, A., Snyder, D., and Gilboa, E. (1996) J Immunol 156, 2918
162. Steinman, R. M., Hawiger, D., and Nussenzweig, M. C. (2003) Annu Rev Immunol 21, 685
163. Dhodapkar, M. V., Steinman, R. M., Krasovsky, J., Munz, C., and Bhardwaj, N. (2001) J Exp Med 193, 233
164. Dhodapkar, M. V., and Steinman, R. M. (2002) Blood 100, 174
165. Baecher-Allan, C., and Anderson, D. E. (2006) Curr Opin Immunol 18, 214
166. Zou, W. (2005) Nat Rev Cancer 5, 263
167. Dannull, J., Su, Z., Rizzieri, D., Yang, B. K., Coleman, D., Yancey, D., Zhang, A., Dahm, P., Chao, N., Gilboa, E., and Vieweg, J. (2005) J Clin Investig 115, 3623
168. Cranmer, L. D., Trevor, K. T., and Hersh, E. M. (2004) Cancer Immunol Immunother 53, 275
169. Heiser, A., Coleman, D., Dannull, J., Yancey, D., Maurice, M. A., Lallas, C. D., Dahm, P., Niedzwiecki, D., Gilboa, E., and Vieweg, J. (2002) J Clin Investig 109, 409
170. Kim, D., Hoory, T., Wu, T. C., and Hung, C. F. (2007) Hum Gene Ther 18, 575
171. Peggs, K. S., Quezada, S. A., Korman, A. J., and Allison, J. P. (2006) Curr Opin Immunol 18, 206
172. Blank, C., and Mackensen, A. (2007) Cancer Immunol Immunother 56, 739
173. Goldberg, M. V., Maris, C. H., Hipkiss, E. L., Flies, A. S., Zhen, L., Tuder, R. M., Grosso, J. F., Harris, T. J., Getnet, D., Whartenby, K. A., Brockstedt, D. G., Dubensky, T. W., Jr., Chen, L., Pardoll, D. M., Drake, C. G. Blood, 110, 186.
174. Yu, H., Kortylewski, M., and Pardoll, D. (2007) Nat Rev 7, 41
175. Groh, V., Wu, J., Yee, C., and Spies, T. (2002) Nature 419, 734
176. Munn, D. H., and Mellor, A. L. (2004) Trends Mol Med 10, 15
177. Rubinstein, N., Alvarez, M., Zwirner, N. W., Toscano, M. A., Ilarregui, J. M., Bravo, A., Mordoh, J., Fainboim, L., Podhajcer, O. L., and Rabinovich, G. A. (2004) Cancer Cell 5, 241
178. Yue, F. Y., Dummer, R., Geertsen, R., Hofbauer, G., Laine, E., Manolio, S., and Burg, G. (1997) Int J Cancer 71, 630
179. Gorelik, L., and Flavell, R. A. (2001) Nat Med 7, 1118
180. Curiel, T. J., Coukos, G., Zou, L., Alvarez, X., Cheng, P., Mottram, P., Evdemon-Hogan, M., Conejo-Garcia, J. R., Zhang, L., Burow, M., Zhu, Y., Wei, S., Kryczek, I., Daniel, B., Gordon, A., Myers, L., Lackner, A., Disis, M. L., Knutson, K. L., Chen, L., and Zou, W. (2004) Nat Med 10, 942
181. Nagaraj, S., Gupta, K., Pisarev, V., Kinarsky, L., Sherman, S., Kang, L., Herber, D. L., Schneck, J., and Gabrilovich, D. I. (2007) Nat Med 13, 828
182. Emens, L. A. (2008) Front Biosci 13, 249

183. Emens, L. A., Reilly, R. T., and Jaffee, E. M. (2005) Cancer Treat Res 123, 227
184. Cohen, A. D., Diab, A., Perales, M. A., Wolchok, J. D., Rizzuto, G., Merghoub, T., Huggins, D., Liu, C., Turk, M. J., Restifo, N. P., Sakaguchi, S., and Houghton, A. N. (2006) Cancer Res 66, 4904
185. Schaft, N., Dorrie, J., Thumann, P., Beck, V. E., Muller, I., Schultz, E. S., Kampgen, E., Dieckmann, D., and Schuler, G. (2005) J Immunol 174, 3087
186. Obeid, M., Tesniere, A., Ghiringhelli, F., Fimia, G. M., Apetoh, L., Perfettini, J. L., Castedo, M., Mignot, G., Panaretakis, T., Casares, N., Metivier, D., Larochette, N., van Endert, P., Ciccosanti, F., Piacentini, M., Zitvogel, L., and Kroemer, G. (2007) Nat Med 13, 54

Dendritic Cell Vaccines for Immunotherapy of Cancer: Challenges in Clinical Trials

Lazar Vujanovic and Lisa H. Butterfield

Abstract Dendritic cells (DCs) are potent activators of immunity. After years of careful laboratory research and painstaking work to define cell culture parameters that allow these cells to be expanded from precursors in vitro, DCs have been tested clinically. Over the last decade, they have demonstrated a clear ability to prime and boost immunity to foreign and self antigens in vitro and in vivo. Clinical trials have also indicated that DC-based vaccines can be effective in promoting clinically relevant antitumor immunity in a small percentage of cancer patients, but these important cells must be better understood for their full clinical potential to be realized.

Introduction

Dendritic cells are the key physiological stimulators for priming naïve cells against specific antigens [1–3]. When an antigen is presented by a sufficiently matured DC with high expression levels of major histocompatibility complex (MHC) class I and II, costimulatory (CD80, CD86) and adhesion molecules (CD54) to deliver a "second signal" and promote stimulatory cytokine and chemokine production [1, 4–7], T cells are optimally activated to mount a protective, cytotoxic response against that antigen. This is in contrast to suboptimal antigen presentation that occurs in an environment lacking adequate costimulation or in a suppressive milieu, such as antigens presented directly by cancer cells, when T cell tolerance or anergy occurs. Utilizing the superior T cell stimulation capacity of different types of activated myeloid DCs has generated clinically relevant responses in human subjects with

L.H. Butterfield (✉)
Department of Medicine, Division of Hematology/Oncology, University of Pittsburgh Cancer Institute
Department of Surgery and Immunology, Research Pavilion, Rm 1.32d, 5117 Centre Avenue, University of Pittsburgh, Pittsburgh, PA, 15213
e-mail: butterfieldl@upmc.edu

J. Lustgarten et al. (eds.), *Targeted Cancer Immune Therapy*,
DOI 10.1007/978-1-4419-0170-5_9, © Springer Science+Business Media, LLC 2009

low grade lymphoma, multiple myeloma, advanced malignant melanoma, and prostate cancer [8–11].

Preclinical Experience of DC-Based Cancer Vaccines and Therapies

The field of tumor immunology has increasingly focused on ways to define, improve, and sustain T cell-mediated immunity to effectively prevent or control tumor development and progression. With the identification of human tumor-associated antigens (TAA) and MHC class I-restricted peptide epitopes subsequently presented to $CD8^+$ T cells, the molecular targets of immune reactivity are clearer. Multiple active specific immunotherapy (e.g., immunization with specific TAA) strategies have been employed, and utilizing the innate adjuvant properties (antigen uptake, processing, and presentation) of autologous DCs appears to be the most effective antigen presentation agent for the priming and maintenance of TAA-specific responses [1, 12, 13].

There are three criteria that are believed to be required for effective antitumor therapy: (1) the ability to activate and expand a sufficient number of high-avidity effector T cells that are capable of recognizing tumor cells; (2) the ability to support the effective trafficking and recruitment of immune cells into tumor lesions, and (3) the ability to maintain antitumor effector or memory cells for an extended period of time. Meeting these three requirements allows the robust recruitment of activated antitumor effectors from the lymph nodes and blood into tumor deposits to eradicate the tumor cells and maintain a population of memory cells available to respond to other metastases. The key to these effects is an increased "type 1" response. The type 1 response is generally characterized by "Th1" and "Tc1." Th1 consists of a $CD4^+$ helper T cell functional phenotype assumed to include the cytokine secretion of interferon (IFN)-γ and interleukin (IL)-2 that supports cytotoxic T cell and natural killer (NK) cell activity, while Tc1 has a functional phenotype of $CD8^+$ T cells (involving the same cytokines) that also possesses cytotoxicity. This is in contrast to a "type 2" response in which the cytokines produced (IL-4, IL-5) support B cells and humoral immunity. Type 1 responses have been associated with spontaneous and therapy-induced regression of tumor lesions [14, 15]. Dendritic cell-based therapies should stimulate high avidity T cells to increase the response to low levels of peptide/MHC complex on the tumor cell surface and Th1 T cell responders capable of mobilizing to the tumor microenvironment that appropriately respond to the disease. To achieve this, DCs need to be sufficiently mature and secrete a dominant balance of Th1-polarizing cytokines to override the inhibitory effects of the tumor microenvironment, such as IL-10 and transforming growth factor (TGF)-β production [13, 16].

A number of DC-based approaches have been tested in vitro and in animal models to evaluate the potential clinical value of DCs. These strategies differ in the source of DCs (directly isolated from blood or solid tumor, monocyte-derived, bone-marrow-derived, $CD34^+$ hematopoietic precursor-derived), type of tumors, TAA(s) targeted, method of antigen loading to DCs (Fig. 1), method of gene introduction

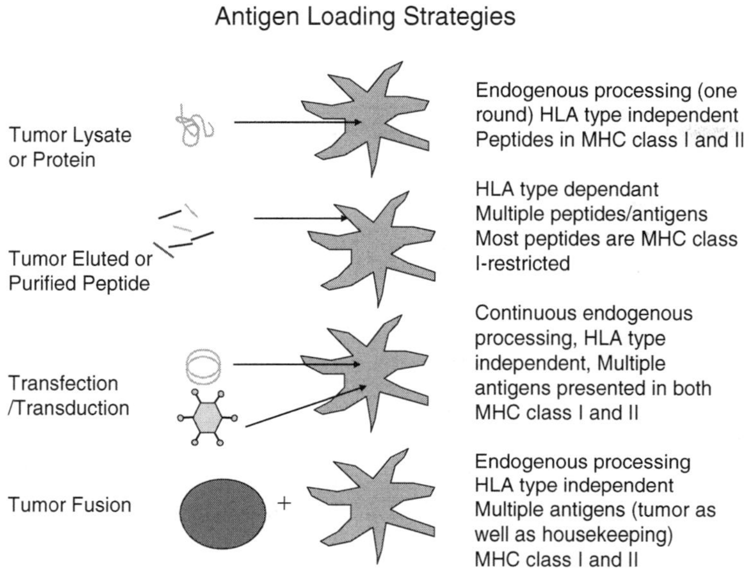

Fig. 1 Antigen loading strategies for DC-based vaccines, and the processing and presentation considerations for each

(e.g., recombinant, retroviral or adenoviral vectors, plasmid transfection, gene gun), and DC maturation stimuli (e.g., cytokines, CpG motifs, microbial membrane motifs). Many of these strategies have shown promise for treating or preventing cancer.

There are several critical differences between promising preclinical results, especially DC studies in murine models, and their translation to the clinic. These include the immunological differences between murine DC studies and those utilizing human cells. First, the cellular sources for DCs are different: murine studies generally prepare DCs from bone marrow aspirates or from splenocytes. These tissues are a source of monocytes that are generally matured in vitro in cultures in the presence of granulocyte macrophage colony-stimulating factor (GM-CSF) and murine IL-4, but the DCs derived from each of these sources are different from the most commonly used human sources: $CD14^+$ peripheral blood monocytes or $CD34^+$ hematopoietic progenitor cells (Fig. 2). Another critical difference is the expression pattern of the toll-like receptor 9 (TLR9). Murine DCs, as in humans, can be separated into two major subsets, myeloid-derived and plasmacytoid DCs (major producers of interferon in response to viral infection). In mice, both types express TLR9 and are capable of responding to stimulatory DNA sequences containing CpG motifs that are highly expressed primarily in nonmammalian DNA. Conversely, in humans, only plasmacytoid DCs express TLR9 and, thus, only they respond to DNA oligonucleotide adjuvant. There are also differences in TLR2 and TLR3 expression patterns, Th1/Th2 predominance determined by IFNα and IL-10 as well as CD1 family genes and their expression [17].

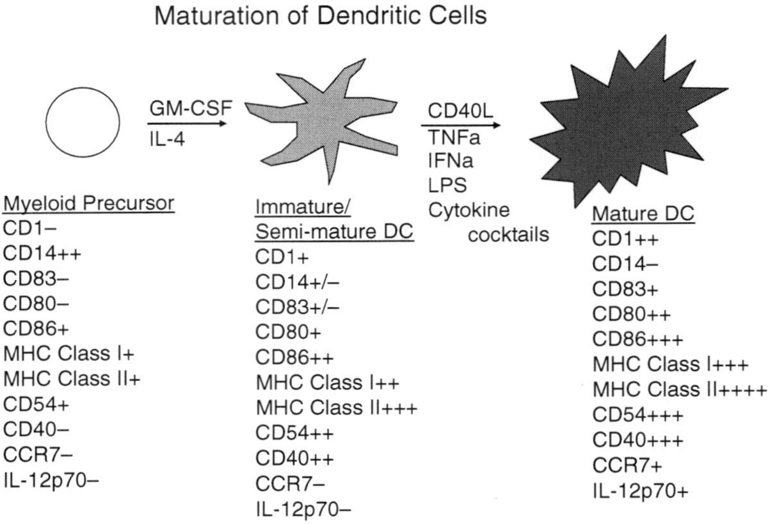

Fig. 2 The cell surface phenotype of human myeloid DC, differentiated in vitro from CD14^{+} loosely adherent monocytic precursors in the presence of GM-CSF and IL-4. Many different reagents are used to mature the DC to different levels with different functional properties

Dendritic cells are exquisitely sensitive to environmental stimuli and their responses to these cues impact the resultant immune response. This sensitivity also impacts the translation of promising in vitro research to clinical testing. They can respond to seemingly subtle cues such as the type of plastic used in a cell culture adherence step and exposure to the culture bags preferred for "closed systems" used in clinical trials. The fetal bovine serum (FBS) often used in preclinical human and murine model cultures is a rich source of foreign antigens. The "reagent grade" FBS used for research laboratory experiments cannot be used in clinical trial "good manufacturing practice" (GMP) compliant procedures (due to the level of endotoxin, a potent DC stimulator), source country (due to Bovine Spongiform Encephalopathy concerns), and lack of full characterization. Most clinical trials for DCs utilize serum-free media, often yielding a DC that differs phenotypically and functionally from the DCs used in preclinical studies.

Shared Antigens

Most DC-based clinical trials load DCs with tumor antigens to restrict the immune responses to be against the tumor. An alternative method is to inject DCs directly into accessible tumor deposits. The T cell repertoire includes cells specific to many self antigens, but these specific T cell precursors are maintained at very low frequencies, often in an anergic or ignorant state [18–20]. When antigens are presented in an immunostimulatory environment, immune effectors specific for the presented antigens can be activated and an immune response can be initiated [21, 22]. The variety of shared TAAs, originally identified in melanoma, but increasingly identified in tumors of other histologies, allows for defined vaccines and careful immunological analysis of tumor responses. Tumors also express "private" or patient-specific antigens that are often mutated (e.g., *Ras* [23], *bcr/abl* rearrangement [24] or *p53* [25, 26]) and may be substantially more potent immunological targets. Exposure to nonmutated self antigens can adversely affect the repertoire of specific T cells (peripheral tolerance) as a normal mechanism to suppress autoimmunity. Mutated antigens may be recognized by a separate population of T cells from their normal counterparts. A strategy utilizing private antigens necessitates either extensive molecular characterization of tumors that is not currently feasible for more than a few subjects, or immunization with complex, uncharacterized tumor-based vaccines such as tumor fusion with DCs, tumor lysate-pulsed DCs, or eluted peptide-pulsed DCs. While this is a promising approach, dissection of antigen-specific immune responses during the study of a vaccine response is problematic. Clinical testing of these shared antigens has led to complete objective clinical responses supporting their use [10, 27–31].

Tumor-Associated Antigen Classification

According to the pattern of expression in neoplastic and normal tissues, TAAs can be classified into four major categories (Table 1). The first category is cancer-testis antigens. These are proteins encoded by genes expressed in various tumors but not in normal tissues other than testis and placenta. Antigens that belong to this group include MAGE, GAGE, and BAGE families, as well as NY-ESO-1 and its alternative ORF products LAGE and CAMEL. The second group represents differentiation or lineage antigens shared between tumors and the normal tissue from which the tumor arose. Most described to date are expressed in melanoma and normal

Table 1 Summary of tumor antigen categories

TAA categories	Antigen characteristic	Genes
Cancer-testis	Expressed in various tumors but not normal tissues except in testis and placenta	MAGE, GAGE, BAGE, NY-ESO-1
Differentiation	Antigens shared between tumors and normal tissues from which they arose	Tyrosinase, Melan-A/MART-1, gp100, TRP-1, and TRP-2; PSA, AFP
Tumor-specific	Antigens generated by point mutations or splicing aberrations in ubiquitous genes	p53, Ras, CDK4, b-catenin, TRP-2/INT2
Widely occurring over-expressed	Proteins over-expressed in histologically different types of tumors	Survivin, MUC1/2, and EphA2

melanocytes, such as tyrosinase, Melan-A/MART-1, gp100, TRP-1, and TRP-2. The third category is tumor-specific antigens. These antigens are generated by point mutations (e.g., p53, Ras, CDK4, *b*-catenin) [32, 33] or tumor-specific splicing aberrations in genes that are ubiquitously expressed (e.g., TRP-2/INT2), and are expressed only in tumors where they were identified (unlike cancer-testis antigens). These molecular changes are associated with neoplastic transformation or progression. The fourth group of antigens is a widely expressed, over-produced TAA. These are proteins that have been detected in different types of tumors, often with no preferential expression by a certain type of cancer, as well as in many normal tissues generally with lower expression levels. Some of the antigens belonging to this group include survivin, MUC1/2, and EphA2.

Peptide-Based Vaccines

The identification of specific peptide epitopes that bind to MHC molecules has allowed the delivery of tumor antigens as synthetic peptides pulsed onto DCs. This has allowed for testing of the activation of specific subsets of $CD8^+$ T cells using inexpensive and quickly synthesized reagents, which has resulted in clinical responses [34]. The principal limitations of peptide-based immunotherapies are clear. In most cases, only a limited number of peptide epitopes have been described and are restricted to the most common human leukocyte antigen (HLA) alleles; therefore, they are only applicable to a subset of potentially treatable patients. This limits patient eligibility (e.g., 40% of Caucasians in North America express the most common allele, HLA-A2) and only provides for oligoclonal, MHC class I-driven, $CD8^+$ T cell responses. The definition of MHC class II-restricted epitopes designed to activate $CD4^+$ T cells has proven to be more cumbersome.

Protein-Loaded and Antigen-Engineered DCS

Dendritic cells loaded or transfected with tumor antigen proteins or genes by DNA or RNA transfection, or transduced with TAA-expressing recombinant viruses, are capable of processing and expressing peptide epitopes in the context of MHC class I and II. Protein loaded DCs take advantage of the natural phagocytic ability of immature DCs and their efficient uptake of exogenous proteins. For transfected DCs, the continuous display of multiple peptide epitopes restricted by several MHC alleles has the advantage of generating polyclonal T cell responses. There are a variety of DC-based genetic immunotherapy strategies that have been characterized in preclinical model systems and tested in a small number of pilot clinical trials. Protein-pulsing with defined, purified proteins or complex lysates of cell lines or autologous tumors has been more commonly tested due to this straightforward methodology.

Another important factor in inducing TAA-specific immunity is the format and uptake pathway of the antigen used. The antigen format used in vaccination impacts which T cell subsets are preferentially stimulated, and the extent of this presentation. Synthetic peptides can be used to stimulate either $CD4^+$ or $CD8^+$ T cell populations. If DCs are loaded with whole TAA protein, the antigen is introduced to the endosomal, MHC class II processing pathway, and derived peptides will primarily stimulate $CD4^+$ T cell responses. On the contrary, if DCs are infected or transfected with TAA cDNA, then the protein may be preferentially expressed in the cytosol where it enters the classical MHC class I antigen processing pathway, and derived peptides may be presented primarily to $CD8^+$ T cells [12, 35, 36].

First Generation Clinical Trials Utilizing DC-Based Cancer Therapy

The early clinical trials of DC-based cancer immunotherapy (Table 2) established the general safety and feasibility of this therapeutic modality and its lack of toxicity compared with other approaches (e.g., chemotherapy, radiation). Further, they demonstrated the clinical potential of this approach for multiple tumor types. These studies have also raised a number of issues that need to be addressed in future trials.

The first reported clinical trial that describing the ability of tumor antigen-pulsed DCs to elicit tumor-specific T cell response and yield a clinical response was published by Hsu et al. in 1996 [9]. In this pilot study, four patients were treated with low-grade follicular B-cell lymphoma resistant to chemotherapy. The DCs were pulsed with target antigens of clonal immunoglobulin (idiotype) expressed by non-Hodgkin's lymphoma. Patients were immunized with 3 monthly DC infusions, followed by subcutaneous booster injections of idiotype protein and keyhole limpet hemocyanin (KLH) 2 weeks later, and a final DC infusion given 5 to 6 months later. No toxicities were observed following the DC immunization protocol. All four patients developed cellular proliferative responses specific to their own idiotype protein, but no humoral responses were detected. More importantly, a sensitive tumor-specific PCR analysis revealed that one patient had a complete tumor regression, a second patient had a partial regression, and a third patient resolved all evidence of disease.

It has been observed that melanoma can occasionally undergo spontaneous regression coincident with strong immune infiltration into tumor deposits [37–39]. This inherent immunogenicity, as well as the molecular characterization of melanoma antigens recognized by T cells, has provided a strong rationale for a variety of melanoma vaccine trials. In one of the earliest trials, Mukherji et al. [40] used intradermal injection of MAGE-1 peptide-pulsed and GM-CSF-treated monocytes to treat three $HLA\text{-}A1^+$ patients with advanced metastatic melanoma. They observed elicitation of autologous melanoma-reactive and peptide-specific $CD8^+$ T cell responses in situ without any immediate or late side effects. Unfortunately, no significant therapeutic responses were seen.

Table 2 Outline of several early DC-based clinical trials

Author	Tumor	APC used	Antigen	Injection route*	TAA-specific CTL response	Objective clinical response	Side effects
Hsu et al.	B-cell lymphoma	Circulating DC precursors	Clonal Immunoglobulin (idiotype)	i.v.	Yes	Yes	None
Mukherji et al.	Melanoma	GM-CSF-treated monocytes	MAGE-A1	i.d.	Yes	No	None
Nestle et al.	Melanoma	Monocyte-derived DCs	MART-1, gp100, Tyrosinase, MAGE-A1, MAGE-3, or tumor lysate	i.n.	Yes	Yes	Mild local injection-site reactions
Banchereau et al.	Melanoma	CD34 progenitor-derived DCs	MART-1, Tyrosinase, MAGE-3, gp100	s.c.	Yes	Yes	Vitiligo

*intravenous (i.v.); intradermal (i.d.); intranodal (i.n.); subcutaneous (s.c.)

While the study performed by Mukherji et al. evaluated monocyte-derived antigen presenting cells (APCs), it may not have formally tested a fully differentiated DC because the culture contained GM-CSF, while it lacked IL-4. The first clinical trial using monocyte-derived DCs was performed by Nestle et al. [10]. Sixteen melanoma patients were treated using autologous monocyte-derived DCs pulsed with a cocktail of gp100, MART-1, tyrosinase, MAGE-1, or MAGE-3 peptides chosen to suit the individual patient's class I HLA molecules. In addition, DCs pulsed with autologous tumor lysate were used to treat another four patients. To provide antigen nonspecific $CD4^+$ T cell-mediated help for the $CD8^+$ T cells, KLH was included during antigen pulsing. Dendritic cells were injected directly into uninvolved lymph nodes. Patients received 6–10 injections of 1×10^6 cells every 1–4 weeks. Toxicity was limited to mild injection-site reactions. Delayed type hypersensitivity (DTH) skin reactions to peptides were reported in 11 cases indica-ting improved immunity, and peptide-specific cytotoxic T lymphocytes (CTL) could be recovered from the skin biopsies of some of these patients. Tumor regression was seen in 5 of the 16 patients, including two complete responses lasting over 15 months. Two of the responding patients received only tumor lysate-pulsed DCs, suggesting an approach applicable to cancers lacking defined tumor antigens or for patients with uncommon HLA types. Tumor regression occurred in skin, soft tissue, lung, and pancreas indicating an impact on the clinical course of metastasizing melanoma, regardless of metastatic site.

In another melanoma clinical trial, Banchereau et al. [41] evaluated immune and clinical responses in 18 patients with metastatic melanoma after injecting them subcutaneously with DCs pulsed with peptides derived from MART-1, tyrosinase, MAGE-A3, and gp100. They utilized $CD34^+$ hematopoietic progenitor cells as an alternative source of DCs to peripheral blood myeloid progenitors. Dendritic cells were administered in a dose-escalation design at the dose level per cohort of 0.1, 0.25, 0.5, and 1×10^6 DCs/kg/injection. Side effects were limited to two patients who developed vitiligo, which is a positive prognostic indicator in melanoma treatment [37]. Enhanced antigen-specific immune responses to at least one of the peptides used for vaccination were seen in 16 of 18 patients. Six of seven patients with immunity to two or fewer antigens had progressive disease 10 weeks after the study ended, while only one of ten patient responded to more than two antigens had tumor progression. Furthermore, seven of the responsive patients had a regression of one or more tumor metastases. This study showed that broad immune responses to multiple tumor antigen-derived peptides correlate with better clinical outcome.

Limited Clinical Results for DC-Based Vaccines

In 2004, Rosenberg et al. published an article on the state of active specific immunotherapy cancer trials [42]. They analyzed 9 years of their data, as well as data from 35 published reports of vaccine trials performed outside of the National Cancer Institute (NCI). Overall, they reviewed 1,306 solid tumor patients using the modified Response Evaluation Criteria in Solid Tumors (RECIST) in which clinical response is defined as at least 50% reduction in the sum of the products of the perpendicular diameters of all lesions without 25% growth of any lesion or the appearance of new lesions. With an overall therapy-induced tumor regression rate of only 3.3% in patients vaccinated with synthetic peptides, "naked" DNA, peptide-pulsed dendritic cells, recombinant vaccinia viruses, recombinant fowlpox viruses, and recombinant adenoviruses expressing various TAA, the results were grim. Of these immunization methods, peptide-pulsed DCs seemed to be the most effective strategy, with 7.1% of treated patients exhibiting tumor regression. While this frequency of response was higher than those frequencies found for other vaccination strategies, the clinical response was still low. Furthermore, the overall vaccine treatments of metastatic melanoma patients, when successful, were predominantly effective in patients with disease at cutaneous or lymphatic sites, but not those with disseminated, visceral disease.

Unlike chemotherapy, immunological vaccines do not follow linear dose-effect kinetics. Instead, these strategies depend on the complex interactions of a number of variables, including the administration method, minimum effective dose, vaccination schedule, immunological adjuvant type, and the existing state of host immunological competence. The slightest discrepancy in any of these variables can affect the patient outcome following therapeutic immunization. The majority of patients treated in these studies were late-stage metastatic patients that were heavily pretreated with conventional chemotherapeutic reagents prior to immunizations. Not only do such tumors have potent immuno-inhibitory functions, but the implemented chemotherapies have also been shown to nonspecifically decrease the number of leukocytes in recipients, making metastatic patients severely immuno-compromised. Such patients would also be expected to have fully entrenched tumor resistance effects in place (e.g., infiltrated regulatory T cells, myeloid derived suppressor cells, immuno-inhibitory cytokines).

There are several other possibilities to explain the poor clinical response to these vaccines. The immune system, while potentially effective, is limited by the frequency of responders that can be stimulated by vaccinations. Even if TAA-specific responses were stimulated by immunization, it is possible that the bulk tumor mass was too large at the time of the treatment for the available effector T cell population to eliminate it efficiently. It is also possible that while the vaccine-targeted antigens are expressed by the tumors, their derivative peptides are not presenting on the cell surface in the context of MHC class I molecules, making the tumor cells effectively invisible to $CD8^+$ T cell recognition. Tumors can down-regulate antigen processing machinery molecules, including β-2-microglobulin. Another possibility is that TAA used for vaccinations were not expressed by targeted tumors because metastatic deposits do not necessarily express the same repertoire of antigens as the primary tumor or that TAA-derived peptides used were not effective at eliciting high-avidity T cell responders. The highest avidity T cells specific for self antigens may have been deleted during development of the immune system by normal negative selection. Therefore, instead of tailoring the vaccine to the individual patient's TAA repertoire, these individuals may have been treated with arguably irrelevant or weakly immunogenic antigens that yield a clinically meaningless immune response. Many trials have shown successful immunization via increased frequency of T cells specific for vaccine presented antigens. Due to the potential limitations under which these clinical trials have been performed to date, novel vaccine strategies need to be developed that have the potential to improve the therapeutic outcome.

Next Generation Clinical Trials

A new generation of clinical trials is underway testing new hypotheses based on the lessons learned from the first. One example is the use of cytokine cocktails and pathogen-derived agonists to mature DCs. The individual constituents of these cocktails have an important impact on DC biology, including the relative level of cell surface molecules (e.g., costimulatory molecules), the amount, timing and duration of cytokine production by DCs (e.g., IL-12p70, IL-12p40, IL-10), DC lifespan, and the trafficking potential or response to chemokine gradients [43]. Early, high level production of IL-12p70 may not be as optimal for T cell activation in vivo as delayed IL-12 production until DCs have arrived from the site of injection to the lymph node. Newer DC vaccines are not simply "mature," but are treated to elicit specific types of "maturity" based on culture conditions.

Another area of investigation is the anatomical site of vaccine injection. In vivo, DCs are exposed to a pathogen at an environment-specific site, believed to mature during their migration to the draining lymph nodes, and ultimately present antigen to lymphocytes. If DCs are fully matured from ex vivo treatment with cytokine and pathogen-derived agonist cocktails at the time of injection, then it may be more efficacious to deliver the DCs to lymph nodes by direct injection, or deliver to the lymphatics. However, the more common intradermal or subcutaneous delivery sites might still be appropriate for partially matured DCs.

Sources of Tumor Antigen

Tumors are not homogenous tissues that can be treated with a single vaccination tactic. They vary in physiological location, TAA repertoire, and other properties. Some types are considered more "immunogenic" and have been an early focus for many DC-based immunotherapy trials. These variations in tumor biology are observed between patients, the tissues affected, and at different time points in the malignant process. Such differences should be taken into account when considering DC preparation and delivery strategies which may need to be tailor-made for specific tumors. For example, when considering inclusion criteria, stage IV cancer patients are not a homogeneous group. When considering autologous tumor-based immunization strategies, there are types of cancer that are not generally surgically removed, so the ability to load DCs with autologous tumor as a source of all potential public and private TAA, as well as normal antigens, may not be feasible. Similarly, some tumor types may have few characterized TAA with few well-defined HLA-matched peptide epitopes. Since the expression of TAA is not uniform among tumors, it may be critical to coadminister several antigens rather than a single one to avoid the possibility that the sole TAA will prove nonimmunogenic or that its epitopes may have been down-regulated on the tumor cell membrane in situ.

Summary

There is a greater understanding of not only direct DC interactions with $CD8^+$ T cells, but also the potential importance of tumor antigen specific $CD4^+$ T cell "help" to promote proper differentiation and ultimate function of the $CD8^+$ effector T cells [44]. There is also an emerging understanding of DC interaction with innate immune effectors, like NK cells. Dendritic cells can interact with these nonantigen-specific effector cells, activating the NK cells, and being similarly activated by them. This broader picture of immunity against heterogeneous tumors will allow for more effective immunity, harnessing optimally activated $CD4^+$ and "helped" $CD8^+$ T cells, as well as NK and NK/T cells.

There have also been substantial improvements in technical aspects of vaccine production, including a broader range of GMP-compliant reagents, the use of more "closed system" methods that allow for improved sterility and serial sampling for "in process testing" of DCs used in vaccines without the risk of contamination. Larger scale closed systems allow for the generation of larger numbers of DCs from leukaphoresis products (5×10^9 to 10^{10} PBMC), which could allow higher doses of DC vaccines and longer term boosting with multiple vaccines to help maintain induced immune responses.

References

1. Banchereau, J., and Steinman, R. M. (1998) Nature 392, 245
2. Steinman, R. M. (1991) Annu Rev Immunol 9, 271
3. Steinman, R. M., Pack, M., and Inaba, K. (1997) Adv Exp Med Biol 417, 1
4. Steinman, R. M., Witmer-Pack, M., and Inaba, K. (1993) Adv Exp Med Biol 329, 1
5. Adema, G. J., Hartgers, F., Verstraten, R., de Vries, E., Marland, G., Menon, S., Foster, J., Xu, Y., Nooyen, P., McClanahan, T., Bacon, K. B., and Figdor, C. G. (1997) Nature 387, 713
6. Tang, H. L., and Cyster, J. G. (1999) Science 284, 819
7. McColl, S. R. (2002) Immunol Cell Biol 80, 489
8. Timmerman, J. M., and Levy, R. (1999) Annu Rev Med 50, 507
9. Hsu, F. J., Benike, C., Fagnoni, F., Liles, T. M., Czerwinski, D., Taidi, B., Engleman, E. G., and Levy, R. (1996) Nat Med 2, 52
10. Nestle, F. O., Alijagic, S., Gilliet, M., Sun, Y., Grabbe, S., Dummer, R., Burg, G., and Schadendorf, D. (1998) Nat Med 4, 328
11. Thurner, B., Haendle, I., Roder, C., Dieckmann, D., Keikavoussi, P., Jonuleit, H., Bender, A., Maczek, C., Schreiner, D., von den Driesch, P., Brocker, E. B., Steinman, R. M., Enk, A., Kampgen, E., and Schuler, G. (1999) J Exp Med 190, 1669

12. Inaba, K., and Inaba, M. (2005) Int J Hematol 81, 181
13. Kapsenberg, M. L. (2003) Nat Rev Immunol 3, 984
14. Lowes, M. A., Bishop, G. A., Crotty, K., Barnetson, R. S., and Halliday, G. M. (1997) J. Invest Derm 108, 914
15. Schwaab, T., Heaney, J. A., Schned, A. R., Harris, R. D., Cole, B. F., Noelle, R. J., Phillips, D. M., Stempkowski, L., and Ernstoff, M. S. (2000) J Urol 163, 1322
16. Adams, S., O'Neill, D. W., and Bhardwaj, N. (2005) J Clin Immunol 25, 177
17. Mestas, J., and Hughes, C. C. (2004) J Immunol 172, 2731
18. Lee, K. H., Wang, E., Nielsen, M. B., Wunderlich, J., Migueles, S., Connors, M., Steinberg, S. M., Rosenberg, S. A., and Marincola, F. M. (1999) J Immunol 163, 6292
19. Lee, P. P., Yee, C., Savage, P. A., Fong, L., Brockstedt, D., Weber, J. S., Johnson, V., Swetter, S., Thompson, J., Greenberg, P. D., Roederer, M., and Davis, M. M. (1999) Nat Med 5, 677
20. Nanda, N. K., and Sercarz, E. (1996) J Exp Med 184, 1037
21. Matzinger, P. (1994) Annu Rev Immunol 12, 991
22. Matzinger, P. (2002) Science 296, 301
23. Peace, D. J., Smith, J. W., Chen, W., You, S. G., Cosand, W. L., Blake, J., and Cheever, M. A. (1994) J Exp Med 179, 473
24 . Bocchia, M., Korontsvit, T., Xu, Q., Mackinnon, S., Yang, S. Y., Sette, A., and Scheinberg, D. A. (1996) Blood 87, 3587
25. Mayordomo, J. I., Loftus, D. J., Sakamoto, H., De Cesare, C. M., Appasamy, P. M., Lotze, M. T., Storkus, W. J., Appella, E., and DeLeo, A. B. (1996) J Exp Med 183, 1357
26. Theobald, M., Biggs, J., Dittmer, D., Levine, A. J., and Sherman, L. A. (1995) Proc Natl Acad Sci USA 92, 11993
27. Banchereau, J., Palucka, K., Dhodpkar, M., Burkeholder, S., Taquet, N., Rolland, A., Taket, S., Coquery, S., Wittkowski, K. M., Bhardwaj, N., Pineiro, L., Steinman, R., and Fay, J. (2001) Cancer Res 61, 6451
28. Butterfield, L. H., Ribas, A., Dissette, V. B., Amarnani, S. N., Vu, H. T., Oseguera, D., Wang, H. J., Elashoff, R. M., McBride, W. H., Mukherji, B., Cochran, A. J., Glaspy, J. A., and Economou, J. S. (2003) Clin Cancer Res 9, 998
29. Rabek, J. P., Hoyt, P. R., Zhang, D. E., Izban, M. G., and Papaconstantinou, J. (1990) Nucleic Acids Res 18, 6677
30. Ribas, A., Glaspy, V., Lee, Y., Dissette, V. B., Seja, E., Vu, H. T., Tchekmedyian, N. S., Oseguera, D., Comin-Anduix, B., Wargo, J. A., Amarnani, S. N., McBride, W. H., Economou, J. S., and Butterfield, L. H. (2004) J Immunother 27, 354
31. Rosenberg, S. A., Zhai, Y., Yang, J. C., Schwartzentruber, D. J., Hwu, P., Marincola, F. M., Topalian, S. L., Restifo, N. P., Seipp, C. A., Einhorn, J. H., Roberts, B., and White, D. E. (1998) J Natl Cancer Inst 90, 1894
32. Jager, D., Stockert, E., Scanlan, M. J., Gure, A. O., Jager, E., Knuth, A., Old, L. J., and Chen, Y. T. (1999) Cancer Res 59, 6197
33. Wang, R. F., Wang, X., Atwood, A. C., Topalian, S. L., and Rosenberg, S. A. (1999) Science 284, 1351
34. Slingluff, C. L., Jr., Petroni, G. R., Yamshchikov, G. V., Barnd, D. L., Eastham, S., Galavotti, H., Patterson, J. W., Deacon, D. H., Hibbitts, S., Teates, D., Neese, P. Y., Grosh, W. W., Chianese-Bullock, K. A., Woodson, E. M., Wiernasz, C. J., Merrill, P., Gibson, J., Ross, M., and Engelhard, V. H. (2003) J Clin Oncol 21, 4016
35. Groothuis, T. A., Griekspoor, A. C., Neijssen, J. J., Herberts, C. A., and Neefjes, J. J. (2005) Immunol Rev 207, 60
36. Villadangos, J. A., Schnorrer, P., and Wilson, N. S. (2005) Immunol Rev 207, 191
37. Nordlund, J. J., Kirkwood, J. M., Forget, B. M., Milton, G., Albert, D. M., and Lerner, A. B. (1983) J Am Acad Dermatol 9, 689
38. Gromet, M. A., Epstein, W. L., and Blois, M. S. (1978) Cancer 42, 2282
39. Tihan, T., and Filippa, D. A. (1996) Cancer 77, 2325
40. Mukherji, B., Chakraborty, N. G., Yamasaki, S., Okino, T., Yamase, H., Sporn, J. R., Kurtzman, S. K., Ergin, M. T., Ozols, J., Meehan, J. et al. (1995) Proc Natl Acad Sci U. S. A. 92, 8078

41. Banchereau, J., Palucka, A. K., Dhodapkar, M., Burkeholder, S., Taquet, N., Rolland, A., Taquet, S., Coquery, S., Wittkowski, K. M., Bhardwaj, N., Pineiro, L., Steinman, R., and Fay, J. (2001) Cancer Res 61, 6451
42. Rosenberg, S. A., Yang, J. C., and Restifo, N. P. (2004) Nat Med 10, 909
43. Mailliard, R. B., Wankowicz-Kalinska, A., Cai, Q., Wesa, A., Hilkens, C. M., Kapsenberg, M. L., Kirkwood, J. M., Storkus, W. J., and Kalinski, P. (2004) Cancer Res 64, 5934
44. Janssen, E. M., Lemmens, E. E., Wolfe, T., Christen, U., von Herrath, M. G., and Schoenberger, S. P. (2003) Nature 421, 852

A "Toll Bridge" for Tumor-Specific T Cells

Eduardo Davila

Abstract Toll-like receptors are among the fundamental molecules that alert the immune system to the presence of an infection by recognizing pathogen-associated molecules. The engagement of TLRs results in the activation of the adaptive immune system and the production of inflammatory molecules and various chemokines. Much of our understanding regarding TLR function stems from the study of innate immune cells, such as dendritic cells and macrophages. However, emerging studies from various groups, including ours, have shown that TLRs are expressed on $CD4^+$ and $CD8^+$ T cells and can function as costimulatory molecules. The engagement of TLRs on various T cell subsets enhances cell survival, proliferation, and/or increases the production of cytokines and effector molecules. These findings reveal a novel role for TLR agonists and may inspire new approaches in the development of immunotherapies and vaccines that are more effective by targeting or manipulating TLR signaling within T cells.

Introduction

Nearly a century ago, Dr. William B. Coley noted that the administration of bacteria into cancer patients stimulated their immune system and that, once activated, the immune system had the capacity to destroy malignant cells along with the infection. He observed significant tumor regression, and in some instances tumor eradiation, in several of his patients following bacterial infection [1]. Based on these observations, he proposed that tumor regression correlated with the activation of the immune system following an infection and designed a mixture of heat-killed bacteria (Streptococci and *Serratia marcescens*) to inoculate patients. He documented successful treatment in a number of patients with malignant soft tissue sarcoma using these formulations.

E. Davila (✉)
Department of Pediatrics and the Stanley S. Scott Cancer Center, Louisiana State University Health Sciences Center, New Orleans, LA 70112
e-mail: edavil@lsuhsc.edu

J. Lustgarten et al. (eds.), *Targeted Cancer Immune Therapy*,
DOI 10.1007/978-1-4419-0170-5_10, © Springer Science+Business Media, LLC 2009

Currently, it is understood that immune system has evolved to detect and respond to infection by recognizing distinct molecular patterns expressed by various microbes. Toll-like receptors (TLRs) are among the fundamental proteins that sense infectious organisms. Expressed primarily on cells of the innate immune system, such as dendritic cells (DCs) and macrophages, TLRs recognize highly conserved pathogen-associated molecular patterns (PAMPs) derived from all known microorganisms, including bacteria, fungi, parasites, and viruses. Each TLR can recognize one or more microbial-derived molecules and can form homo- or heterodimers that presumably aid in the detection of a broader array of microbial components (Table 1).

The engagement of TLRs functions as a "danger signal" for the immune system, initiating a cascade of signaling events that trigger host defenses. The ligation of TLRs commences molecular signals through the toll-interleukin (IL)-1 receptor (TIR) domains, which can interact with cytoplasmic adaptor proteins including Myeloid-differentiation factor 88 (MyD88), TIR domain-containing adaptor protein/MyD88 adaptor like (TIRAP/MAL), and TIR domain-containing adaptor-inducing interferon (IFN)-β (TRIF) [2]. Depending on the specificity of the TLR stimulation, i.e., which TLRs are stimulated, the resulted activation of TLR signaling pathways and transcription factors vary greatly, including NF-κB, JNK/c-jun, IRF3, IRF7, and p38. These factors subsequently regulate the expression of various genes involved in the elimination of the infectious microbe [2].

T Cell-Based Tumor Immunotherapy

Our understanding of how the immune system recognizes malignant cells has led to the improvement of immune-based therapies to treat cancer. One form of immunotherapy uses tumor-specific T lymphocytes to kill malignant cells after recognizing tumor antigens (TA), preferentially expressed by tumor cells. Effective T cell-based immunotherapy, leading to increased cancer patient survival, depends on the activation of professional antigen presenting cells (APCs), as well as the successful stimulation and generation of sufficient numbers of tumor-reactive T cells. Further, the long-term persistence of these tumor-specific T cell responses is necessary to prevent tumor recurrences.

The role of TLR agonists is principally believed to occur by stimulating TLRs on professional APCs to efficiently activate T cell-mediated immunity to cancer cells [2, 3]. One of the most distinguishing features of TLR agonists is their aptitude to induce the expression of costimulatory molecules (e.g., CD80 and CD86) and major histocompatability molecules I (MHC I) and MHC II on APCs. Moreover, TLR-stimulated APCs produce high amounts of inflammatory cytokines (e.g., IL-12 and IFN-γ) and chemokines [2, 4] necessary for optimal activation of $CD4^+$ T helper and $CD8^+$ T cells. Stimulation of TLRs on DCs has also been shown to prolong cell survival by inducing the expression of antiapoptotic molecules and maintaining T cell responses [5].

Although the activation of TLR signals within APCs is clearly important for generating potent T cell responses, emerging data from numerous groups, including ours,

Table 1 Effects of TLR engagement on different T cell subsets

TLR	Cellular localization	Ligand	Effects of TLR engagement on T cells	T cell subset	Ref
TLR1/2	Surface intracellular	Lipopeptides Lipoproteins Peptidoglycan Heat shock proteins	Augments production of IFN-γ, perforin, granzyme B, IL-2 Increases proliferation Decreases antigen threshold Upregulates the expression of antiapoptotic molecules	CD4 and CD8 γδ T cell T_{memory}	[15, 16, 17, 36, 46, 58]
TLR3	Intracellular	dsRNA polyI:C	Augments production of IFN-γ	γδT cell	[14]
TLR4	Surface	Lipopolysaccharides	Upregulates the expression of CD69 and CD25	CD4 and CD8 Treg	[10, 59]
TLR5	Surface	Flagellin	Augments production of IFN-γ and IL-2 Suppress Treg function?	CD4 and CD8 Treg	[11, 21]
TLR2/6	Surface intracellular	Diacyl lipoproteins	Increases proliferation	CD8	[16]
TLR7	Intracellular	ssRNA	Augments production of IFN-γ and IL-4	CD4	[21]
TLR8	Intracellular	ssRNA	Reverses Treg function	Treg	[19]
TLR9	Intracellular	Unmethylated CpG DNA	Augments production of IL-2 Increases proliferation Radioprotection	CD4	[20, 25, 8, 29, 30, 60, 85]
TLR10	Unknown	Unknown	Unknown	–	–
TLR11	Surface	*T gondii* Profilin	Unknown	–	–
TLR12	Surface	Uropathogenic bacteria	Unknown	–	–
TLR13	Unknown	Unknown	Unknown	–	–

indicate that T cells also receive costimulatory signals through TLRs. We hypothesize that cancer vaccines aimed at generating potent antitumor responses have failed to control tumor progression somewhat due to (1) suboptimal T cell activation, partially a result from low T cell receptor (TCR) affinity to TA; (2) the short-term duration of antitumor T cell responses; and (3) suppressor mechanisms that down-regulate immune responses. Based on published reports and compelling preliminary data, we believe that the ligation of TLRs on APCs and tumor-specific T cells facilitates the generation of potent antitumor immunity. In this chapter, we present both theoretical and experimental arguments in support of this hypothesis.

T Cell Activation and Differentiation

The initial response of a T cell to an antigen is characterized by three well-defined phases (Fig. 1). In the first phase, the naïve clonal precursor receives signals from the priming APCs and from signals, such as cytokines, present in the microenvironment. Several groups have shown that various signals received during priming are "hard-wired" into the T cell and passed onto clonal progeny [6]. Upon activation, T cells undergo a series of rapid divisions, increasing their number by up to 1,000-fold. Within several hours following activation, T cells upregulate the expression levels of effector and cytolytic molecules including IFN-γ, perforin, granzyme B, and Fas-ligand. However, because T cell activation also commits the cell to an apoptotic pathway [7, 8], this initial response is followed by a sharp contraction in T cell numbers, in which most (90–95%) effector T cells die. The few cells that survive persist as effector memory (T_{EM}) or long-lived central memory T cells (T_{CM}). Upon reencounter with the cognate antigen, T_{EM} exhibits rapid effector function, in the form of cytokine secretion and cytotoxicity, and undergo an additional phase of rapid expansion within hours of stimulation, whereas T_{CM} cells produce IL-2 and require a longer period of antigen activation [9, 10].

Identifying the signals that influence the magnitude, duration, and promote the generation of memory T cells is critical for developing effective T cell-based cancer vaccines. We postulate that TLR engagement on T cells occurs in vivo and functions to enhance tumor-specific T cell responses by promoting T cell expansion, facilitating memory development, and enhancing cytolytic function.

Effects of Toll-Like Receptor Engagement on T cells

Regulation of TLR Expression on T Cell Subsets

At least 13 TLRs have been identified in mammalian cells that recognize molecular products/signals from all the main classes of pathogens. The expression of TLRs on human and mouse T cells has been analyzed by quantitative PCR and flow cytometry.

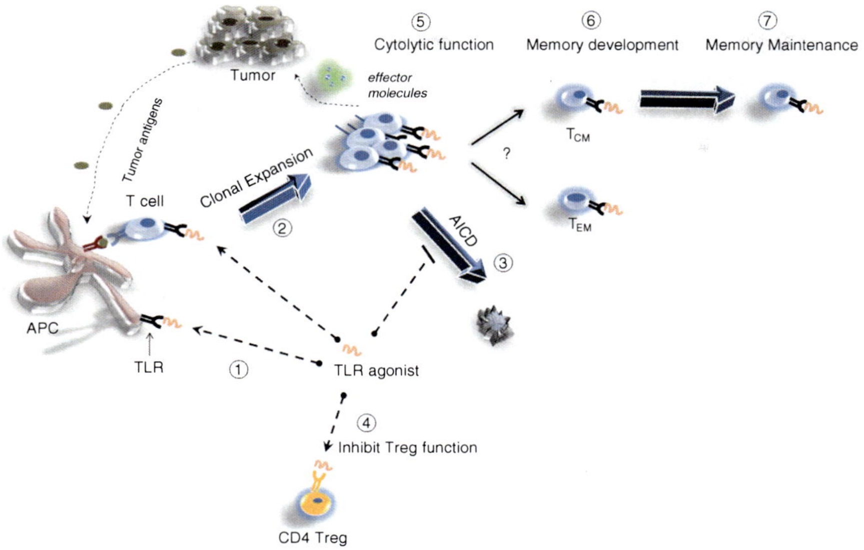

Fig. 1 Model describing the costimulatory effects of TLR engagement on T cell subsets. TLR agonists enhance tumor-reactive CD4 and CD8 T cell responses through numerous mechanisms: (1) TLR stimulation on professional antigen presenting cells increases the expression levels of peptide/MHC complexes, costimulatory molecules (CD80/CD86), as well as cytokines and chemokines necessary for the optimal activation of CD4 and CD8 T cells. (2) T cell activation induces the expression of distinct TLRs on T cell subsets. In CD4 helper and CD8 cytolytic T cells, TLR engagement augments clonal expansion by enhancing cell division. (3) The induction of antiapoptotic molecules by TLR stimulation decreases activation-induced cell death and passive death. (4) The expression of distinct TLRs is maintained on CD4$^+$ CD25$^+$ Treg cells and the TLR engagement in Tregs can inhibit their suppressive function. (5) TLR engagement on tumor-specific T cells enhances the production of effector molecules, such as IFN-γ, perforin, granzyme B, and Fas ligand, resulting in greater lysis of tumor cells. The enhanced killing of tumor cells by TLR-stimulated CD8 T cells results in the release of vast amounts of tumor antigens, leading to antigen cross-presentation and epitope spreading and the priming of new tumor-specific CD8 T cells. (6) The ligation of TLRs on effector T cells facilitates the development of effector (T_{EF}) and/or central memory (T_{CM}) T cells by promoting longevity and enhancing T cell division. Unlike naïve T cells, memory T cells maintain TLR expression and continuous exposure to TLR agonists may help promote memory T cell longevity

These studies revealed that TLR expression is dependent on the activation status (naïve, activated, or memory) of the T cell and that the TLR expression pattern varies amongst different T cell subsets (CD4$^+$, CD8$^+$, and γδ) [11–15]. The effects of TLR engagement on various T cell subpopulations are summarized in Table 1. The costimulatory effects of TLR agonists on human and mouse T cell responses are significantly enhanced and, in some cases, only observed following T cell activation with antigen, anti-CD3 antibodies, or concavalin A [16–18]. However, in the absence of concomitant T cell activation, the costimulatory effects of TLRs are minimal or absent. One possible explanation for these observations is that T cell activation induces the expression of TLRs or other molecules, such as adopter proteins, involved in

TLR signaling [16]. We recently demonstrated that TLR2 gene transcription and protein expression are upregulated following T cell activation, whereas TLR1 and MyD88 expression was not affected [16]. Alternatively, because TLRs are localized to intracellular compartments, TCR-mediated signals may induce their translocation to the cell surface [11]. Although T cell activation enhances the expression and function of certain TLRs, distinct T cell subpopulations constitutively express high levels of TLRs. For example, memory ($CD45RO^+$) T cells express TLR2 [13], whereas $CD28^-$ $CD4^+$ T cells express TLR4 [19], and $CD25^+$ $CD4^+$ regulatory T cells (Treg) express TLR4 and TLR8 [20]. Therefore, it appears that prior to T cell activation (naïve T cells), TLR expression is relatively low or absent and localized to intracellular compartments. However, upon an encounter with antigen, the expression levels of TLRs or TLR-related signaling molecules increase. Following activation, TLR expression decreases in some cell subsets, whereas, in other T cell subpopulations, such as memory T cells and Tregs, TLR expression is retained.

Potential Impact on Clonal Expansion

The ligation of certain TLRs on T cells may influence T cell expansion by enhancing cell division. In supporting reports from several groups indicate that the engagement of TLR1/2, TLR5, TLR7/8, and TLR9 directly on $CD4^+$ T-helper cells enhances IL-2 production and augments T cell proliferation in vitro (Table 1) [13, 21–23]. Further, TLR-mediated signals have been shown to modulate the expression levels of CD25 (IL-2Rα chain), as well as the duration of the IL-2R expression, indicating that one mechanism through which TLR engagement enhances T cell responses is by modifying cytokine production and cytokine receptor expression [17]. Bendigs et al. showed that TLR stimulation on $CD4^+$ T cells bypassed the need for CD28 ligation in vitro, further highlighting the potent costimulatory potential of TLR ligation on T cells [21]. Additionally, recent studies by our group and by Cottolarda and colleagues demonstrated that the engagement of TLR2 on $CD8^+$ T cells decreased the antigen threshold required to induce cell division in vitro [16, 17].

The engagement of TLRs on $CD4^+$ and $CD8^+$ T cells may lessen the severe contraction phase following antigenic exposure by modulating the expression of apoptosis-related molecules. Two distinct mechanisms regulate T cell apoptosis following activation. The first is activation-induced cell death (AICD), which occurs in repetitively stimulated T cells and is believed to be important in limiting the intensity of an immune response to prevent collateral damage or autoimmunity. The elimination of activated T cells is mediated through the fatty acid synthase (Fas)/Fas ligand (FasL) death pathway [24]. However, AICD not only plays a critical role in controlling the overall number of activated T cells, but is also involved in establishing tolerance to TAs [25]. In some cases, T cells avoid AICD by expressing high levels of the antiapoptotic Fas-associated death domain-like IL-1β-converting enzyme-inhibitory protein (FLIP), which interferes with the formation of the death-inducing signaling complex. Previously, we showed that injection of the TLR9 ligand into mice increased the numbers of $CD4^+$ and $CD8^+$ T cells, and that T cells from these mice were more resistant against serum deprivation- and activation-induced cell death ex vivo [26]. We detected significantly elevated levels of FLIP in both $CD4^+$ and $CD8^+$ T cells obtained from TLR-treated mice when compared with T cells isolated from control mice. However, it was unclear from these initial studies whether these effects were the result of direct TLR9 stimulation on T cells or through the stimulation of innate immune cells, such as DCs.

The second mechanism of T cell apoptosis – termed passive cell death – occurs when activated T cells are deprived of growth and survival factors, namely cytokines (e.g., IL-2, IL-7, IL-15). Several B-cell leukemia (Bcl) family members, including the antiapoptotic molecules such as bcl-2 and bcl-x_L and the proapoptotic molecules such as bim, bax, and bid, play a critical role in modulating passive cell death [27, 28]. Gelman et al. reported that costimulation of TLR3 or TLR9 on $CD4^+$ T cells increased T cell survival and was associated with the enhanced expression of Bcl-x_L [29, 30]. Similarly, we documented that TLR9 engagement on $CD4^+$ T cells augmented the levels of Bcl-2 and Bcl-x_L and maintained elevated levels of these molecules despite exposure to genotoxic stress (γ-radiation) [31]. In $CD8^+$ T cells, the engagement TLR2 increased the expression of bcl-x_L and another antiapoptotic molecule, A1 [17]. In addition, previous work from our group showed that $CD8^+$ and $CD4^+$ T cells obtained from TLR9 ligand-injected mice, specifically in the absence of exogenous antigen, showed increased expression levels of bcl-2 and bcl-x_L compared with T cells obtained from control mice [26]. Given the important role of apoptosis-related molecules have on generating and sustaining long-lived tumor-specific T cell responses, Rosenberg and colleagues reported that over-expression of Bcl-2 in tumor-specific T cell populations enhanced survival and was accompanied by tumor regression of an established melanoma tumor in mice [28].

Altogether, these data suggest that the ligation of certain TLRs on T cells positively influences the duration and extent of T cell response by enhancing proliferation and decreasing apoptosis. Therefore, strategies aimed at modulating TLR signals within tumor-specific T cells represent a useful approach to augment antitumor responses.

CTL Effector Function

Gaining a better understanding of the molecular pathways that influence T cell differentiation and effector function is important for the development of potent T cell-based immunotherapies. Transcription factors (TF) play a critical role in this process [32]. The transcription factor T-bet (Tbx21) and EOMES modulate $CD8^+$ T cell cytotoxicity and the expression of IFN-γ, perforin, and granzyme B (referred to as effector genes) [32–34]. In the absence of these TF, $CD8^+$ T cells fail to effectively transition from a naïve phenotype into an effector or memory cell [35, 36]. T-bet expression is induced by signals mediated through the TCR and the IFN-γR, and function downstream of Signal Transducers and Activators of Transcription 1 (Stat). While T-bet expression is induced rapidly following TCR stimulation and amplified by IFN-γR signals [32], it remains unknown whether other signals, such as TLR signals, received by a T cell during activation can influence the expression of these TF.

Recent studies conducted in our laboratory, as well as those conducted by various groups, have shown that TLR2 engagement on $CD8^+$ T cells enhances IFN-γ, granzyme B, and perforin production suggesting cross-talk between TLR and T-bet signals [4, 13, 16, 17, 37, 38]. Furthermore, TLR2-ligated $CD8^+$ T cells, but not $MyD88^{-/-}CD8^+$ or $TLR2^{-/-}$ $CD8^+$ T cells, showed enhanced cytolytic activity. In the absence of the TLR2 ligand, wild type $CD8^+$ and $TLR2^{-/-}CD8^+$ T cells demonstrated similar levels of cytotoxicity. In the absence of antigen, TLR agonists alone do not costimulate T cell responses, suggesting that TLR signals enhance T cell receptor signals. Interestingly, in $MyD88^{-/-}CD8^+$ T cells show a reduced capacity for cytokine production and cytolytic activity as compared with wild type T cells, highlighting an important role for MyD88 in T cells. We examined the expression levels T-bet and EOMES in response to TLR2-stimulation. The increased levels of IFN-γ, granzyme B, and perforin transcripts in TLR2-engaged $CD8^+$ T cells and production of IFN-γ correlated with an increase in T-bet mRNA and protein (but not EOMES) expression. The increased T-bet expression correlated with increased binding to the promoters of effector genes as detected by chromatin immunoprecipitation assay. Noteworthy, the production of effector molecules in $T\text{-}bet^{-/-}$ and $IFN\text{-}\gamma R^{-/-}$ $CD8^+$ T cells was reduced as compared with wild-type (WT) $CD8^+$ T cells and absent in $Stat1^{-/-}$ $CD8^+$ T cells following TLR2 stimulation, indicating a critical role for these molecules in the TLR-mediated upregulation of effector molecules (not shown).

Recent studies conducted in monocytes and DCs confirm a connection with the TLR-induced expression of T-bet [39, 40]. We propose that TLR signals received by T cells during an antigen encounter (during priming or at recall phase) partially enhance effector function in increasing the activity or expression levels of certain TF (e.g., T-bet) which amplify the expression of effector molecules.

These data demonstrate a novel role for TLRs and may explain why vaccines containing certain TLR agonists are more effective at generating T cell responses than others. Further, these findings are important in understanding of the host T cell response to certain infections expressing distinct PAMPs.

Memory T Cell Development, Persistence, and Migration

The precise signals that a naïve T cell incorporates during priming to successfully transition to a memory cell are not fully understood [6, 41–45]; however, TLR signals play a critical role in this process. Pasare and Medzhitov demonstrated that memory T cell development is significantly impaired in mice lacking the common TLR adapter protein MyD88, indicating a critical role for TLR signaling in the induction of immunological memory [46]. While this study highlighted the importance of TLR signals for memory T cell generation, the exact role of TLR agonists remains unknown. One possibility is that TLR-activated APCs provide an environment that facilitates memory T cell development.

Alternatively, TLR agonists may contribute to the generation and persistence of memory cells by stimulating TLRs directly on T cells, resulting in enhanced proliferation or cell survival [16, 17, 29, 31]. We propose that during priming, one of the instructive signals a T cell receives is through signals emanating from TLRs and that the fate and function of the T cell is partially programmed into clonal progeny by this signal. In support of this assertion, several reports have indicated that TLRs are constitutively expressed and functional on memory-phenotype T cells. Komai-Koma et al. documented that TLR2 stimulation on CD45RO$^+$ T-helper cells enhanced cytokine production and resulted in heightened T cell responses upon reencounter with antigen [13]. In another study, Zanin-Zhorov et al. [47] showed that TLR2 ligation on CD45RO$^+$ T cells regulated the expression of CXCR4 and CCR7 and consequently altered their migration patterns, suggesting that TLR-dependent signals within T cells could regulate their localization to distinct tissues. Moreover, a recent report by Fan and Malik demonstrated that TLR4 stimulation directly influenced the homing capacity of leukocytes [48]. Finally, it remains unknown whether TLR engagement on T cells impacts other parameters of memory T cells such as recall responses and delineation into T_{EF} and T_{CM}. The diverse phenotypes of T_{CM} (CD62L$^+$ CCR7$^+$) and T_{EM} (CD62L$^-$CCR7$^-$) T cells influence their distinct capacity to migrate to lymphoid and nonlymphoid tissue [49]. Moreover, T_{CM} and T_{EM} subsets differ in their ability to respond to antigen restimulation, with T_{EM} primarily producing effector molecules (IFN-γ, TNF) and T_{CM} cells principally producing IL-2 [10]. Although the exact nature of these signals in memory T cells is unknown, these data imply that the expression of TLRs on memory T cell subsets may influence tissue localization and may affect the functional capacity of different memory cells to react to antigenic stimulation. Defining the signals that promote the development and maintenance of a memory T cell subset that mediate the most effective protection against tumors are important factors to be considered in the development of immunotherapies and vaccines. Furthermore, determining how best to trigger TLR signals within distinct memory T cell populations will aid in the generation of T cells with potent cytolytic activity.

Modulating Regulatory CD4$^+$ T Cell Function

The suppression of tumor immunity by CD4$^+$ CD25$^+$ regulatory T cells (Tregs) represents another obstacle in generating effective antitumor T cell responses [50] because they suppress CD8$^+$ T cell activity without killing them in contact-dependent and independent mechanisms. Studies conducted by several groups have shown that Treg downplay CD8$^+$ T cell responses through the production of immunosuppressive soluble factors, such as IL-10, tumor growth factor-β, as well as other negative signals mediated by APCs [51]. Although this form of lymphocyte regulation is beneficial in controlling autoimmune disorders, the suppressive effects of Treg cells hinder the generation of tumor-specific T cells [52, 53]. In support of this assertion, it has been shown that the timely depletion of Treg cells enhances antitumor immunity [52, 53]. Other studies have found that CD25$^+$ T cell depletion prior to vaccination or before the infusion of tumor-specific T cells enhances antitumor immunity with prolonged tumor-specific T cell activity [54, 55]. Because Treg cells suppress cell-mediated immunity, these studies indicate that in tumor-bearing patients, depletion of Treg cells or inhibition of their regulatory action before vaccination should improve vaccine efficacy.

Several studies demonstrate a role for TLR-MyD88 signals in modulating the activity of Treg cells. For example, the engagement of TLR2 on activated Treg cells induces proliferation and results in downregulation of FoxP3 expression and their suppressive activity [53, 56]. Peng et al. demonstrated that the addition of TLR8 agonist (poly-G oligodeoxynucleotides or single stranded-RNA) to Treg cells reverted their suppressive effects [20]. Likewise, the TLR4 agonist, lipopolysaccharide (LPS), was reported to inhibit the activity of murine Treg cells, by a yet unidentified mechanism [12, 13, 57]. In contrast to the modulatory effects of TLR2 and TLR8 agonists on $CD4^{+}$ Tregs, stimulation of TLR5 on human Tregs was reported to enhance their suppressive activity [12]. The diverse effects of TLR agonists indicate that targeting specific TLRs on APCs and T cells is a novel and promising strategy to optimize protective and long-lasting tumor immunity by inhibiting the suppressive effects of Treg cells.

Does TLR Engagement on T Cells Occur In Vivo?

Although there is data demonstrating the costimulatory capacity of TLRs on T cells in vitro, the biological significance of TLR engagement on T cells has not been well studied. Further, the physiological importance of how TLR stimulation on T cells affects tumor immunity has only lately been investigated. We recently examined the effects of TLR2 ligation on $CD8^{+}$ T cells on their cytolytic activity in vivo. We found that in mice injected with OT-1 $CD8^{+}$ T cells plus TLR2 ligand, the vast majority of Ova-pulsed target cells were killed [16]. Because cells from $MyD88^{-/-}$ mice do not respond to TLR2 agonists, these findings indicated that enhanced cytolytic activity by $CD8^{+}$ T cells occurred as a result of TLR ligation directly on T cells. To confirm that TLR engagement on transferred OT-1 T cells was responsible for augmenting cytolytic activity, we generated $TLR2^{-/-}$OT-1 and examined their cytolytic potential in response to TLR2 signals. As expected, we found that TLR2 agonist did not increase $TLR2^{-/-}$OT-1 T cell cytotoxicity [16]. These findings confirmed that TLR2 engagement on T cells occurs in vivo and results in enhanced cytolytic activity.

Based on the enhanced killing by TLR2-stimulated T cells, we examined whether TLR2 engagement on $CD8^{+}$ T cells (OT-1) enhanced the antitumor activity in a therapeutic model of B16-Ova melanoma. We observed significant tumor regression in mice receiving OT-1 T cells and TLR2 ligand in WT and $MyD88^{-/-}$ tumor-bearing mice. In contrast, $MyD88^{-/-}$ mice receiving $TLR2^{-/-}$OT-1 T cells and TLR2 ligand showed minimal therapeutic efficacy as compared with mice injected with $TLR2^{-/-}$OT-1 T cells alone [16].

In more recent studies, we used the bona fide tumor antigen-specific "pmel" CD8 T cells, which recognize the weakly immunogenic $gp100_{25-33}$ expressed on human and mouse melanoma cells. In mice that received only TLR2 ligand or PBS, without adoptive cell transfer (ACT) tumor growth kinetics were greater as compared with mice that received ACT (Fig. 2). In addition, mice treated with TLR2 ligand alone demonstrated comparable tumor growth kinetics as mice treated with PBS, indicating that the stimulation of TLR2 on APCs was insufficient to suppress

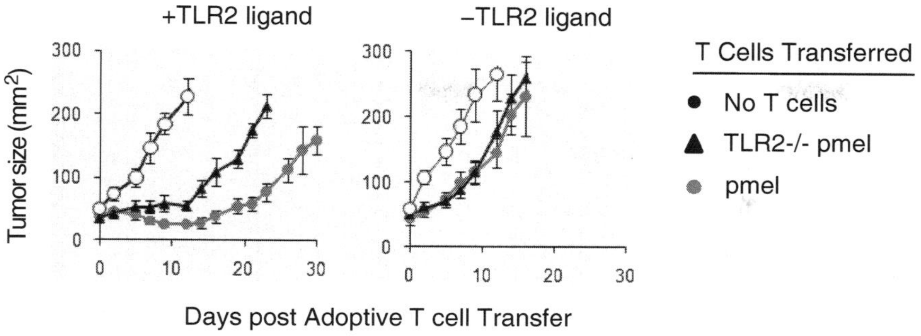

Fig. 2 TLR2 engagement on tumor antigen-specific T cells occurs in vivo and enhances antitumor activity against an established melanoma tumor. Wild-type mice were injected (s.c.) with B16-Ova tumor cells. When tumors reached 50 mm^2, mice were injected (i.v.) with 1×10^6 pmel or $TLR2^{-/-}$pmel CD8 T cells. Mice were injected peritumorally with TLR2 ligand or PBS every 7 days, starting on the same day that mice received T cells. Tumor sizes (mm^2) were calculated by measuring perpendicular by longitudinal diameter

tumor development. In sharp contrast, pmel CD8 T cells, in combination with TLR2 ligand, were able to effectively treat large, established B16 melanoma (Fig. 2). However, mice receiving $TLR2^{-/-}$pmel CD8 T cells and TLR2 ligand also showed delayed tumor growth, as compared with control mice that did not receive CD8 T cells. Importantly, tumor growth in mice receiving pmel CD8 T cells was significantly slower than in mice receiving $TLR2^{-/-}$pmel T cells. In the absence of TLR2 ligand, tumor growth was similar in mice receiving pmel and $TLR2^{-/-}$pmel CD8 T cells. These findings emphasize the physiological significance of TLR2 engagement on TA-specific T cells and could make possible new approaches for the development of effective immunotherapies by manipulating TLR signaling within CTLs.

The physiological significance of MyD88 signals in T cells is also highlighted in recent studies by Turka and colleagues. Turka and colleagues showed that replacing WT $CD4^+$ T cells with $MyD88^{-/-}$ $CD4^+$ T cells resulted in severe toxoplasmic encephalitis and most mice succumbed to infection [58]. In contrast, mice harboring MyD88 signaling-competent $CD4^+$ T cells offered enhanced immunity against *Toxoplasma gondii*. There is also accumulating evidence suggesting that TLR agonists perpetuate autoimmune T cell responses and are involved in the immunopathological process of certain inflammatory diseases. For example, it has been reported that TLR9 agonists, found in the synovium of rheumatoid arthritis patients, can costimulate T cells of multiple specificities including self-antigens, resulting in enhanced cytolytic function and IFN-γ production [59]. Sobek et al. observed that activation of T cells with TLR2 agonists sustained pathogen-induced chronic inflammatory joint disease by inducing T cell proliferation and interferon IFN-γ secretion [18]. Similarly, Ronaghy et al. found that TLR9 agonists injected directly into joints of mice increased NF-κB activation and IFN-γ production [60].

Collectively, these findings strongly suggest that, in addition to stimulating TLRs on APCs, the engagement of certain TLRs directly on $CD4^+$ or $CD8^+$ T cells occurs in vivo and can promote T cell responses and inflammation.

When TCR and TLR Signals Collide

The integration of novel signaling cascades (i.e., TLR) that can enhance the production of effector molecules in CD8 T cells has not been studied extensively. Understanding these mechanisms will emerge as a critical step to promote CTL-mediated effector functions, which could be used as a strategy to enhance immune responses against cancer. Hence an important objective is to clarify the hierarchical sequence of events mediated by TLR-MyD88 signals in tumor-reactive CD8 T cells leading to increased CTL antitumor activity.

TLR2 engagement on CD8 T cells has been shown to reduce the activation threshold [16]. We examined if TLR2 stimulation enhanced T cell activation to weakly immunogenic TA by enhancing TCR affinity or avidity. However, we did not detect changes between TLR2-stimulated and on TLR-stimulated T cells. In addition, we tested whether activation of the TLR2 signaling cascade altered proximal TCR signals. The initial events following TCR engagement include phosphorylation of tyrosine residues in p56lck, ZAP-70, and linker for T cell activation (LAT). We found that TLR2 engagement on pmel T cells did not increase the magnitude nor the duration of any of these phosphorylated intermediates, indicating that the costimulatory effects of TLR2 occurred downstream of proximal TCR signals. TLR2 signals are known to activate multiple signal transduction pathways simultaneously in different cell types. These signals include the activation of p38, Janus-kinase (JNK), protein kinase C (PKC) isoforms, and phosphoinositide-3 kinase (PI3K). Because these signaling intermediates are also activated following TCR stimulation, we speculate that TLR2 signals may serve to enhance CTL effector responses by amplifying downstream TCR signals. This hypothesis is further supported by the observation that TLR2 agonists don't influence T cell responses in the absence of concomitant TCR stimulation. These potential changes are currently under investigation.

Synergistic Effects of TLR Stimulation with Anticancer Chemotherapy or Radiation Therapy

Current studies reveal that TLR agonists can be combined with radiotherapy (RT) or chemotherapy (CT) to enhance antitumor T cell responses. For example, Delattre and colleagues demonstrated that a combination therapy of RT and TLR9 agonist induced complete tumor remission in one-third of the animals bearing malignant glioma [61]. Milas and colleagues demonstrated that the local administration of TLR9 ligand increased the radioresponse of the nonimmunogenic fibrosarcoma tumor [62, 63]. Further, this group demonstrated that TLR9 agonist improved the response of the chemotherapeutic drug docetaxel against murine tumors (fibrosarcoma and a mammary carcinoma).

Although the mechanisms through which TLR agonists function in combination with cancer therapies remain undefined, several mechanisms have been proposed. First, tumor cells killed by RT or CT likely could provide an excellent source of TA for APCs to uptake and present to T cells, and this process could be enhanced following TLR engagement on APCs [64]. Second, RT has been shown to enhance the expression levels of the death receptor Fas/CD95, MHC I, and costimulatory molecules on certain tumor cells [65–67] and may enhance T cell-mediated immunity [68, 69]. Third, RT and CT destroy immune cells, including Treg cells, thus creating a "vacancy" in the T cell compartment [26, 70–72]. When combined with adoptive transfer techniques or vaccination regimens using TA, this vacancy allows for the rapid and preferential expansion of tumor-specific T cells [73–78].

Alternatively, TLR stimulation might enhance the antitumor effects of CT or RT by protecting T cell against the toxic effects of these therapies [79–85]. We recently demonstrated that TLR9 engagement imparts a radioprotective effect on activated $CD4^+$ T cells [31]. This radioprotective effect was manifested in vitro by decreased apoptosis, increased cell-cycle arrest, and an increased rate of DNA double-strand break repair, specifically following TLR9 stimulation directly on $CD4^+$ T cells. Additionally, TLR9 engagement on T cells was responsible for the increased activation of checkpoint kinases Chk1 and Chk2 and expression of the antiapoptotic molecules bcl-2 and bcl-x_L. In vivo, TLR9-stimulated T cells displayed higher radioresistance than TLR9-stimulated $MyD88^{-/-}$ T cells and responded to antigenic stimulation after total body irradiation. In another study, Sohn et al. reported that TLR9 agonists protected primary mouse spleen cells from the cell death induced by γ-radiation. Radioprotection was accompanied by increased expression levels of bcl-x_L and Bcl-2. These findings indicate that TLR engagement on T cells reduces RT-induced apoptosis and helps maintain T cell function, potentially allowing for combinatorial immunotherapy and RT against tumors.

Exploiting TLR Signals Within T Cells to Enhance Antitumor Immunity

The inclusion of TLR agonists to T cell-based therapies has shown promising results in treating several tumor types in both the preclinical and clinical setting. Currently, our laboratory is experimentally addressing what we consider several major obstacles in the generation of effective and long-lasting antitumor T cell responses. First, we hope to generate sufficient numbers of tumor-reactive T cells by augmenting T cell proliferation and reducing cell death following T cell activation. The second obstacle is the short-term duration and suboptimal production of effector molecules. Third, we aim to protect tumor-specific T cells against the toxic effects of radiation therapy and CT. To address these challenges, we are investigating the effects of amplifying TLR-MyD88 signals within tumor-specific $CD8^+$ T cells using molecular approaches to enhance TLR signaling. Fourth, by selecting a specific cocktail of TLR agonists, we intend to prevent some of the suppressor mechanisms that downregulate Treg suppressive activity while simultaneously activating tumor-reactive $CD8^+$ T cells. We theorize that by addressing these issues, we will be able to promote the preferential expansion and facilitate the persistence of tumor-specific T cells, leading to the prevention of tumor recurrences or metastatic diseases.

Summary

Beyond stimulating innate immune cells, TLR agonists costimulate T cell responses by ligating TLRs directly on T cells. These findings have immediate implications for the enhancement of tumor immunity through the activation of TLRs on tumor-specific T cell responses or through the suppression of regulatory T cell activity. Upcoming studies should focus on deciphering the molecular pathways involved in linking TCRs and TLRs. Further, a detailed analysis aimed at resolving the diverse outcome of ligating certain TLRs on different T cell subsets will also help enhance the effectiveness of vaccines or adoptive transfer protocols aimed at inducing potent tumor-specific immune responses.

Acknowledgments This work was supported by a National Institutes of Health (NIH) Center for Biomedical Research Excellence Grant (1P20RR021970) and the Louisiana Cancer Research Consortium NIH grant number 1R01CA140917–0109 as a source of support.

References

1. Coley, W. B. (1893) Clin Orthop Relat Res 1991, 3
2. Akira, S., and Hemmi, H. (2003) Immunol Lett 85, 85
3. Iwasaki, A., and Medzhitov, R. (2004) 5, 987
4. Ghosh, T. K., Mickelson, D. J., Fink, J., Solberg, J. C., Inglefield, J. R., Hook, D., Gupta, S. K., Gibson, S., and Alkan, S. S. (2006) Cell Immunol 243, 48
5. Prins, R. M., Craft, N., Bruhn, K. W., Khan-Farooqi, H., Koya, R. C., Stripecke, R., Miller, J. F., and Liau, L. M. (2006) J. Immunol 176, 157
6. Masopust, D., Kaech, S. M., Wherry, E. J., and Ahmed, R. (2004) Curr Opin Immunol 16, 217
7. Russell, J. H., White, C. L., Loh, D. Y., and Meleedy-Rey, P. (1991) Proc Natl Acad Sci USA 88, 2151
8. Russell, J. H. (1995) Curr Opin Immunol 7, 388
9. Sprent, J., and Tough, D. F. (1994) Lymphocyte life-span and memory. Science 265, 1395
10. Sallusto, F., Geginat, J., and Lanzavecchia, A. (2004) Annu Rev Immunol 22, 745
11. Babu, S., Blauvelt, C. P., Kumaraswami, V., and Nutman, T. B. (2006) J Immunol 176, 3885
12. Crellin, N. K., Garcia, R. V., Hadisfar, O., Allan, S. E., Steiner, T. S., and Levings, M. K. (2005) J Immunol 175, 8051
13. Komai-Koma, M., Jones, L., Ogg, G. S., Xu, D., and Liew, F. Y. (2004) Proc Natl Acad Sci USA 101, 3029
14. Mansson, A., Adner, M., and Cardell, L. O. (2006) Respir Res 7, 36
15. Wesch, D., Beetz, S., Oberg, H. H., Marget, M., Krengel, K., and Kabelitz, D. (2006) J Immunol 176, 1348
16. Asprodites, N., Zheng, L., Geng, D., Velasco-Gonzalez, C., Sanchez-Perez, L., and Davila, E. (2008) FASEB J in press

17. Cottalorda, A., Verschelde, C., Marcais, A., Tomkowiak, M., Musette, P., Uematsu, S., Akira, S., Marvel, J., and Bonnefoy-Berard, N. (2006) Eur J Immunol 36, 1684
18. Sobek, V., Birkner, N., Falk, I., Wurch, A., Kirschning, C. J., Wagner, H., Wallich, R., Lamers, M. C., and Simon, M. M. (2004) Arthritis Res Ther 6, R433
19. Raffeiner, B., Dejaco, C., Duftner, C., Kullich, W., Goldberger, C., Vega, S. C., Keller, M., Grubeck-Loebenstein, B., and Schirmer, M. (2005) Arthritis Res Ther 7, R1412
20. Peng, G., Guo, Z., Kiniwa, Y., Voo, K. S., Peng, W., Fu, T., Wang, D. Y., Li, Y., Wang, H. Y., and Wang, R. F. (2005) Science 309, 1380
21. Bendigs, S., Salzer, U., Lipford, G. B., Wagner, H., and Heeg, K. (1999) Eur J Immunol 29, 1209
22. Caron, G., Duluc, D., Fremaux, I., Jeannin, P., David, C., Gascan, H., and Delneste, Y. (20050 J Immunol 175, 1551
23. Matsuguchi, T., Takagi, K., Musikacharoen, T., and Yoshikai, Y. (2000) Blood 95, 1378
24. Greil, R., Anether, G., Johrer, K., and Tinhofer, I. (2003) J Leukoc Biol 74, 311
25. Tschopp, J., Irmler, M., and Thome, M. (1998) Curr Opin Immunol 10, 552
26. Davila, E., Velez, M. G., Heppelmann, C. J., and Celis, E. (2002) Blood 100, 2537
27. Chao, D. T. and Korsmeyer, S. J. (1998) Annu Rev Immunol 16, 395
28. Charo, J., Finkelstein, S. E., Grewal, N., Restifo, N. P., Robbins, P. F., and Rosenberg, S. A. (2005) Cancer Res 65, 2001
29. Gelman, A. E., Zhang, J., Choi, Y., and Turka, L. A. (2004) J Immunol 172, 6065
30. Gelman, A. E., LaRosa, D. F., Zhang, J., Walsh, P. T., Choi, Y., Sunyer, J. O., and Turka, L. A. (2006) Immunity 25, 783
31. Zheng, L., Asprodites, N., Keene, A. H., Rodriguez, P., Brown, K. D., and Davila, E. (2008) Blood 111, 2704
32. Glimcher, L. H., Townsend, M. J., Sullivan, B. M., and Lord, G. M. (2004) Nat Rev Immunol 4, 900
33. Kabelitz, D. (2007) Curr Opin Immunol 19, 39
34. Pearce, E. L., Mullen, A. C., Martins, G. A., Krawczyk, C. M., Hutchins, A. S., Zediak, V. P., Banica, M., DiCioccio, C. B., Gross, D. A., Mao, C. A., Shen, H., Cereb, N., Yang, S. Y., Lindsten, T., Rossant, J., Hunter, C. A., and Reiner, S. L. (2003) Science 302, 1041
35. Intlekofer, A. M., Takemoto, N., Wherry, E. J., Longworth, S. A., Northrup, J. T., Palanivel, V. R., Mullen, A. C., Gasink, C. R., Kaech, S. M., Miller, J. D., Gapin, L., Ryan, K., Russ, A. P., Lindsten, T., Orange, J. S., Goldrath, A. W., Ahmed, R., and Reiner, S. L. (2005) Nat Immunol 6, 1236
36. Sullivan, B. M., Juedes, A., Szabo, S. J., von, H. M., and Glimcher, L. H. (2003) Proc Natl Acad Sci USA 100, 15818
37. Mokuno, Y., Matsuguchi, T., Takano, M., Nishimura, H., Washizu, J., Ogawa, T., Takeuchi, O., Akira, S., Nimura, Y., and Yoshikai, Y. (2000) J Immunol 165, 931
38. Schwarz, K., Storni, T., Manolova, V., Didierlaurent, A., Sirard, J. C., Rothlisberger, P., and Bachmann, M. F. (2003) Eur J Immunol 33, 1465
39. Lighvani, A. A., Frucht, D. M., Jankovic, D., Yamane, H., Aliberti, J., Hissong, B. D., Nguyen, B. V., Gadina, M., Sher, A., Paul, W. E., and O'Shea, J. J. (2001) Proc Natl Acad Sci USA 98, 15137
40. Lugo-Villarino, G., Ito, S., Klinman, D. M., and Glimcher, L. H. (2005) Proc Natl Acad Sci USA 102, 13248
41. Farber, D. L. (1998) J Immunol 160, 535
42. Masopust, D., and Ahmed, R. (2004) Immunol Res 29, 151
43. Opferman, J. T., Ober, B. T., and shton-Rickardt, P. G. (1999) Science 283, 1745
44. Van Stipdonk, M. J., Lemmens, E. E., and Schoenberger, S. P. (2001) Nat Immunol 2, 423
45. Van Stipdonk, M. J., Hardenberg, G., Bijker, M. S., Lemmens, E. E., Droin, N. M., Green, D. R., and Schoenberger, S. P. (2003) Nat Immunol 4, 361
46. Pasare, C., and Medzhitov, R. (2004) Immunity 21, 733
47. Zanin-Zhorov, A., Nussbaum, G., Franitza, S., Cohen, I. R., and Lider, O. (2003) FASEB J 17, 1567

48. Fan, J., and Malik, A. B. (2003) Nat Med 9, 315
49. Masopust, D., Vezys, V., Marzo, A. L., and Lefrancois, L. (2001) Science 291, 2413
50. Curiel, T. J. (2007) J Clin Invest 117, 1167
51. Curotto de Lafaille, M. A., and Lafaille, J. J. (2002) Curr Opin Immunol 14, 771
52. Lanzavecchia, A., and Sallusto, F. (2001) Cell 106, 263
53. Sutmuller, R. P., den Brok, M. H., Kramer, M., Bennink, E. J., Toonen, L. W., Kullberg, B. J., Joosten, L. A., Akira, S., Netea, M. G., and Adema, G. J. (2006) J Clin Invest 116, 485
54. Casares, N., Arribillaga, L., Sarobe, P., Dotor, J., Lopez-Diaz de, C. A., Melero, I., Prieto, J., Borras-Cuesta, F., and Lasarte, J. J. (2003) J Immunol 171, 5931
55. Morse, M. A., Hobeika, A. C., Osada, T., Serra, D., Niedzwiecki, D., Lyerly, H. K., and Clay, T. M. (2008) Blood 112, 610
56. Liu, H., Komai-Koma, M., Xu, D., and Liew, F. Y. (2006) Proc Natl Acad Sci USA 103, 7048
57. Caramalho, I., Lopes-Carvalho, T., Ostler, D., Zelenay, S., Haury, M., and Demengeot, J. (2003) J Exp Med 197, 403
58. LaRosa, D. F., Stumhofer, J. S., Gelman, A. E., Rahman, A. H., Taylor, D. K., Hunter, C. A., and Turka, L. A. (2008) Proc Natl Acad Sci USA 105, 3855
59. van der Heijden, I., Wilbrink, B., Tchetverikov, I., Schrijver, I. A., Schouls, L. M., Hazenberg, M. P., Breedveld, F. C., and Tak, P. P. (2000) Arthritis Rheum 43, 593
60. Ronaghy, A., Prakken, B. J., Takabayashi, K., Firestein, G. S., Boyle, D., Zvaifler, N. J., Roord, S. T., Albani, S., Carson, D. A., and Raz, E. (2002) J Immunol 168, 51
61. Meng, Y., Carpentier, A. F., Chen, L., Boisserie, G., Simon, J. M., Mazeron, J. J., and Delattre, J. Y. (2005) Int J Cancer 116, 992
62. Mason, K. A., Ariga, H., Neal, R., Valdecanas, D., Hunter, N., Krieg, A. M., Whisnant, J. K., and Milas, L. (2005) Clin Cancer Res 11, 361
63. Mason, K. A., Neal, R., Hunter, N., Ariga, H., Ang, K., and Milas, L. (2006) Radiother Oncol 80, 192
64. Larsson, M., Fonteneau, J. F., and Bhardwaj, N. (2001) Trends Immunol 22, 141
65. Klein, H., Mehlhorn, H., and Ruger, W. (1996) Parasitol Res 82, 468
66. Sheard, M. A., Vojtesek, B., Janakova, L., Kovarik, J., and Zaloudik, J. (1997) Int J Cancer 73, 757
67. Sheard, M. A. (2001) Int J Cancer 96, 213
68. Chakraborty, M., Abrams, S. I., Camphausen, K., Liu, K., Scott, T., Coleman, C. N., and Hodge, J. W. (2003) J Immunol 170, 6338
69. Garnett, C. T., Palena, C., Chakraborty, M., Tsang, K. Y., Schlom, J., and Hodge, J. W. (2004) Cancer Res 64, 7985
70. Cho, B. K., Rao, V. P., Ge, Q., Eisen, H. N., and Chen, J. (2000) J Exp Med 192, 549
71. Ge, Q., Palliser, D., Eisen, H. N., and Chen, J. (2002) Proc Natl Acad Sci USA 99, 2983
72. Goldrath, A. W., Bogatzki, L. Y., and Bevan, M. J. (2000) J Exp Med 192, 557
73. Dudley, M. E., Wunderlich, J. R., Robbins, P. F., Yang, J. C., Hwu, P., Schwartzentruber, D. J., Topalian, S. L., Sherry, R., Restifo, N. P., Hubicki, A. M., Robinson, M. R., Raffeld, M., Duray, P., Seipp, C. A., Rogers-Freezer, L., Morton, K. E., Mavroukakis, S. A., White, D. E., and Rosenberg, S. A. (2002) Science 298, 850
74. Dummer, W., Ernst, B., LeRoy, E., Lee, D., and Surh, C. (2001) J Immunol 166, 2460
75. Dummer, W., Niethammer, A. G., Baccala, R., Lawson, B. R., Wagner, N., Reisfeld, R. A., and Theofilopoulos, A. N. (2002) J Clin Invest 110, 185
76. Hellstrom, K. E. and Hellstrom, I. (1978) Proc Natl Acad Sci USA 75, 436
77. Hellstrom, K. E., Hellstrom, I., Kant, J. A., and Tamerius, J. D. (1978) J Exp Med 148, 799
78. Hu, H. M., Poehlein, C. H., Urba, W. J., and Fox, B. A. (2002) Cancer Res 62, 3914
79. Bohnhorst, J., Rasmussen, T., Moen, S. H., Flottum, M., Knudsen, L., Borset, M., Espevik, T., and Sundan, A. (2006) Leukemia 20, 1138
80. Jozsef, L., Khreiss, T., and Filep, J. G. (2004) FASEB J 18, 1776
81. Kuo, C. C., Liang, S. M., and Liang, C. M. (2006) J Biol Chem 281, 38200

82. Sester, D. P., Brion, K., Trieu, A., Goodridge, H. S., Roberts, T. L., Dunn, J., Hume, D. A., Stacey, K. J., and Sweet, M. J. (2006) J Immunol 177, 4473
83. Sohn, W. J., Lee, K. W., Choi, S. Y., Chung, E., Lee, Y., Kim, T. Y., Lee, S. K., Choe, Y. K., Lee, J. H., Kim, D. S., and Kwon, H. J. (2006) Mol Immunol 43, 1163
84. Yi, A. K., Chang, M., Peckham, D. W., Krieg, A. M., and Ashman, R. F. (1998) J Immunol 160, 5898
85. Yi, A. K., Peckham, D. W., Ashman, R. F., and Krieg, A. M. (1999) Int Immunol 11, 2015

Engineering Adult Stem Cells for Cancer Immunotherapy

Wesley Burnside and Yan Cui

Abstract Stem cells are rare populations of multipotent and undifferentiated progenitors, demonstrating an unlimited self-renewal capacity and high plasticity. After isolation from embryonic or adult tissues, stem cells can be expanded and manipulated ex vivo for therapeutic use. With recent advances in our understanding of stem cell biology, their pluripotency and longevity, and especially, the realization of their tumoritropic migratory property, stem cells are thought to be ideal candidates as vehicles for long-term and tissue-specific transgene delivery for cancer therapeutics. Stem cell-based approaches directly modifying, attracting, or enhancing the function of immune effector cells, such as T cells or APCs, and enhancing tumor killing have been proven feasible. However, the clinical efficacy of the engineered adult stem cells for specific and targeted cancer treatment has yet to be attested. With increased venues of stem cell generation, separation, ex vivo expansion, and improvement in targeted gene delivery vehicles, it is expected that broadened applications and improved clinical outcome of adult stem cell-based cancer treatment could be realized in the near future. Here, we review the rationale and current status of adult stem cell-based cancer immune therapy in experimental models and early clinical trials and extend our discussion to prospects for clinical application.

Introduction

Forty-five years ago, landmark studies, describing the existence of self-renewing cells of the blood-forming system in mouse bone marrow by McCulloch and Till, marked the origins of stem cell research [1, 2]. By defining the self-renewal and differentiation hallmark properties of stem cells, these studies established the scientific bases of bone marrow transplantation (BMT) practice initiated in 1950s.

Y. Cui (✉)
Department of Medicine, Gene Therapy Program, Stanley S. Scott Cancer Center, Louisiana State University Health Sciences Center, 533 Bolivar Street, CSRB 601F, New Orleans, LA 70112
e-mail: ycui@lsuhsc.edu

J. Lustgarten et al. (eds.), *Targeted Cancer Immune Therapy*,
DOI 10.1007/978-1-4419-0170-5_11, © Springer Science+Business Media, LLC 2009

However, it wasn't until the 1970s did the successful isolation and characterization of the bone marrow hematopoietic stem cells (HSC) occur [3, 4]. Throughout this period, BMT continues to be used for treating inherent immunodeficiency, hematological malignancy, and hematopoietic defects. Similar to BMT, hematopoietic stem cell transplantation (HSCT) is currently the therapy of choice for leukemia and lymphoma treatment.

In addition to simply utilizing the capacity of HSC to replace the entire diseased immune system of the host with unmanipulated stem cells, HSCs can also be engineered to correct genetically defective stem cells or to enhance their immunostimulatory capacity for tumor immunotherapy. Incorporation of modified or engineered stem cells into HSCT as therapeutic interventions has been proven beneficial as demonstrated by the successful transplant of adenosine-deaminase (ADA)-gene modified bone marrow stem cells into children with severe immunodeficiency due to ADA deficiency [5]. The real excitement and proven clinical success of stem cell-based gene therapy in curing inherited genetic defects came with reports of the transplantation of IL-2Rγ chain or ADA gene modified HSCs completely corrected the X-linked or ADA deficiency-related immunological diseases, respectively [6–8]. Therefore, stem cell-based therapies present us with opportunities to fully exploit their self-renewal and differentiation capacity in that they can be integrated into specific tissue/organ and give rise to cells of the desired lineage for the production of therapeutic transgene(s). Some of the engineered stem cells do maintain their self-renewal potency, serving as a constant source for continuous generation of daughter cells. With the rapid advance in stem cell research and better understanding of stem cell biology and improved protocols for their ex vivo and in vivo expansion, there exist an increased appreciation of adult stem cells' tissue diversity and plasticity, including mesenchymal stem cells (MSC). As a result, engineering stem cells for clinical cancer treatment hold high promises. However, major obstacles for the safe and effective clinical use of embryonic stem cells or progenies derived from ESC are the immune rejection and the potential risk of tumor formation [9]. So far, various types of adult stem cells, including HSC and MSC, both derived from bone marrow, have shown promise in enhancing antitumor immunity in experimental and clinical cancer therapies. As HSCs and MSCs are predominently used in experimental and clinical cancer research due to their availability from adult donors, we will focus mainly on the status and application of these two types of adult stem cells in this review.

Stem Cell Biology

Stem cells are self-renewing progenitors varying in differentiation potency depending on the developmental stage and tissue origin from which they are generated. Totipotency refers to the capacity of a stem cell to divide and differentiate into any type of cells of the particular organism. An example of a totipotent cell is a fertilized egg.

Pluripotency refers to the ability of a stem cell to differentiate into the cells or tissues of any of the three germ layers – ectoderm, mesoderm, and endoderm. An example of this is an embryonic stem cell. Multipotency indicates a stem cell that can only produce cells of closely related lineage subsets, such as HSC [10]. Overall, stem cells can be categorized into two major types according to their sources: embryonic stem cells (ESC) and adult stem cells (ASC). Most of the ASCs are progenitors already committed to a specific lineage or confined to limited and related lineages. ASCs can be obtained from various types of mature tissues including brain, bone marrow, heart, skin, guts, and liver [11–13]. These cells are not only capable of replicating infinitely, but also differentiating into daughter cells that possess a restricted and specialized lineage. During the past few years, there has been a rapid expansion and the exploration of these ASCs, resulting in the realization of their fundamental roles in tissue repair, as well as their great potential for regenerative medicine and cancer treatment. Although the cell surface marker characteristics of each ASC type are not yet well defined, their isolation and characterization, to a certain extent, rely on functional confirmation of the self-renewal and differentiation potentials, the two hallmark characteristics of stem cells.

ESC

ESCs are generated from the inner cell mass of a blastocyst formed a few days after the fertilization. They are totipotency or pluripotency and, theoretically, have unlimited capacity of expansion and self-renewal. Thus, they can give rise to any tissue types of a particular organism. However, the pluripotency of ESCs also appears to contribute to the risks of teratomas formation, tumors that contain all types of tissues associated with inappropriate differentiation occurred in vivo [9]. Different from ASCs, ESCs proliferate through symmetric divisions, i.e., generating identical daughter cells, whereas ASCs divide asymmetrically [11].

HSC

HSCs, derived in the bone marrow, were the earliest stem cells studied and are the most commonly used/manipulated stem cells in clinical application. As multipotent stem cells, they give rise to cells of the hematopoietic and lymphoid lineages [14]. The most primitive, undifferentiated human HSCs with long-term engraftment, self-renewal, and multipotent differentiation potency are characterized as $CD34^{+}$/$CD38^{-/low}$$Thy\text{-}1^{+}$/$c\text{-}Kit^{-/low}$/$Lin^{-}$/$CD133^{+}$/$VEGF\text{-}R2^{+}$ [14, 15]. They can be obtained from bone marrow (BM), mobilized peripheral blood, cord blood, or even placenta [16, 17]. Primitive murine HSCs are usually harvested from mouse BM and characterized as Lin^{-}/$Sca\text{-}1^{+}$/$Thy\text{-}1^{low}$/$c\text{-}Kit^{+}$ population [14].

MSC

The identification and characterization of MSC was initiated by Owen et al. and Friedenstein during the period from the 1980s to 1990s [18, 19]. These cells are derived from bone stroma localized in perivasuclar niches of the bone cavity with diverse differentiation potential. They can give rise to mesoderm-type cells including osteoblasts, chondrocytes, adipocytes, myoblasts, and potentially other nonmesoderm type cells, such as neuronal cells or hepatocytes. Although still a subject of debate, MSCs appear to have the highest plasticity in lineage differentiation among all adult stem cells. They are also supportive stroma population for the growth and differentiation of HSC and hematopoiesis [20, 21]. The characteristic cell surface markers for defining MSC are still a subject to final acceptance by the scientific community. Overall, MSCs are generally shown to be negative for CD34, CD45, CD14 and positive for some of the markers such as Stro-1, CD29, CD73, CD90, CD105, CD166, and CD44 [22].

Umbilical Cord Blood Stem Cells

Umbilical cord blood stem cells (UCB-SC) are harvested from cord blood upon delivery. Recent studies also showed that they can be obtained from the placenta shortly after birth using the $CD34^{+}$ marker [16]. UCB-SCs appear to have a higher level of engraftment potency and multipotent differentiation capacity compared with HSCs. They can differentiate into cells of hematopoietic lineages, mesenchymal progenitors, neural stem cell progenitors, hepatocytes, and endothelial cells in vitro or in vivo [17]. Their clinical application potential might be limited due to the requirement of matched HLA type to minimize the risk of graft rejection.

Adult Tissue-Resident Stem Cells

Recently, there is increased interest and improvement in identification and functional studies of tissue-resident stem cells. These specialized stem cells are committed to tissue specificity and colocalize with supporting cells within the specific niche of each tissue/organ. They are critical sources for tissues replenishment and homeostatic maintenance of mature cell population throughout the adult life [12]. Neural stem cells, cardiac stem cells, and endothelial progenitors, for instance, are among the extensively studied tissue-resident stem cells that have demonstrated promising potentials for regenerative medicine [12].

Overall, HSC and MSC are, thus far, the mostly accessible and explored stem cell populations for experimental and clinical cancer treatment. This review will mainly focus on their application for cancer immune therapy.

HSC for Tumor Immune Therapy-Arming Stem Cells

For more than four decades, HSCT has been effectively used for disease treatment especially in the treatment of blood disorders including severe combined immune deficiency and hematological malignancy. In fact, cancer treatment by autologous HSC was among one of the first clinical applications of stem cell-based gene therapy. Currently, HSCT has been the treatment of choice for hematological malignancy such as leukemia, multiple myloma, Hodgkin's lymphoma, and non-Hodgkin's lymphoma, either alone, or in combination with other conventional or novel regimens [23–25].

It is now clear that a critical requirement of effective cancer immunotherapy is to generate good quantity and quality of tumor-specific T cells for complete tumor elimination. An effective approach is the direct targeting of antigen-specific T cells, or indirectly enhancing the immune stimulatory function of antigen presenting DCs within the tumor microenvironment and lymphoid tissues. Besides direct engineering of mature T cells and DCs, their modification can also be achieved via engineering their presurcusors – HSCs to fully utilize the self-renewal and differentiation properties of stem cells. Recent major advancements in gene transfer technology and rapid expansion of stem cell research, incorporating engineered HSC into the conventional HSCT and adjuvant immunotherapy regimens, represent a promising opportunity for augmenting antitumor immunity. Indeed, recently immune gene therapy for cancer has been focused on the use of gene transfer to increase the immunogenicity of tumor cells and antitumor immunity of the host via ex vivo or in vivo engineering of T cells, antigen presenting cells, or HSC [26–28].

HSCT for Hematological Malignancy and Solid Tumors: GVL and GVT

The initial incorporation of HSCT into the treatment of patients with hematological diseases was based on the premise that HSCs are capable of replacing the diseased HSC and reconstituting the entire hematopoietic lineage populations to restore the function of the defective hematopoietic and the immune system after myeloablation. Thus, HSCT also allows patients to tolerant high-dose chemotherapy or irradiation treatment for tumor eradication and has been established as standard procedure for leukemia, multiple myloma, Hodgkin's lymphoma, and non-Hodgkin's lymphoma [23–25]. Lately, autologous HSCT has also been incorporated into the therapeutic regimen of patients with advanced metastastic breast cancers and other metastatic diseases receiving chemotherapy and radiation therapy to provide additional protective benefits [29, 30]. Clinical results tend to suggest that HSC transplantation in combination with high-dose chemotherapy or irradiation therapy constituted a major development in treating some high-risk patients with advanced metastatic tumors such as breast, ovarian, prostate, colorectal, brain, lung cancers, and melanoma by facilitating hematopoietic recovery and antitumor immunity [29, 31–36].

Currently, both autologous (stem cells of self origin) and allogenic (stem cells from other individuals) HSCT have been employed clinically. However, their use is primarily dependent on the quality and availability of stem cells and on the compatibility or matching of the major MHC molecules (human leukocyte antigen-HLA) between donors and recipients. The use of autologous HSCs is associated with the risk of contaminating disease (*tainted*) blood cells; whereas, the use of allogenic HSCs from healthy donors eliminates this risk. However, an HLA-match donor stem cell is required to prevent the rejection of cell transplantation. Since a perfect match of HLA type between the donor and recipient is very unusual, allogenic HSCT is often associated with graft-versus-host-disease (GVHD). GVHD is an inflammatory disease usually mediated by T cells reaction to foreign peptides presented on the MHC of the host. This occurs as the result of donor-derived T cells or NK cells attack the recipient's tissues, either in the form of acute or chronic GVHD. Acute GVHD is usually deadly which occurs within the first 3 months of the transplantation with severe damages in the skin, intestine, and the liver. Chronic GVHD is milder and nonlethal which develops and persists after allogeneic transplant associated with treatment-related complications.

On the contrary, GVHD may also be beneficial for treating hematological malignancy as has been shown clinically that the development of GVHD correlates well with the clinical response of graft-versus-leukemia (GVL) or graft-versus-tumor (GVT). This is believed to be contributed by a therapeutic immune reaction of the grafted donor T lymphocytes and NK cells against the recipient's diseased bone marrow. Among the tumor patients who received allogeneic HCST, those with either acute or, particularly, chronic GVHD appear to have a lower risk of cancer relapse [37, 38]. Similarly, this lower rate of relapse is also demonstrated as the increased success of tumor treatment of patients received allogeneic transplants compared with those from identical twins. These suggest that allogenic HSCT by itself is a form of immunotherapy and has been employed as a standard procedure for the treatment of hematological malignancy to improve the prognosis [39]. Interestingly, the major GVL benefit is more evident in HSCT patients who do not receive the highest immuno-suppressive regimens, and GVL appears to be always associated with GVHD. Therefore, it will be particularly beneficial if specific interventions can be developed to induce GVL or GVT in the absence of GVHD. The potential separation of GVL from undesirable GVHD is the subject of intensive study and is beyond the topic of this review.

DC-Targeted Immune Therapy from Engineered HSC

As professional APCs and the critical regulators bridging innate and adaptive immunity, dendritic cells (DCs) play critical roles in activating T cell-mediated cellular immunity and B cell-mediated humoral immunity. Many preventive and therapeutic tumor vaccination approaches have heavily focused on engineering DCs for immune activation. Previous chapters have provided extensive reviews on the current status of ex vivo DC manipulation for tumor vaccines; therefore, it will not be the subject of discussion here. Overall, initial clinical trials with ex vivo manipulated DCs, serving as proof-of-principle, demonstrated their capacity in immune activation and provided the impetus for further development of more effective novel DC-targeted vaccines.

One particular approach to enhance the efficacy of DC vaccine that has not been studied extensively is DC targeting in vivo. Strategies for targeting antigens to DCs in vivo present a major advantage of vaccines in that these DCs are naturally located in the proper lymphoid compartment for appropriated interaction with T cells. More importantly, their numbers and activation status can be further enhanced by DC stimulatory cytokines and adjuvant. It has been demonstrated that in vivo DC targeting can be mediated either by antibody-guided antigen delivery to DC-specific receptors, such as mannose or CD205 receptors, or HSC engineering-mediated transgene delivery. Since DCs are normally derived from hematopoietic stem/progenitors, modification of HSC with genes of specific antigen followed by transplantation would provide a constant progenitor reservoir for continued generation of antigen expressing DCs in vivo. Using lentiviral vector (LV) modified HSC in combination with HSCT, we demonstrated that specific antigen gene modified HSC by LV reconstituted host lymphoid-hematopoietic system and provided a constant pool of antigen gene-carrying DC progenitors [40–42]. Upon appropriate maturation and activation by DC stimulatory cytokines in vivo, a significant number of antigen expressing DCs was generated in vivo which subsequently promoted a marked activation of antitumor immunity, resulting in prolonged tumor-free survival of mice bearing preestablished tumors [27, 43, 44]. Therefore, using LV-mediated gene transfer to HSC in the context of stem cell transplantation and DC activation adjuvant may offer new avenues toward generating/redirecting desired antigen-specific immune responses in experimental models and clinical applications.

It is important to point out that antigen presentation by DCs results in either immune activation or tolerance depending on the maturation and activation status of DCs: tolerance is induced when antigen presenting DCs are immature, semi-mature, or of the so-called "steady-state" phenotype; whereas, immune activation is induced when antigen presenting DCs are mature and activated [45–49]. Therefore, targeted antigen delivery to DCs in the absence of additional DC activation regimen resulted in antigen-specific tolerance induction [50]. Most importantly, incorporating appropriate DC maturation and activation regimens together with in vivo DC targeting approach is essential for the successful promotion of antitumor immune responses. The importance of adjuvant-mediated immune activation in the face of conventional DC vaccine or this HSC-mediated in vivo DC targeting to stimulate strong antitumor immunity is demonstrated both experimentally and clinically [27, 28, 51].

T Cell-Targeted Immune Therapy Using Engineered HSC

Adoptive transfer of tumor-specific T cells, also called adoptive cell transfer (ACT) therapy, has been used for cancer treatment either as a monotherapy or more recently in combination with other therapeutic regimens [52–54]. Overall, these studies demonstrated that ACT using ex vivo expanded T cells from patient's tumor infiltrating lymphocytes or peripheral blood lymphocytes temporarily suppressed tumor progression but failed to provide lasting therapeutic effect, partly due to low T cell frequency and their poor durability. These shortcomings could be moderately improved either by establishing a lymphophenia status of the hosts by low dose irradiation or chemotherapy or improving ex vivo T cell expansion protocol for generating larger numbers of tumor antigen-specific T cells. However, a recent study indicated that ex vivo expanded effector memory T cells are intrinsically associated with poor survival capacity and clinical efficacy [55]. Therefore, alternative strategies of generating tumor antigen-specific T cells may prove more productive.

Recently, empowered with advanced molecular biology techniques, T cell receptor α and β chains with defined tumor antigen specificity have been cloned from tumor antigen-specific T cells. It is proposed that introducing these TCR α and β chains to mature T cells or T cell precursors, such as HSC, for enforced expression will result in engineered T cells redirected to the desired tumor antigen specificity. Successful transferring of functional TCR α and β chains from one T cell to another by Demibic et al. in 1986 confirmed the feasibility of this approach in redirecting T cell antigen specificity [56]. Subsequent studies by various groups with murine and human T cells in experimental models, as well as in clinical trials for melanomas, further demonstrated the function and effectiveness of these engineered T cells in combating tumor and infectious pathogens [57–59]. However, T cell engineering using mature T lymphocytes encountered a problem of low frequency of cells expressing engineered TCR αβ chains due to stringent competition with endogenous α and β chains for proper pairing. To curtail this problem, engineering HSC with exogenous TCR α and β chains followed by their differentiation to mature T cells is more plausible. Indeed, T cells generated in mice transplanted with TCR α and β chain gene transduced HSC confirmed that endogenous TCR rearrangement is prevented during T cell development in the thymus due to the suppression of RAG gene expression, thus alleviating the potential TCR mispairing [60]. Moreover, these engineered mature T cells express functional exogenous TCR with specific cytolytic activity against the defined tumor antigen and, consequently, suppress the growth of established tumors in an antigen-specific manner [60]. More meaningfully, the function of these antigen-specific effectors and their antitumor immunity could be further enhanced by subsequent vaccination with tumor antigens resulting in complete elimination of established tumors. Therefore, introducing specific TCR to HSC for engineering and redirecting T cells to antitumor specificity in the context of HSCT is a promising combination approach to further augment host antitumor immunity in vivo.

MSC for Immune Therapy

MSCs are easily obtained from patients' marrow aspirate and can be expended in culture for as many as 50 doublings, i.e., more than 1×10^{15} fold expansion within 10 weeks. Like most other ASCs, MSCs are believed to be important in maintaining tissue homeostasis by replenishing and repairing injured tissues. One of the unique properties of MSCs and other ASCs, realized over the past few years, is their preferential migratory property toward sites of pathology, including wounds and ischaemia, and injury. Interestingly, it is proposed that the microenvironment of a solid tumor is similar to that of damaged or stressed tissues and, thus, MSCs may preferentially migrate toward site of primary and metastastic tumors and potentially contribute to the tumor stroma formation [61–63]. This led to a rapid expansion of the MSC research for the past few years and numerous studies revealed that MSCs not only preferentially migrate to established tumor site, but also could track minor metastases in the pulmonary and brain tissues. This preferential migration of MSC toward tumors is thought to resemble their migration process toward the inflamed or injured tissue sites. It is speculated that this tumoritrophic property is mediated by chemokine receptors, such as CXCR4/CXCL12, on MSC surface and various chemotactic cytokines and inflammatory signals from the tumor or wound, supporting the theory that tumors resemble that of an unresolved wound [61, 64, 65]. Currently, the molecular mechanism and specific chemotactic signals contributing to the tumoritrophic migration of MSC are under intensive investigation. Notwithstanding, this tumoritrophic property of MSCs makes them ideal candidates of cancer therapy for targeted delivery of therapeutic genes to tumor and tumor microenvironment [64, 66].

Immunotherapy Through Tumor Attraction and Cytokine Production

Based on the observed tumoritrophic property of MSCs, various MSC-based immunotherapy approaches have been developed and tested. Most of the MSC-based therapy, combining gene therapy-mediated transgene delivery with stem cell-based cellular therapy, relies on local delivery of MSC for treating localized diseases because they exhibit poor capacity in crossing capillary barriers when delivered systemically or to noninjured tissues. Interestingly, a recent study showed that total body irradiation appears to increase the homing of MSC to different organs and, thus, may enhance their systemic migratory ability [67]. To further utilize and enhance their tumoritrophic migratory capacity, MSCs were pretreated with proinflammatory cytokine, such as TNF-α or IL-1β, prior to injection, which appeared to up-regulate their integrin and extracellular adhesion molecules and enhanced their in vivo migration and adhesion ability toward tumor [67]. Furthermore, Tomchuck et al. observed that TLR stimulation, especially TLR3, enhanced the migratory capacity of MSC, which can be blocked by a specific antibody neutralizing the TLR3 signaling [68].

The antitumor effects of engineered MSC are mostly based on cytokine-mediated direct tumor suppression or activation of immune response. Injection of MSC modified to express IFN-β to mice bearing established tumors resulted in MSC incorporation into tumor microenvironment and suppression of tumor progression through the local toxic effects of IFN-β in melanoma, lung, breast cancer, and glioma animal models [69–71]. Expression of immune stimulatory cytokines, such as IL-2, IL-12, and interferon-β (IFN-β) in MSC activated a systemic immune responses against tumor, possibly involving IFN-γ-mediated immune responses in some cases [69, 72–75]. Furthermore, engineered bone marrow derived neural stem cells, a more committed type of MSCs, expressing IL-4 or IL-12 or IL-23 also showed to induce systemic immune responses against gliomas, suppressed tumor progression, and improved tumor-free survival in mice and rat glioma models [76–78]. Overall, MSCs have been shown as ideal vehicles for targeted delivery of immunostimulatory genes to tumor and tumor microenvironment to enhance antitumor immune responses.

MSC in the Context of HSCT

It has been well documented that MSCs are weakly immunogenic or potentially immunosuppressive as they express very low level of MHC II molecules and undetectable MHC I molecule. Recent studies showed that MSCs inhibited proliferation of both $CD4^+$ and $CD8^+$ T cells in mixed lymphocyte reaction culture in a cell-dose dependent manner. Simultaneous infusion of MSC from donor or irrelevant origin at the time of allogeneic skin graft implantation prolonged graft survival, and further investigation suggested that the suppressive mechanism of MSCs to allo-antigen-mediated immune activation is likely mediated by suppressing DC migration, maturation, and antigen presentation [82]. Similar studies using human MSC also demonstrated that they suppressed T cell proliferation by licensing monocyte or $CD34^+$ progenitor to differentiate into regulatory DCs [79–81].

With this observed inherent immuosuppressive nature, MSCs have then been considered of great therapeutic value for potentially facilitating allogeneic transplantation across HLA-barriers, meliorating graft rejection, and GVHD. This was first confirmed in a Baboon skin allograft transplant experiment that systemic injection of donor MSCs prior to allogenic skin graft implantation significantly suppressed the graft rejection [83]. Similar clinical studies by Lee et al. in 2002 and Fouillard et al. in 2003 demonstrated that coinfusion of MSCs with HSCs for allogenic HSCT reduced hematological pathology and GVHD [84, 85]. Therefore, a multicenter clinical trial of coinfusing HSCs and MSCs from HLA-identical sibling donors was coordinately performed by Lazarus et al. for patients with hematological malignancy undergoing myeloablative HSCT treatment. It was observed that in most patients who received MSCs 4 h before HSCT showed a rapid hematopoietic recovery and 50% of the patients did not develop symptoms related to acute GVHD [86]. Similarly, Koc et al. also observed that coinfusion of autologous MSC with HSC in myeloablative HSCT for hematological diseases improved bone marrow and hematopoietic recovery [89]. The potential correlation of improved HSC engraftment and immune recovery with MSC-mediated GVHD suppression was confirmed in an NOD/SCID mice model of human stem cell engraftment in that human MSC from unrelated individual enhanced HSC engraftment by suppressing T cell activation-mediated GVHD [87, 88]. Recently, cotransplant of IL-7 gene transduced MSC along with the allogenic HSCT also seemed to prevent host from GVHD and enhance immune reconstitution [90]. On the contrary, a different study with MSCs in nonmyeloablative HSCT setting revealed that the origin of MSC appeared to be a critical determining factor for the effectiveness of allograft rejection in that MSC of host origin during HSCT-induced tolerance and prolonged engraftment, whereas MSC of donor origin stimulated a memory T cell response and resulted in enhanced allograft rejection [91]. These experimental and clinical results suggest that cotransfer of MSC during HSCT is at least a safe procedure and might have potential benefits in enhancing hematological recovery and reducing transplantation-associated side effects, including GVHD. However, it is still unknown whether the observed immunosuppressive effects of MSCs on GVHD or overall immune activation may introduce any potentially negative effects on antitumor immunity, such as the GVL or GVT effects discussed earlier.

Requirement and Consideration for Stem Cell Engineering for Therapeutic Use

Because of the self-renewal and differentiation potential of stem cells, the required long-term expression and preferably in restricted progeny of interests are the major considerations of stem cell gene therapy. This requires the efficient transduction of the stem cells and maintenance of the transgene expression within the host with a high level of engraftment. All viral and nonviral vectors have been tested for gene delivery to HSCs. So far, it appears that onco-retroviral and LVs are most efficient and reliable in gene delivery to HSCs because of their capacity in transgene integration for long-term expression. Early studies mainly employed retroviral vectors for transgene delivery to stem cells, which resulted in the successful gene therapy trial by Cavazzana-Calvo et al., and was the first direct proof that stem cell gene therapy could provide cure for a genetic disease, X-linked SCID [6]. Subsequently, ADA-SCID was also corrected by stem cell-based gene therapy [7]. However, these excitements were overshadowed by the incidences of leukemia development in some of the cured SCID patients [95, 96]. Extensive investigations to understand the cause of leukemia and other potential risks associated with retroviral-mediated gene transfer revealed that MLV-based retroviral vectors preferentially target the 5′ region of the active gene for their integration, making them more susceptible in activating a downstream oncogene via transcriptional read-through [92, 93]. In fact, it is now believed that both the retroviral gene delivery vectors and the oncogenic nature of the transgene, such as IL-2Rγc, used in the early clinical trials contributed to the leukemia development [8, 94–96].

With the development and significant improvement of LV system during the past decade, HIV-1-based vectors have been used more regularly as gene delivery vehicles to stem cells. Unlike conventional onco-retrovirus, HIV-1-based LVs are able to transduce HSCs that are not actively dividing [97]. Furthermore, LVs have been demonstrated to be less prone to transcriptional activation of downstream genes via read-through [98]. More importantly, with the further development of self-inactivating LVs, transgene expression can be transcriptionally controlled by tissue-specific or drug inducible promoters [40, 99, 100]. The promise of LV-based gene therapy in clinical use is demonstrated by the recent safe and successful trials of LV-mediated gene delivery to T cells for patients with HIV [101] and β-globin gene to HSC for the treatment of β-thalassemia [102]. Overall, the development and significant improvement in LVs during the past decade make them promising vectors for HSC-based gene therapy with broadened potential clinical application. Other vector systems, such as adeno-associated virus, as delivery vehicles to HSCs have also been studied extensively with limited success [103].

Transgene delivery to MSC is less problematic. Many viral- or nonviral-based gene delivery approaches proved to be efficient in delivery transgene to MSCs. Because MSCs are usually slow dividing cells, their long-term transgene expression may not always be an essential requirement for the therapeutic nature that they are involved. For instance, adenovirus-mediated gene delivery has been shown to work efficiently for MSC-based cancer immune therapy because they provide local high level transgene expression and additional immunostimulatory signals to further enhance the immune activation.

Together, safe and effective modification of stem cells for targeted or restricted transgene expression in defined lineages and long-term expression is important and might be one of the determining factors on the effectiveness of stem cell-based gene therapy in clinics.

Summary

The ultimate goal of cancer treatment is the complete elimination of all macroscopic and microscopic tumors. So far, we have mainly relied on enhancing the function of immune cells, such as effector T cells and professional antigen presenting DCs, to identify and eradicate microscopic and metastatic tumors. HSC, as precursors of DCs and T cells, represent ideal candidates for cancer immunotherapy. Recent advances in stem cell research and our better understanding of tumoritrophic migratory property of MSC generate excitement and promise of MSC as trangene delivery vehicles for promoting antitumor immunity. Current experimental and early clinical results support the feasibility of engineered stem cells for generating super effectors and antitumor immunity for cancer eradication. Therefore, with more intensive and rapid advancement of stem cell research, engineered stem cells offer great promise for developing novel, safe, and effective immunotherapy protocols for successful cancer treatment.

Acknowledgments We would like to thank Ms. Alexandra Wesley-Smith for her editorial assistance.This work is supported by funds from the Louisiana Gene Therapy Consortium, Stanley S. Scott Cancer Center and grants from the National Institutes of Health to YC (CA112065 and P20RR021970).

References

1. Till, J. E., and Mc, C. E. (1961) Radiat Res 14, 213
2. Becker, A. J., Mc, C. E., and Till, J. E. (1963) Nature 197, 452
3. Thomas, E. D., Lochte, H. L., Jr., Lu, W. C., and Ferrebee, J. W. (1957) N Engl J Med 257, 491
4. Spangrude, G. J., Heimfeld, S., and Weissman, I. L. (1988) Science 241, 58
5. Bordignon, C., Notarangelo, L, D., Nobili, N., Ferrari, G., Casorati, G., Panina, P., Mazzolari, E., Maggioni, D., Rossi, C., and Servida, P. (1995) Science 270, 470
6. Cavazzana-Calvo, M., Hacein-Bey, S., de Saint Basile, G., Gross, F., Yvon, E., Nusbaum, P., Selz, F., Hue, C., Certain, S., and Casanova, J.L. (20000 Science 288, 669
7. Aiuti, A., Slavin, S., Aker, M., Ficara, F., Deola, S., Mortellaro, A., Morecki, S., Andolfi, G., Tabucchi, A., and Carlucci, F. (2002) Science 296, 2410
8. Hacein-Bey-Abina, S., Le Deist, F., Carlier, F., Bouneaud, C., Hue, C., De Villartay, J. P., Thrasher, A. J., Wulffraat, N., Sorensen, R., and Dupuis-Girod, S. (2002) N Engl J Med 346, 1185
9. Byrne, J. A., Mitalipov, S. M., Wolf, D. P. (2006) Curr Stem Cell Res Ther 1, 127
10. Lakshmipathy, U., and Verfaillie, C. (2005) Blood Rev 19, 29
11. Serakinci, N., and Keith, W. N. (2006) Eur J Cancer 42, 1243
12. Mimeault, M., Hauke, R., and Batra, S. K. (2007) Clin Pharmacol Ther 82, 252
13. Corsten, M. F., and Shah, K. (2008) Lancet Oncol 9, 376
14. Kondo, M., Wagers, A. J., Manz, M. G., Prohaska, S. S., Scherer, D. C., Beilhack, G. F., Shizuru, J. A., and Weissman, I. L. (2003) Annu Rev Immunol 21, 759
15. Civin, C. I., Trischmann, T., Kadan, N. S., Davis, J., Noga, S., Cohen, K., Duffy, B., Groenewegen, I., Wiley, J., and Law, P. (1996) J Clin Oncol 14, 2224
16. Matikainen, T., and Laine, J. (2005) Toxicol Appl Pharmacol 207, 544
17. Weiss, M. L., and Troyer, D. L. (2006) Stem Cell Rev 2, 155
18. Friedenstein, A. J. (1980) Haematol Blood Transfus 25, 19
19. Owen, M. (1980) Arthritis Rheum 23, 1073
20. Jiang, Y., Vaessen, B., Lenvik, T., Blackstad, M., Reyes, M., and Verfaillie, C. M. (2002) Exp Hematol 30, 896
21. Orlic, D., Kajstura, J., Chimenti, S., Jakoniuk, I., Anderson, S. M., Li, B., Pickel, J., McKay, R., Nadal-Ginard, B., and Bodine, D. M. (2001) Nature 410, 701
22. Abdallah, B. M., and Kassem, M. (2008) Gene Ther 15, 109
23. Popat, U., Carrum, G., and Heslop, H. E. (2003) Cancer Treat Rev 29, 3
24. Nabhan, C., Mehta, J., and Tallman, M. S. (2001) Bone Marrow Transplant 28, 219
25. Maris, M., Sandmaier, B. M., Maloney, D. G., McSweeney, P. A., Woolfrey, A., Chauncey, T., Shizuru, J., Niederwieser, D., Blume, K. G., and Forman, S. (2001) Transfus Clin Biol 8, 231
26. Pardoll, D. M. (2000) Clin Immunol 95, S44
27. Cui, Y., Kelleher, E., Straley, E., Fuchs, E., Gorski, K., Levitsky, H., Borrello, I., Civin, C. I., Schoenberger, S. P., and Cheng, L. (2003) Nat Med 9, 952
28. Zhang, X., Zhao, P., Kennedy, C., Chen, K., Wiegand, J., Washington, G., Marrero, L., and Cui, Y. (2008) Cancer Gene Ther 15, 73
29. Negrin, R. S., Atkinson, K., Leemhuis, T., Hanania, E., Juttner, C., Tierney, K., Hu, W. W., Johnston, L. J., Shizurn, J. A., and Stockerl-Goldstein, K. E. (2000) Biol Blood Marrow Transplant 6, 262
30. Gerrero, R. M., Stein, S., and Stadtmauer, E. A. (2002) Drugs Aging 19, 475
31. Imamura, M., Asano, S., Harada, M., Ikeda, Y., Kato, K., Kato, S., Kawa, K., Kojima, S., Morishima, Y., and Morishita, Y. (2006) Int J Hematol 83, 164
32. Hale, G. A. (2005) Expert Rev Anticancer Ther 5, 835
33. Rizzo, J. D., Elias, A. D., Stiff, P. J., Lazarus, H. M., Zhang, M. J., Oblon, D. J., Pecora, A. L., Hale, G. A., and Horowitz, M. M. (2002) Biol Blood Marrow Transplant 8, 273
34. Frickhofen, N., Berdel, W. E., Opri, F., Haas, R., Schneeweiss, A., Sandherr, M., Kuhn, W., Hossfeld, D. K., Thomssen, C., and Heimpel, H. (2006) Bone Marrow Transplant 38, 493

35. McNiece, I., Jones, R., Bearman, S. I., Cagnoni, P., Nieto, Y., Franklin, W., Ryder, J., Steele, A., Stoltz, J., and Russell, P. (2000) Blood 96, 3001
36. Nieto, Y., Shpall, E. J., McNiece, I. K., Nawaz, S., Beaudet, J., Rosinski, S., Pellom, J., Slat-Vasquez, V., McSweeney, P. A., and Bearman, S. I. (2004) Clin Cancer Res 10, 5076
37. Baron, F., Maris, M. B, Sandmaier, B. M., Storer, B. E., Sorror, M., Diaconescu, R., Woolfrey, A. E., Chauncey, T. R., Flowers, M. E., and Mielcarek, M. (2005) J Clin Oncol 23, 1993
38. Toze, C. L., Galal, A., Barnett, M. J., Shepherd, J. D., Conneally, E. A., Hogge, D. E., Nantel, S. H., Nevill, T. J., Sutherland, H. J., and Connors, J. M. (2005) Bone Marrow Transplant 36, 825
39. Bachanova, V., and Weisdorf, D. (2008) Bone Marrow Transplant 41, 455
40. Cui, Y., Golob, J., Kelleher, E., Ye, Z., Pardoll, D., and Cheng, L. (2002) Blood 99, 399
41. Trono, D. (2000) Gene Ther 7, 20
42. Miyoshi, H., Smith, K. A., Mosier, D. E., Verma, I. M., and Torbett, B. E. (1999) Science 283, 682
43. Weigel, B. J., Nath, N., Taylor, P. A., Panoskaltsis-Mortari, A., Chen, W., Krieg, A. M., Brasel, K., and Blazar, B. R. (2002) Blood 100, 4169
44. Merad, M., Sugie, T., Engleman, E. G., and Fong, L. (2002) Blood 99, 1676
45. Hawiger, D., Inaba, K., Dorsett, Y., Guo, M., Mahnke, K., Rivera, M., Ravetch, J. V., Steinman, R. M., and Nussenzweig, M. C. (2001) J Exp Med 194, 769
46. Heath, W. R., and Carbone, F. R. (2001) Annu Rev Immunol 19, 47
47. Steinman, R. M., Hawiger, D., Liu, K., Bonifaz, L., Bonnyay, D., Mahnke, K., Iyoda, T., Ravetch, J., Dhodapkar, M., and Inaba, K. (2003) Ann N Y Acad Sci 987, 15
48. Banchereau, J., Paczesny, S., Blanco, P., Bennett, L., Pascual, V., Fay, J., and Palucka, A. K. (2003) Ann N Y Acad Sci 987, 180
49. Mahnke, K., Knop, J., and Enk, A. H. (2003) Trends Immunol 24, 646
50. Kimura, T., Koya, R. C., Anselmi, L., Sternini, C., Wang, H. J., Comin-Anduix, B., Prins, R. M., Faure-Kumar, E., Rozengurt, N., and Cui, Y. (2007) Mol Ther 15, 1390
51. Engell-Noerregaard, L., Hansen, T. H., Andersen, M. H., Thor Straten, P., Svane, I. M. (2008) Cancer Immunol Immunother 58, 1–14
52. Ganss, R., Ryschich, E., Klar, E., Arnold, B., and Hammerling, G. J. (2002) Cancer Res 62, 1462
53. Yee, C., Thompson, J. A., Byrd, D., Riddell, S. R., Roche, P., Celis, E., and Greenberg, P. D. (2002) Proc Natl Acad Sci USA 99, 16168
54. Dudley, M. E., and Rosenberg, S. A. (2003) Nat Rev Cancer 3, 666
55. Leen, A. M., Rooney, C. M., and Foster, A. E. (2007) Annu Rev Immunol 25, 243
56. Dembic, Z., Haas, W., Weiss, S., McCubrey, J., Kiefer, H., von Boehmer, H., and Steinmetz, M. (1986) Nature 320, 232
57. Kessels, H. W., Wolkers, M. C., van den Boom, M. D., van der Valk, M. A., and Schumacher, T. N. (2001) Nat Immunol 2, 957
58. Xue, S. A., Gao, L., Hart, D., Gillmore, R., Qasim, W., Thrasher, A., Apperley, J., Engels, B., Uckert, W., and Morris, E. (2005) Blood 106, 3062
59. Morgan, R. A., Dudley, M. E., Wunderlich, J. R., Hughes, M. S., Yang, J. C., Sherry, R. M., Royal, R. E., Topalian, S. L., Kammula, U. S., and Restifo, N. P. (2006) Science 314, 126
60. Yang, L., and Baltimore, D. (2005) Proc Natl Acad Sci USA 102, 4518
61. Dvorak, H. F. (1986) N Engl J Med 315, 1650
62. Hall, B., Andreeff, M., and Marini, F. (2007) Handb Exp Pharmacol 180, 263
63. Kaplan, R. N., Psaila, B., and Lyden, D. (2006) Cancer Metastasis Rev 25, 521
64. Aboody, K. S., Najbauer, J., and Danks, M. K. (2008) Gene Ther 15, 739
65. Spaeth, E., Klopp, A., Dembinski, J., Andreeff, M., and Marini, F. (2008) Gene Ther 15, 730
66. Jorgensen, C., Djouad, F., Apparailly, F., and Noel, D. (2003) Gene Ther 10, 928
67. Klopp, A. H., Spaeth, E. L., Dembinski, J. L., Woodward, W. A., Munshi, A., Meyn, R. E., Cox, J. D., Andreeff, M., and Marini, F. C. (2007) Cancer Res 67, 11687
68. Tomchuck, S. L., Zwezdaryk, K. J., Coffelt, S. B., Waterman, R. S., Danka, E. S., and Scandurro, A. B. (2008) Stem Cells 26, 99

69. Studeny, M., Marini, F. C., Dembinski, J. L., Zompetta, C., Cabreira-Hansen, M., Bekele, B. N., Champlin, R. E., and Andreeff, M. (2004) J Natl Cancer Inst 96, 1593
70. Hall, B., Dembinski, J., Sasser, A. K., Studeny, M., Andreeff, M., and Marini, F. (2007) Int J Hematot 86, 8
71. Kanehira, M., Xin, H., Hoshino, K., Maemondo, M., Mizuguchi, H., Hayakawa, T., Matsumoto, K., Nakamura, T., Nukiwa, T., and Saijo, Y. (2007) Cancer Gene Ther 14, 894
72. Eliopoulos, N., Francois, M., Boivin, M. N., Martineau, D., and Galipeau, J. (2008) Cancer Res 68, 4810
73. Nakamura, K., Ito, Y., Kawano, Y., Kurozumi, K., Kobune, M., Tsuda, H., Bizen, A., Honmou, O., Niitsu, Y., and Hamada, H. (2004) Gene Ther 11, 1155
74. Elzaouk, L., Moelling, K., and Pavlovic, J. (2006) Exp Dermatol 15, 865
75. Nakamizo, A., Marini, F., Amano, T., Khan, A., Studeny, M., Gumin, J., Chen, J., Hentschel, S., Vecil, G., and Dembinski, J. (2005) Cancer Res 65, 3307
76. Benedetti, S., Pirola, B., Pollo, B., Magrassi, L., Bruzzone, M. G., Rigamonti, D., Galli, R., Selleri, S., Di Meco, F., and De Fraja, C. (2000) Nat Med 6, 447
77. Ehtesham, M., Kabos, P., Kabosova, A., Neuman, T., Black, K. L., and Yu, J. S. (2002) Cancer Res 62, 5657
78. Yuan, X., Hu, J., Belladonna, M. L., Black, K. L., and Yu, J. S. (2006) Cancer Res 66, 2630
79. Li, Y. P., Paczesny, S., Lauret, E., Poirault, S., Bordigoni, P., Mekhloufi, F., Hequet, O., Bertrand, Y., Ou-Yang, J. P., and Stoltz, J. F. (2008) J Immunol 180, 1598
80. Jiang, X. X., Zhang, Y., Liu, B., Zhang, S. X., Wu, Y., Yu, X. D., and Mao, N. (2005) Blood 105, 4120
81. Nauta, A. J., Kruisselbrink, A. B., Lurvink, E., Willemze, R., and Fibbe, W. E. (2006) J Immunol 177, 2080
82. English, K., Barry, F. P., and Mahon, B. P. (2008) Immunol Lett 115, 50
83. Bartholomew, A., Sturgeon, C., Siatskas, M., Ferrer, K., McIntosh, K., Patil, S., Hardy, W., Devine, S., Ucker, D., and Deans, R. (2002) Exp Hematol 30, 42
84. Lee, S. T., Jang, J. H., Cheong, J. W., Kim, J. S., Maemg, H. Y., Hahn, J. S., Ko, Y. W., and Min, Y. H. (2002) Br J Haematol 118, 1128
85. Fouillard, L., Bensidhoum, M., Bories, D., Bonte, H., Lopez, M., Moseley, A. M., Smith, A., Lesage, S., Beaujean, F., and Thierry, D. (2003) Leukemia 17, 474
86. Lazarus, H. M., Koc, O. N., Devine, S. M., Curtin, P., Maziarz, R. T., Holland, H. K., Shpall, E. J., McCarthy, P., Atkinson, K., and Cooper, B. W. (2005) Biol Blood Marrow Transplant 11, 389
87. Groh, M. E., Maitra, B., Szekely, E., and Koc, O. N. (2005) Exp Hematol 33, 928
88. Maitra, B., Szekely, E., Gjini, K., Laughlin, M. J., Dennis, J., Haynesworth, S. E., and Koc, O. N. (2004) Bone Marrow Transplant 33, 597
89. Koc, O. N., Day, J., Nieder, M., Gerson, S. L., Lazarus, H. M., and Krivit, W. (2002) Bone Marrow Transplant 30, 215
90. Li, A., Zhang, Q., Jiang, J., Yuan, G., Feng, Y., Hao, J., Li, C., Gao, X., Wang, G., and Xie, S. (2006) Gene Ther 13, 1178
91. Nauta, A. J., Westerhuis, G., Kruisselbrink, A. B., Lurvink, E. G., Willemze, R., and Fibbe, W. E. (2006) Blood 108, 2114
92. Mitchell, R. S., Beitzel, B. F., Schroder, A. R., Shinn, P., Chen, H., Berry, C. C., Ecker, J. R., and Bushman, F. D. (2004) PLoS Biol 2, 234
93. Rohdewohld, H., Weiher, H., Reik, W., Jaenisch, R., and Breindl, M. (1987) J Virol 61, 336
94. Hacein-Bey-Abina, S., von Kalle, C., Schmidt, M., Le Deist, F., Wulffraat, N., McIntyre, E., Radford, I., Villeval, J. L., Fraser, C. C., and Cavazzana-Calvo, M. (2003) N Engl J Med 348, 255
95. Woods, N. B., Bottero, V., Schmidt, M., von Kalle, C., and Verma, I. M. (2006) Nature 440, 1123
96. Hacein-Bey-Abina, S., Von Kalle, C., Schmidt, M., McCormack, M. P., Wulffraat, N., Leboulch, P., Lim, A., Osborne, C. S., Pawliuk, R., and Morillon, E. (2003) Science 302, 415

97. Chang, A. H., and Sadelain, M. (2007) Mol Ther 15, 445
98. Zaiss, A. K., Son, S., and Chang, L. J. (2002) J Virol 76, 7209
99. Zufferey, R., Dull, T., Mandel, R. J., Bukovsky, A., Quiroz, D., Naldini, L., and Trono, D. (1998) J Virol 72, 9873
100. Kafri, T., van Praag, H., Gage, F. H., and Verma, I. M. (2000) Mol Ther 1, 516
101. Levine, B. L., Humeau, L. M., Boyer, J., MacGregor, R. R., Rebello, T., Lu, X., Binder, G. K., Slepushkin, V., Lemiale, F., and Mascola, J. R. (2006) Proc Natl Acad Sci USA 103, 1737
102. Bank, A., Dorazio, R., and Leboulch, P. (2005), Ann N Y Acad Sci 1054, 308
103. Srivastava, A. (2005) Hum Gene Ther 16, 792

Animal Models for Evaluating Immune Responses of Human Effector Cells *In Vivo*

Faisal Razzaqi, Wesley M. Burnside, Lolie Yu, and Yan Cui

Abstract Studying the responses of the human immune system to specific antigens in vivo for vaccine development has been limited by ethical and practical concerns. Up to now all of the in vivo preclinical testing for cancer vaccine development have been performed in various animal models. Although successful stimulation of antitumor immunity has been demonstrated by many therapeutic maneuvers in animal models, the outcome of subsequent clinical applications is less encouraging due to, at least in part, the limitations of currently used animal models, the most important of which is the inability to accurately mimic the human immune system in initiating and maintaining the immune responses. Therefore, an animal model that mimics or consists of crucial components of the functional human immune system will be valuable for vaccine development and testing. The first breakthrough came with the discovery of the severe combined immunodeficiency (SCID) mouse and its ability to sustain engrafted human cells, albeit at a low level. Since that discovery, several new strains of mice have been developed to improve human leukocyte, including stem cell, engraftment and their differentiation to functional human immune cells. The most recent models consist of mice with a mutation of the interleukin-2 receptor γ chain (IL2Rγ_c^{null}) in the NOD/SCID background. This IL2Rγ_c^{null} genotype led to mice with significantly decreased innate immunity that allows increased levels of human cell engraftment and multilineage development of human immune cells. With further improvements, these mouse models may help in the understanding of the complex human immune responses to cancers and infectious diseases and assist in preclinical evaluation of vaccine regimens.

Y. Cui (✉)
Department of Medicine, Gene Therapy Program, Stanley S. Scott Cancer Center, Louisiana State University Health Sciences Center, 533 Bolivar Street, CSRB 601F, New Orleans, LA 70112
e-mail: ycui@lsuhsc.edu

J. Lustgarten et al. (eds.), *Targeted Cancer Immune Therapy*,
DOI 10.1007/978-1-4419-0170-5_12,

Introduction

Cancer is still one of the deadliest diseases despite great improvements made over the last decade in prevention, early diagnosis, and treatment of localized diseases with new chemotherapies and targeted molecular therapy [1]. In particular, the treatment of disseminated disease remains a formidable task which requires a targeted approach to distinguish cancer cells from normal tissues. Because of the defensive nature of the immune system in discriminating and eliminating non-self entities including cancers, immunotherapy with high specificity, efficiency, and minimal toxicity holds promise for treating tumor dissemination. Although both antibody-mediated and cytotoxic T cell-mediated elimination of non-self entities are important for controlling and treating infectious diseases, cytotoxic T cell-mediated tumor killing appears to be more effective for tumor immunotherapy. Therefore, appropriate evaluation of human T cell, and possibly B cell, effector function in animal models for vaccine development is valuable. Since the antigen presenting cells (APC), especially dendritic cells (DCs), are an important initiator and regulator of innate and adaptive immune responses, the presence of this subpopulation along with B and T cells is equally important [2–6]. Interestingly, it has been shown that the rate of certain cancers is increased in the immunodeficient population [7] and also in the elderly, most likely secondary to waning immunity [8]. Therefore, understanding the development, longevity, and interaction of different subsets of the immune effectors, including T, B, and DCs, during tumorigenesis and immune responses in an animal model is invaluable for clinical treatment [9].

Initial in vivo studies on tumorigenesis and infectious diseases were performed on animals such as dogs, rodents, and nonhuman primates. Due to the physiological differences from humans, these models are associated with certain limitations. Therefore, therapies that work well in these animal models may not always show similar effects in humans. Nonhuman primates share the most physiological similarities with humans; however, cost and other ethical issues limit their use for cancer studies [10, 11]. In fact, mouse has been the most popularly used model system for cancer studies, including tumor immunology and preclinical immunotherapy studies, due to the low cost for maintenance, high productivity, and our better understanding in their genetics with the entire genome having been sequenced [12]. Nevertheless, many immune therapies that have demonstrated preclinical efficacy in mice showed disappointing clinical outcome.

In attempts to reconstruct or mimic the human immune activation process in mice, various approaches have been developed to transplant human cells to immunodeficient mice or to engineer mice that express human major histocompatibility complex (MHC) or human leukocyte antigens (HLA) to generate the so-called humanized mice. Over the last 25 years, significant progress has been made to allow reliable engraftment and development of human immune cells in those mice to a point that the potential reconstruction of a functional human immune system containing the essential elements for *in vivo* evaluation of the responses of human immune cells is possible. In this chapter, we discuss mouse models that have been humanized by transplantation and engraftment of human stem cells for potential use in vaccine development.

First Models for Human Immune Cell Engraftment

In 1983, Bosma *et al.* reported a mouse with the *scid* mutation that resembled the human SCID illness [13]. This mouse strain has a mutated *prkdc* gene which is involved in T cell receptor (TCR) and immunoglobulin (Ig) gene rearrangement [14]. This mutation leads to the near absence of mature T and B cells leaving the mouse susceptible to pathogens and also foreign cell establishment, such as human exografts. The latter was demonstrated in 1988 by Mosier *et al.* with the successful transfer of human peripheral blood leukocytes (PBL) after injection and their production of immunoglobulin and response to tetanus toxoid [15]. Although not perfect, this model demonstrated the potential of studying the function of human immune cells in mouse, which is invaluable for vaccine development for not only infectious diseases, but also cancers. Subsequent studies showed that efficacy, as well as other potential problems, appeared to vary depending on the number of human PBL used. For instance, Bankert *et al.* found that injecting SCID mice with high numbers of human cells (5×10^7 to 1×10^8) led to their early death because of graft versus host disease (GVHD) or tumor development [16]. On the contrary, other groups, including Mosier's, found that GVHD development in SCID mice injected with human PBL was a relatively rare event among more than 2,800 mice tested [17, 18]. However, the injected human T cells did not appear to repopulate the secondary lymphoid organs such as the spleen and lymph nodes of the SCID mice. It was also noticed that for the mice that developed lymphomas, the majority of them received human PBLs from Epstein–Barr virus (EBV) positive donors. Therefore, although the SCID mouse was an important step in the evolution of xenogeneic cell transfer, the development of GVHD or lymphomas as well as the lack of consistency clearly indicated a need for improvement.

To further improve the engraftment of human immune cells by providing them with appropriate lymphoid structures, SCID mice transplanted with human fetal tissues including thymus (SCID-hu Thy), liver (SCID-hi Liv), bone (SCID-hu BM), or a combination of these tissues under the kidney capsule were developed as the so-called SCID-hu models [19, 20, 21]. McCune *et al.* were the first to describe human stem cell engraftment in *scid* mice using this method [21]. Interestingly, the implanted fetal thymus can establish in the kidney capsule and vascularize, which histologically resembles normal human thymus. Upon subsequent intravenous infusion of human fetal liver (FL) cells which contain hematopoietic stem cells, these cells were capable of migrating to and seeding in the transplanted thymus. Analyses at a later time point revealed that the thymic structure established in the kidney capsule of the SCID mice consisted of normal ratios of human T cell subsets indicating proper human T cell development. In agreement with this, mature human T cells were also detected in the peripheral blood of these SCID mice, albeit at low levels. However, the duration of the existence of human T cells in these mice was rather short, which appeared around 27 days posttransplant and became undetectable by day 64 [21]. Importantly, human immunoglobulin was also detected in the sera of these mice confirming the presence or development of human B cells. As further evidence of immune reconstitution, these SCID-hu mice did not have the opportunistic infections that usually lead to early demise of SCID mice, a phenomenon attributed to the defense mounted by the transplanted human immune system. These exciting data generated with the SCID-hu model further validate the potential engraftment of human stem cells and the development of immune effector populations in animal models. However, the limited availability of human fetal tissues and ethical issues prevents the broad application of the SCID-hu model. Thus, the challenges for generating a mouse model that supports reliable and lasting engraftment of human hematopoietic cells, especially stem cells and their differentiation, in the absence of additional human fetal tissues remain.

Improvement in Animal Models for Human Leukocyte and Stem Cell Engraftment

Although progress was made, the residual immunity in the mouse models so far continued to impede the engraftment of human cells. To curb this problem, great efforts have been invested to manipulate the microenvironment of these immunodeficient mice or to generate new mouse strains for sustained human hematopoietic cell engraftment. In the following, we review the advantages and disadvantages of various mouse models and specific maneuvers.

Overall Suppression of NK Activity

Although the SCID mice are deficient in endogenous T and B cells, they possess normal immunological components of innate immunity such as NK cells, complement, macrophages, and granulocytes. The existence of the innate immunity, especially NK cells, is believed to be a major contributor to the low level of human cell engraftment in SCID mice which is in the range of 0.5–5% [22]. Early studies with athymic mice which lack functional T cells indicated that their resistance to parental or MHC mismatched grafts involves NK activity [23, 24]. This was further supported by the observation that reducing NK activity with various methods enhanced engraftment of BM graft or human lymphoid cells [24, 25]. Furthermore, the involvement of NK cells in graft rejection and suppression of the long-term engraftment of human cells in SCID mice may be more severe due to their increased levels of NK cell activity to compensate for the diminished adaptive immunity [26]. Therefore, a mouse lacking NK activity could be helpful in enhancing human cell engraftment for evaluating the function of these immune cells. The inbred nonobese diabetic (NOD) mouse with low NK cell activity, poor myeloid differentiation, and lacking C5 complement represents an attractive candidate [27–31]. Therefore, these NOD mice were crossed with the SCID mice to generate the NOD/SCID strain, which possess defective adaptive immunity and suppressed NK activity. Indeed, experimental results showed that the NOD/SCID mouse strain seemed to be a better candidate for achieving higher levels of human cell engraftment and for studies of human immune cell function [26, 32]. On the contrary, despite low but residual NK activity, the engraftment of human immune cells in these mice was still not as high as expected. Several strategies have been applied to temporarily curb the NK cell-mediated innate immunity, such as pretreatment of mice with an NK-depleting antibody or low, nonlethal dose irradiation [33–35]. It is shown that NOD/SCID mice treated with the NK-depleting antibody supported greater engraftment of human $CD45^+$ ($hCD45^+$) cells in the peripheral blood compared with untreated NOD/SCID mice. In an effort to suppress NK activity for extended duration and to further enhance human cell engraftment, the creation of new strains of mice with low to no NK cell activity has also been explored.

$\beta 2m^{null}$ *Mice*

One of the immunodeficient mouse models that have been created to support sustained human cell engraftment is the $\beta 2m^{null}$ mouse which lacks cell surface MHC class I expression. Because of the crucial role of MHC I expression in NK and CD8 T cell development, the $\beta 2m^{null}$ mice lack functional NK and $CD8^+$ T cells [36, 37]. To completely eliminate their adaptive immunity, this mouse was further crossed with the NOD/SCID strain resulting in the NOD/SCID/$\beta 2m^{null}$ strain which should provide superior engraftment of human cells because of combined defects of adaptive immunity and innate immunity. To compare the engraftment efficiency of the various derivative strains of SCID mice, Christianson *et al.* injected 2×10^7 human peripheral blood mononuclear cells (PBMC) to SCID, NOD/SCID, or NOD/SCID/$\beta 2m^{null}$ mice intraperitoneally [38]. Four weeks after the injection, the percentage of total $hCD45^+$ cells in the spleens of NOD/SCID/$\beta 2m^{null}$ mice was ~43%, while that in NOD/SCID mice was ~18% and ~3% in SCID mice. Furthermore, the engraftment of human $CD4^+$ T cells was also greatly improved in the NOD/SCID/$\beta 2m^{null}$ mice demonstrating increased human hematopoietic cell engraftment over NOD/SCID and SCID mice [38]. However, neither B cell engraftment nor human Ig levels in NOD/SCID/$\beta 2m^{null}$ mice were significantly different than the other strains used. Furthermore, the NOD/SCID/$\beta 2m^{null}$ mice had a high incidence of thymic lymphomas with shortened lifespan.

It is helpful to point out that early experiments regarding human cell transfer used PBL or PBMC which are not a significant source of stem cells. Engraftment of these mice with the above sources really refers to the population of recipient organs by the transferred cells and their further expansion, i.e. mainly T and B cells.

Other sources including FL cells and the sources mentioned below contain hematopoietic stem cells. Engraftment in this case refers to the population of recipient organs by these stem cells and then their differentiation into the various components of the hematopoietic system.

The IL2R$\gamma_c^{-/-}$ Mouse

Given the illustrated crucial roles of IL2Rγ_c in the signaling of common γ chain cytokines IL-2, IL-4, IL-7, IL-9, IL-15, and IL-21 and its essential role in lymphopoiesis, several groups developed mice with targeted mutations of the IL2Rγ_c locus around 1995 [39–43]. These mice, known as *IL2R*$\gamma^{-/-}$ or $\gamma_c^{-/-(\text{null})}$, were defective in T, B, and NK cell development. They were further crossed with other immunodeficient mice such as NOD/*scid* or *Rag2*$^{-/-}$ mice, which have mutations of the recombination-activating gene 2 or DNA-PK gene with severe blockade in the development of T and B cells [43]. The resulting crossed mice led to several new models for human cell engraftment due to their deficiency in both adaptive and innate immunity. These new mice include the NOD/LtSz-*scid IL2R*$\gamma^{-/-}$ and NOD/Shi-*scid IL2R*$\gamma^{-/-}$, as well as BALB/c-*Rag2*$^{-/-}$*IL2R*$\gamma^{-/-}$, and H2d-*Rag2*$^{-/-}$*IL2R*$\gamma^{-/-}$. The original strains NOD/Ltz-*scid* and NOD/Shi-*scid* are similar in that they have significantly reduced NK cell activity compared with C.B.-17-*scid* mice, with NOD/Ltz-*scid* mice exhibiting slightly lower activity than that of the NOD/Shi-*scid*. Elimination of the *IL2R*γ_c gene in either NOD/Ltz-*scid* or NOD/Shi-*scid* strain further suppressed their NK activity. It is also shown that NOD/LtSz-*scid IL2R*$\gamma^{-/-}$ mice, referred to as NOD/SCID/γ_c^{null}, have detectible NK cells (8.8%), but no NK cell activity [44].

The NOD/SCID/IL2R$\gamma_c^{-/-}$ Mouse

The real major advance of human stem cell engraftment and multilineage leukocyte differentiation in a mouse model was made by the observation of Ito *et al.* demonstrating the superior human cell engraftment in the NOD/SCID/γ_c^{null} mice in the absence of additional human fetal tissues compared with other mouse strains [44]. Infusion of 1×10^5 cord blood CD34$^+$ stem cells (CB-SC) to NOD/SCID/γ_c^{null} mice resulted in higher level of hCD45$^+$ cells in the peripheral blood (8.5%) than NOD/SCID mice treated with (1.5%) or without (1%) NK-depleting antibody. Furthermore, NOD/SCID/γ_c^{null} mice showed sustained human leukocyte engraftment with 40% hCD45$^+$ cells in the peripheral blood at 8 and 12 weeks compared with less than 5% in NOD/SCID mice treated with NK-depleting antibody. Four months after transplantation, bone marrow and spleens of these human stem cell engrafted NOD/SCID/γ_c^{null} mice contained 75% hCD45$^+$ cells, whereas the percentage of hCD45$^+$ cells in the bone marrow and spleens of NOD/SCID mice treated with

NK-depleting antibody was 10%, and less than 5% when antibody untreated. Furthermore, among the $hCD45^+$ populations in the bone marrow of these NOD/SCID/γ_c^{null} mice, the presence of $hCD19^+$, $hCD33^+$, and $hCD3^+$ cells was observed, suggesting multilineage differentiation of transplanted stem cells [44]. Therefore, NOD/SCID/γ_c^{null} mice showed greatly improved human cell engraftment and more importantly, supported better multilineage human cell differentiation compared with NOD/SCID mice.

Around the same time as the studies of Ito *et al.* Yahata and colleagues performed a similar study by transplanting 8×10^4 to 2×10^5 CB-SC into NOD/SCID and NOD/SCID/γ_c^{null} mice [45]. At 6 weeks posttransplant, human B cells ($CD19^+$ $CD45^+$), but not T cells ($CD3^+$ $CD45^+$), were detected in both strains of mice. By 13 weeks however, human T cells were detected in NOD/SCID/γ_c^{null} mice, which reached a level of about 67.5% by 19 weeks, whereas human T cell development was not detected in NOD/SCID mice. This study also showed that overall, human leukocyte engraftment in NOD/SCID/γ_c^{null} was much higher (54%) compared with NOD/SCID (6.8%) mice and only NOD/SCID/γ_c^{null} mice supported human T cell development. Subsequent studies by other groups further confirmed the consistent engraftment of human CB-SC and the *de novo* development of mature human T, B, and NK cells from the transplanted stem cells in NOD/SCID/γ_c^{null} mice [46].

Other Immunodeficient Mouse Models

A more recent but less utilized model, BALB/c-$Rag2^{-/-}IL2R\gamma_c^{-/-}$, was also shown to support human stem cell engraftment and differentiation into various immune cells after transplantation of CB-SC [47]. Their differentiation into mature human T cells, B cells, and DCs and production of immunoglobulins, IgM and IgG, were detected 4–26 weeks after transplant. Moreover, lymph nodes of the CB-SC engrafted mice reached a size similar to those in wild type mice. More importantly, the human T cells developed in these mice can be activated to proliferate by antigens and they support HIV-1 replication *in vivo*, which subsequently resulted in $CD4^+$ T cell depletion [48, 49].

Stem Cell Sources and Route of Stem Cell Delivery

As the NOD/SCID/γ_c^{null} mice appear to be one of the best and most popularly used humanized mouse model so far that provide reliable human stem cell engraftment and differentiation, we will mainly focus our discussions in the following sections on results obtained with this mouse model regarding the various maneuvers employed that appear to affect the level of human immune cell engraftment and differentiation.

NOD/SCID/γ_c^{null} Mice Support Human Cell Engraftment from a Variety of Stem Cell Sources

Human CD34$^+$ stem cells can be obtained from different sources such as bone marrow aspirate (BM-SC), cord blood or placenta (CB-SC), peripheral blood leukophoresis especially after G-CSF treatment for their mobilization (PBSC), and human fetal tissues such as thymus or liver. Although they all bear the CD34 stem cell marker, their stem cell potency in repopulating hosts and differentiation to various progeny appear to differ experimentally and clinically. To examine the differences of human CB-SC, PBSC, and BM-SC in engraftment and differentiation, Matsumura *et al.* transplanted these three kinds of stem cells at varying numbers to NOD/SCID/γ_c^{null} mice [50]. Fourteen weeks later, the percent of hCD45$^+$ cells in the bone marrow, spleen, and peripheral blood of these NOD/SCID/γ_c^{null} mice was examined. Interestingly, on average, mice that received CB-SC had the highest levels of human cell engraftment at 66.7%, 63.7%, and 47.5% in the bone marrow, spleen, and peripheral blood, respectively. Those that received PBSC showed human cell engraftment at 45.4%, 13.8%, and 10.7% in the above tissues, while those in BM-SC group had hCD45$^+$ cell levels of 22.5%, 14%, and 8.1% in the bone marrow, spleen, and peripheral blood, respectively. Furthermore, the experimenters were specifically interested in the hCD5$^+$ subset of B cells. This subset is usually present in fetal spleen and umbilical cord blood but is diminished in adult bone marrow and peripheral blood. CD34$^+$ stem cells from all three sources appeared to be equally capable of developing into B cell subsets as demonstrated by their equal ratios of CD5$^+$ to CD19$^+$ B cells [50]. Studies by Shultz's group using PBSC in NOD/SCID/γ_c^{null} mice further confirmed the capacity of mobilized hematopoietic stem cells to engraft NOD/SCID/γ_c^{null} mice at reasonable levels and to differentiate into mature T and B cells, which could be further augmented by treating the mice with Fc-conjugated IL-7, a cytokine that supports T and B cell development [51]. These studies demonstrated that human PBSC are capable of engrafting and differentiating into human immune effectors in NOD/SCID/γ_c^{null} mice, which has significant clinical implication as PBSC are easier to obtain and are being used more frequently clinically for transplantation. Promising experimental results obtained from this hPBSC-NOD/SCID/γ_c^{null} mouse model have a high likelihood of reflecting potential clinical outcome in patients.

Routes of Human Stem Cell Injection Have Moderate Effects on Their Engraftment in NOD/SCID/γ_c^{null} Mice

To explore other potential means of further improving human stem cell engraftment in NOD/SCID/γ_c^{null} mice, stem cell delivery to mice at various stages of their life has been tested. Interestingly, some studies have shown that injection of human stem cells during the neonatal period results in a higher level of human cell engraftment [52].

This is possibly because the endogenous hematopoietic-lymphoid system in NOD/SCID/γ_c^{null} neonates is immature and expands during the first few weeks of their life [47], thereby the injected human stem cells may participate in their hematopoiesis and expand along with their endogenous stem cell population. Our results in comparing human cell engraftment in neonates and adult mice demonstrated faster engraftment in the neonates with detectible human cells in the peripheral blood one week after injection. However, the challenge of using neonates lies in the technical difficulty of cell delivery into the blood stream. Some investigators reported using facial vein injection for this purpose, which is sophisticated and technically challenging due to the small size of neonates and their vasculature [53]. To explore other more practical and reproducible means of delivery, we compared routes of intrahepatic, intracardiac, or intraperitoneal stem cell delivery into nonirradiated 2-day old NOD/SCID/γ_c^{null} neonates. Human cell engraftment at 1 and 2 weeks postinjection was examined. Interestingly, the neonates that received human stem cells via intrahepatic route consistently showed detectible human cells in their liver, peripheral blood, and bone marrow. Those that received stem cells via intraperitoneal or intracardiac route showed inconsistent results with some showing low levels and others nondetectible levels of human cells. Therefore, these results suggest that intrahepatic delivery of human stem cells to neonates during the early phase of their hematopoiesis is a relatively easy and consistent means of improving human cell engraftment in NOD/SCID/γ_c^{null} mice for preclinical use of this model.

Multilineage Differentiation of Human Stem Cells in NOD/SCID/γ_c^{null} Mice to Functional Effectors

As discussed earlier, the major advances made in this field with the development of NOD/SCID/γ_c^{null} mice lie in their superior capacity of not only supporting human cell engraftment, but also more importantly, their support of human stem cell differentiation into multilineage immune effector populations. It is known that proper initiation of immune responses involves intimate interaction of T and B effector cells with APCs such as DCs. Early humanized animal models, including the NOD/SCID mice, are capable of supporting the survival of transferred human B cells and their expansion for extended period of time. However, they appear to be incapable of supporting the survival or function of infused human T cells, at least in maintaining their naïve phenotype at a relatively steady number or in supporting differentiation of naïve T cells from transplanted human stem cells [44–46].

With the development of the NOD/SCID/γ_c^{null} mouse model, the capacity of these mice in supporting *de novo* development of human T cells from transplanted CB-SC was examined extensively by many investigators [45, 46, 52]. The first sign of successful T cell development is the existence of human $CD3^+$ cells in the bone marrow, spleen, thymus, and peripheral blood of stem cell engrafted NOD/SCID/γ_c^{null} mice [46, 52]. Further examination of human cells in the thymus confirmed the coexistence of human $CD4^+$ $CD8^+$ double positive T cells, which express TCR-$\alpha\beta$

chains, and small numbers of $CD4^+$ or $CD8^+$ single positive mature T cells, indicating the *de novo* development of human immature T cells and their differentiation to maturation [46]. The *de novo* human T cell development was further confirmed by the TREC assay analysis in the mature T cells harvested in the periphery as TREC was formed during intrathymic TCR rearrangement [51]. It is noteworthy that TCR analysis of the mature T cells showed adequate generation of both αβ and γδ T cells, as well as a broad spectratyping of TCR CDR3β among the αβ T cells indicating diversified TCRβ utilization [51]. It is also important to know that the $hCD3^+$ T cells that developed in the spleen of NOD/SCID/γ_c^{null} mice primarily expressed $hCD45RA^+$ (naïve T cells), rather than $hCD45RA^+$/$hCD45RO^+$ (activated T cells) or $hCD45RO^+$ (memory T cells) [54]. The function of these mature human T cells was further examined by stimulating the splenocytes of these mice with a mitogen phytohemagglutinin (PHA), IL-2, or even alloantigens. Upon PHA and IL-2 stimulation, *in vivo* proliferation of human $CD3^+$ T cells from the spleen of these mice was increased from approximately 17% to 93% as determined by flow cytometry [46]. *In vitro* proliferation assay via ^{3}H-thymidine incorporation revealed a 30- to 40-fold increase in proliferation upon their stimulation by PHA and IL-2 [45]. Another study also showed that these T cells proliferated vigorously upon mixing with alloantigen specific human cell lines but not with cell lines that did not share HLA with the effector cells or unstimulated controls [52]. Interestingly, these activated T cells produced many effector cytokines such as interferon-γ (IFN-γ), tumor necrosis factor-α (TNF-α), IL-10, IL-15, and IL-4 to the culture supernatant as determined by ELISA [46]. Lastly, the proper cytolytic activity of these activated human cells was demonstrated via different cytotoxic assays [52]. This demonstrated cytotoxic activity could be inhibited by anti-HLA antibodies demonstrating its MHC-dependency. Furthermore, an assay to determine the FAS-perforin-dependent cytolytic activity of these *in vivo* derived human T cells revealed that the cytolytic activity of these human T cells developed in NOD/SCID/γ_c^{null} mice was only slightly lower than that of T cells from a healthy donor [46].

Similarly, the *de novo* development of human B cells and immunoglobulin production in human stem cell engrafted NOD/SCID/γ_c^{null} mice was examined. Overall, systemic existence of human B lineage populations was observed with immature populations predominant in the bone marrow and mature cells in the spleen. Histological analysis on the structure of secondary lymphoid tissues revealed that follicle-like structures were present in the spleen and mesenteric lymph nodes [52]. Blood sera contained high levels of IgG, IgM, and IgA, which reached 600 μg/mL (for IgM). Upon immunization with ovalbumin (OVA), these mice produced significant levels of OVA-specific IgG and IgM compared with those nonimmunized mice 2 weeks postimmunization. More interestingly, the intestinal tract stained positive for cells expressing IgA suggesting that mucosal immunity was also reconstituted.

Although DCs do not directly participate in cytolytic activity most of the time for pathogen elimination, DCs are crucial players for regulating the immune response for bridging innate immunity and adaptive immunity, as well as initiating adaptive immune response to foreign pathogens [55]. Therefore, appropriate presence of human DCs for appropriate activation of human T and B cells in engrafted

NOD/SCID/γ_c^{null} mice is important and valuable in understanding the immune response to human diseases, including cancer [56]. To this end, Palucka *et al.* carried out extensive characteristic analyses on human DC subsets derived in NOD/SCID mice transplanted with either CB-SC, FL, or PBSC [57]. Particularly, hCD45$^+$ HLA-DR$^+$ cells displaying DC morphology were observed within the skin. Antibody staining revealed that these cells expressed Langerin suggesting successful differentiation of stem cells into Langerhans cells in these mice. In the marrow compartment a distinct human DC population was observed which bore surface markers of either HLA-DR$^+$ CD11c$^+$ myeloid DCs (3.5%) or HLA-DR$^+$ CD11c$^-$CD123$^+$ plasmacytoid DCs (2.7%). The majority of human leukocytes in the spleen bear the B-cell phenotype, and there were rare myeloid and plasmacytoid DCs based on flow cytometry and immunofluorescent microscopy. Furthermore, low levels of these DC subsets were also found in the peripheral blood of these mice. To further confirm the immune stimulatory function of these DCs, both myeloid DCs and plasmacytoid DCs were enriched from the bone marrow samples. Myeloid DCs were plated with allogeneic human CD4$^+$ T cells and demonstrated significant capacity in stimulating T cell proliferation. The ability of producing interferon-α (IFN-α) upon incubation with live influenza virus by these plasmacytoid DCs was also confirmed, whereas B-cells or *ex vivo* generated myeloid DCs were incapable of producing IFN-α. To demonstrate the function and immune responsiveness of these DC subsets *in vivo*, these humanized mice were injected with live influenza virus or specific antigens. Indeed, mice that were challenged with live influenza virus, their serum human IFN-α reached 300–900 pg/ml in 16 h. In comparison, the serum IFN-α was less than 50 pg/ml in nonhumanized mice that were challenged with the virus or humanized mice that were not exposed to virus. Furthermore, the human myeloid DCs upon encountering specific antigen challenges showed maturation as evidenced by the up-regulation of CD40, CD80, and CD83 and their increased migration to the spleen [57].

Besides the well studied differentiation and function of human B (CD19$^+$) cells, T (CD3$^+$) cells and DCs in transplanted NOD/SCID/γ_c^{null} mice, development of human myeloid (CD33$^+$), platelets (hCD41a$^+$), and erythrocytes (hGPA$^+$) was also observed in the bone marrow, spleen, thymus, and peripheral blood of these mice [52]. Together, these studies demonstrated that the NOD/SCID/γ_c^{null} mice provide a better supportive environment for not only human stem cell engraftment, but also their differentiation and development of a potentially complete hematopoietic system which is capable of initiating a functional cell-mediated or humoral immune response systemically and possibly at the mucosal level, as well.

Use of Humanized Mice as an Experimental Model to Evaluate Human Immune Responses

The premise of this humanized mouse model in preclinical evaluation of human immune responses rests on appropriate function of those engrafted and differentiated human immune cells to specific pathogens and antigens in a similar manner as they would have in patients. With the demonstrated robust reconstitution of a human hematopoietic-lymphoid system in these humanized mice, they were put under a stringent test to determine whether those human immune cells would be similar in their responsiveness to real pathogenic challenges to that when encountered clinically.

Functional Immune Response of Differentiated Human Immune Cells Against EBV in the Humanized Mice

The first study that clearly demonstrated the antigen specific adaptive immunity of human immune cells against an infectious pathogen in humanized mice was performed by Melkus *et al.* where the SCID-hu model was used [58]. These NOD/SCID mice were first introduced with human FL and thymic tissues under the kidney capsule followed by the transplantation of autologous $CD34^+$ stem cells, which were designated as BLT (bone marrow, liver, thymus) mice. Similar to the stem cell engrafted NOD/SCID/γ_c^{null} mice, these BLT mice support the development of significant levels of human T cells, B cells, monocytes, macrophages, and DCs in a variety of organs with a well structured human thymic tissue under the kidney capsule and mouse spleen and lymph nodes containing human immune cells within the organized germinal center-like structures. Upon infection of these BLT mice with the clinically relevant infectious pathogen EBV, a rapid increase in the percentages of memory phenotype of human T cells as $CD45RA^-CD27^+$ was observed, similar to the pattern of human T cell expansion in humans with acute EBV infection [58]. More importantly, human T cells isolated from these EBV infected BLT mice showed antigen specific γ-interferon production via an enzyme-linked immunosorbent spot (ELI-SPOT) only when they were restimulated by an autologous EBV infected lymphoblastoid cell line (LCL). Furthermore, their EBV specific γ-interferon production was blocked when the LCL was pretreated with antibodies directed at human MHC I or MHC II molecules. These results demonstrated that the human immune cells within the BLT mice can properly interact with each other in supporting EBV infection and in initiating an MHC-restricted immune response.

To further examine the interaction of human DCs and T cells in the BLT mice during innate immunity, the mice were injected with the superantigen toxic shock syndrome toxin 1 (TSST-1) which specifically activates and expands human $V\beta2^+$ T cells. Shortly after TSST-1 injection, a significant increase in human IFN-γ, IL-10, IL-2, and IL-6 in the serum of these mice has been observed, which reaches a peak at around 18 h postinjection [58]. This increase in T cell effector cytokine production correlated well with subsequent expansion of human $V\beta2^+$ T cells, but not irrelevant human $V\beta17^+$ T cells, in the peripheral blood, bone marrow, and spleen. Again, these observed responses of effector cytokine production and T cell expansion very much resemble the clinical responses observed in humans [58]. As DCs were the initiators of these immune responses, their existence and phenotype in the spleen and bone marrow of these mice were examined. Interestingly, before TSST-1 challenge or in control mice that did not receive TSST-1, splenic and bone marrow DCs all showed immature resting phenotype. Strikingly, upon TSST-1 injection, marked up-regulation of CD40, CD80, CD83, and CD86, an indication of maturation and activation was observed 18 h postinjection in the human DCs localized in the spleen, but not in the bone marrow [58]. Furthermore, the observed DC maturation and activation post-TSST-1 injection appeared to be dependent on T cell-DC interaction because in mice that are devoid of human T cells, human DCs could not be matured and activated by TSST-1 injection [58]. Therefore, these results clearly demonstrate that the established human immune components in the humanized mice can closely recapitulate various aspects of functional human immune responses against clinical relevant infectious pathogens.

Functional Human Immune Responses Against HIV in the Humanized Animal Models

Another research area that urgently needs humanized animal models that closely resemble the function of the human immune system is AIDS research. In fact, this has been one of the primary driving forces for the extensive studies and rapid development of these models. Therefore, upon confirmation of appropriate engraftment and differentiation of essential human immune components in the humanized NOD/SCID/γ_c^{null} mice, testing the immune responses against HIV in these mice was a rational move [54]. Watanabe *et al.* infected NOD/SCID/γ_c^{null} mice that were engrafted with CB-SC and had successful development of human T, B, and DCs and other myeloid subpopulations in the bone marrow, PBL, and spleen, with CCR5- and CXCR4-tropic HIV-1 strains. Both HIV-1 strains appeared to replicate well in the humanized mice with high levels of viral DNA and detectable level of viral antigen p24 of the Gag protein in multiple lymphoid tissues [54]. More importantly, some of the HIV-1 infected mice showed significant levels of human antibodies against a variety of HIV-1 specific antigens including HIV Env gp120 and Gag p24 [54]. This is clearly different from the animal models used previously where HIV-1 infection completely depleted all the preestablished human cells in immunodeficient mice and no anti-HIV antibody responses could be detected [59, 60].

The excitement on the potential use of these humanized mouse models for HIV studies and vaccine development is further substantiated by the studies performed in the Garcia laboratory using the BLT model [61]. Because intrarectal transmission remains as an important route of HIV infection in the USA, the potential HIV infection and pathogenesis in these BLT mice upon intrarectal inoculation of HIV-1 was examined. Similar to humanized NOD/SCID/γ_c^{null} mice, high levels of human immune cells repopulated primary and secondary lymphoid tissues of the BLT mice, including the gastrointestinal (GI) tract and gut-associated lymphoid tissues (GALT) [61]. Upon intrarectal inoculation of HIV-1 to these BLT mice, an increase in plasma viral load and human anti-HIV p24 IgG was detected in the majority of mice [61]. Furthermore, coinciding with the increased HIV viral load and specific antibody, a deletion of human CD4+ T cells in the peripheral blood with parallel increases in CD8+ T cells was clearly evident [61]. Interestingly, the remaining human CD8+ T cells in the GI tract bore an effector memory phenotype of CD27−CD45RA− with increased levels of granzyme and perforin [61]. All of these closely resemble the clinical symptoms and pathogenesis of intrarectal HIV transmission and suggest that this can serve as a good model system for studying host-HIV interaction and for evaluation of potential immunological intervention for HIV treatment.

Together, these studies demonstrated that humanized mouse models can be effectively utilized for HIV infection, evaluation of human anti-HIV immune response, HIV pathogenesis, and the development of HIV vaccines for therapeutic measures.

Future Directions

As discussed above, the humanization of mice has become more reliable and also more representative of the actual human body. To date, the mouse models based on the IL2R$\gamma_c^{-/-}$ phenotype have demonstrated the best engraftment and development of functional human immune cells *in vivo*. Most of the studies performed so far heavily rely on the high stem cell potency of CB-SC or FL tissues. This will be a limiting factor for broader application of this humanized mouse model. Therefore, improving the engraftment efficiency of PBSC in this humanized mouse model is definitely needed for vaccine development and preclinical evaluation of individualized therapeutic regimens. A particular way for the improvement is to generate transgenic NOD/SCID/γ_c^{null} or BALB/c-*Rag2*$^{-/-}$*IL2R*$\gamma_c^{-/-}$ mice expressing human growth factors [62]. Since these growth factors can enhance engraftment and are vital to development of hematopoietic cells, their presence in these mouse models could prolong engraftment and augment differentiation. Further depletion of innate immunity using a variety of techniques could also improve engraftment. In addition, the introduction of HLA genes to these humanized mice may more accurately mimic the environment present in humans and allow for proper cell-to-cell interaction [62]. As seen by the experiments mentioned above, the introduction of human thymic tissue prior to transplantation provides added benefits. Mouse thymus lacks the human MHC expression and therefore prevents the development of a true human repertoire profile. This could lead to lack of tolerance induction and possibly GVHD as we observed in some of our studies. By introducing human thymic tissue, a scaffold is provided for the developing human cells to encounter the same interactions they would in a human. Expanding this by implanting other human tissues or artificial lymph nodes [63] may facilitate study of the secondary lymph organs and the adaptive immune responses for translational research, including preclinical testing of cancer immune therapy and new vaccines for infectious diseases.

Summary

The ability to study human diseases *in vivo* makes great contributions for developing effective clinical protocols for treating numerous diseases. Although early animal models provided valuable information, they have some inherent issues in mimicking the true human body, especially for a functional human immune system. The discovery of an immunodeficient mouse in 1983 led to the engraftment of human immune cells into these mice. Extensive studies over the past 20 years with the development of new mouse strains, especially the NOD/SCID/γ_c^{null} and BALB/c-*Rag2*$^{-/-}$*IL2R*$\gamma_c^{-/-}$ strains, have made it possible to establish a functional human immune system in these mice. More importantly, these human immune cells developed in the humanized mice are susceptible to pathogenic infections and are capable of mounting immune responses against these infections. Therefore, these humanized mouse models, although not yet being extensively utilized in the field of cancer research, represent an exciting and promising resource for potential preclinical vaccine testing against human cancers and infectious pathogens in translation research.

Acknowledgments This work is supported by funds from the Louisiana Gene Therapy Consortium, Stanley S. Scott Cancer Center and grants from the National Institutes of Health to YC (CA112065 and P20RR021970).

References

1. Espey, D. K., Wu, X. C., Swan, J., Wiggins, C., Jim, M. A., Ward, E., Wingo, P. A., Howe, H. L., Ries, L. A. G., Miller, B. A., Jemal, A., Ahmed, F., Cobb, N., Kaur, J. S., and Edwards, B. K. (2007) Cancer 110, 2119
2. Banchereau, J., and Palucka, A. K. (2005) Nat Rev Immunol 5, 296
3. Mellman, I., and Steinman, R. M. (2005) Cell 106, 255
4. Jego, G., Palucka, A. K., Blanck, J. P., Chalouni, C., Pascual, V., and Banchereau, J. (2003) Immunity 19, 225
5. Fernandez, N. C., Lozier, A., Flament, C., Ricciardi-Castagnoli, P., Bellet, D., Suter, M., Perricaudet, M., Tursz, T., Maraskovsky, E., and Zitvogel, L. (1999) Nat Med 5, 405
6. Kadowaki, N., Antonenko, S., Ho, S., Rissoan, M. C., Soumelis, V., Porcelli, S. A., Lanier, L. L., and Liu, Y. J. (2001) J Exp Med 193, 1221
7. Euvrard, S., Kanitakis, J., and Claudy, A. (2003) N Engl J Med 348, 1681
8. Hakim, F. T., Flomerfelt, F. A., Boyiadzis, M., and Gress, R. E. (2004) Curr Opin Immunol 16, 151
9. Gilboa, E., Nair, S. K., and Lyerly, H. K. (1998) Cancer Immunol Immunother 46, 82–87
10. Lane, M. A. (2000) Exp Gerontol 35, 533
11. Nath, B. M., Schumann, K. E., and Boyer, J. D. (2000) Trends Microbiol 8, 426
12. Frese, K. K., and Tuveson, D. A. (2007) Nat Rev Cancer 7, 645
13. Bosma, G. C., Custer, R. P., and Bosma, M. J. (1983) Nature 301, 527
14. Legrand, N., Weijer, K., and Spits, H. (2006) J Immunol 176, 2053
15. Mosier, D. E., Gulizia, R. J., Baird, S. M., and Wilson, D. B. (1988) Nature 335, 256
16. Bankert, R. B., Umemoto, T., Sugiyama, Y., Chen, F. A., Repasky, E., and Yokota, S. (1989) Curr Top Microbiol Immunol 152, 201
17. Pfeffer, K., Heeg, K., Bubeck, R., Conradt, P., and Wagner, H. (1989) Curr Top Microbiol Immunol 152, 211

18. Mosier, D. (1991) Adv Immunol 50, 303
19. Namikawa, R., Weilbaecher, K. N., Kaneshima, H., Yee, E. J., and McCune, J. M. (1990) J Exp Med 172, 1055
20. Roncarolo, M. G., Carballido, J. M., Rouleau, M., Namikawa, R., and de Vries, J. E. (1996) Semin Immunol 8, 207
21. McCune, J. M., Namikawa, R., Kaneshima, H., Shultz, L. D., Lieberman, M., and Weissman, I. L. (1988) Science 241, 1632
22. Lapidot, T., Pflumio, F., Doedens, M., Murdoch, B., Williams, D. E., and Dick, J. E. (1992) Science 255, 1137
23. Kaiser, S., Kagi, D., Ihorst, G., and Kapp, U. (2006) Clin Exp Immunol 145, 332
24. Christianson, S. W., Greiner, D. L., Schweitzer, I. B., Gott, B., Beamer, G. L., Schweitzer, P. A., Hesselton, R. M., and Shultz, L. D. (1996) Cell Immunol 171, 186
25. Kiessling, R., Hochman, P. S., Haller, O., Shearer, G. M., Wigzell, H., and Cudkowicz, G. (1977) Eur J Immunol 7, 655
26. Shultz, L. D., Schweitzer, P. A., Christianson, S. W., Gott, B., Schweitzer, I. B., Tennent, B., McKenna, S., Mobraaten, L., Rajan, T. V., Greiner, D. L., and Leiter, E. H. (1995) J Immunol 154, 180
27. Kataoka, S., Satoh, J., Fujiya, H., Toyota, T., Suzuki, R., Itoh, K., and Kumagai, K. (1983) Diabetes 32, 247
28. Greiner, D. L., Hesselton, R. A., and Shultz, L. D. (1998) Stem Cells 16, 166
29. Serreze, D. V., and Leiter, E. H. (1988) J Immunol 140, 3801
30. Serreze, D. V., Gaskins, H. R., and Leiter, E. H. (1993) J Immunol 150, 2534
31. Baxter, A. G. and Cooke, A. (1993) Diabetes 42, 1574
32. Prochazka, M., Gaskins, H. R., Shultz, L. D., and Leiter, E. H. (1992) Proc Natl Acad Sci USA 89, 3290
33. Pearson, T., Greiner, D. L., and Shultz, L. D. (2008) Curr Top Microbiol Immunol 324, 25
34. Sandhu, J., Shpitz, B. Gallinger, S., and Hozumi, N. (1994) J Immunol 152, 3806
35. Shpitz, B., Chambers, C. A., Singhal, A. B., Hozumi, N., Fernandes, B. J., Roifman, C. M., Weiner, L. M., Roder, J. C., and Gallinger, S. (1994) J Immunol Methods 169, 1
36. Zijlstra, M., Bix, M., Simister, N. E., Loring, J. M., Raulet, D. H., and Jaenisch, R. (1990) Nature 344, 709
37. Liao, N. S., Bix, M., Zijlstra, R., Jaenisch, R., and Raulet, D. H. (1991) Science 253, 199
38. Christianson, S. W., Greiner, D. L., Hesselton, R., Leif, J. H., Wagar, E. J., Schweitzer, I. B., Rajan, T. V., Gott, B., Roopenian, D. C., and Shultz, L. D. (1997) J Immunol 158, 3578
39. Cao, X., Shores, E. W., Hu-Li, J., Anver, M. R., Kelsail, B. L., Russell, S. M., Drago, J., Noguchi, M., Grinberg, A., Bloom, E. T., Paul, W. E., Katz, S. I., Love, P. E., and Leonard, W. J. (1995) Immunity 2, 223
40. DiSanto, J. P., Müller, W., Guy-Grand, D., Fischer, A., and Rajewsky, K. (1995) Proc Natl Acad Sci USA 92, 377
41. Ohbo, K., Suda, T., Hashiyama, M., Mantani, A., Ikebe, M., Miyakawa, K., Moriyama, M., Nakamura, M., Katsuki, M., Takahashi, K., Yamamura, K., and Sugamura, K. (1996) Blood 87, 956
42. Jacobs, H., Krimpenfort, P., Haks, M., Allen, J., Blom, B., Démollière, C., Kruisbeek, A., Spits, H., and Berns, A. (1999) J Exp Med 190, 1059
43. Shultz, L. D., Ishikawa, F., and Greiner, D. (2007) Nat Rev Immunol 7, 118
44. Ito, M., Hiramatsu, H., Kobayashi, K., Suzue, K., Kawahata, M., Hioki, K., Ueyama, Y., Koyanagi, Y., Sugamura, K., Tsuji, K., Heike, T., and Nakahata, T. (2002) Blood 100, 3175
45. Yahata, T., Ando, K., Nakamura, Y., Ueyama, Y., Shimamura, K., Tamaoki, N., Kato, S., and Hotta, T. (2002) J Immunol 169, 204
46. Hiramatsu, H., Nishikomori, R., Heike, T., Ito, M., Kobayashi, K., Katamura, K., and Nakahata, T. (2003) Blood 102, 873
47. Traggiai, E., Chicha, L., Mazzucchelli, L., Bronz, L., Piffaretti, J. C., Lanzavecchia, A., and Manz, M. G. (2004) Science 304, 104

48. Rozemuller, H., Knaän-Shanzer, S., Hagenbeek, A., van Bloois, L., Storm, G., and Martens, A. C. M. (2004) Exp Hematol 32, 1118–1125
49. Berges, B. K., Wheat, W. H., Palmer, B. E., Connick, E., and Akkina, R. (2006) Retrovirology 3, 76
50. Matsumura, T., Kametani, Y., Ando, K., Hirano, Y., Katano, I., Ito, R., Shiina, M., Tsukamoto, H., Saito, Y., Tokuda, Y., Kato, S., Ito, M., Motoyoshi, K., and Habu, S. (2003) Exp Hematol 31, 78
51. Shultz, L. D., Lyons, B. L., Burzenski, L. M., Gott, B., Chen, X., Chaleff, S., Koth, M., Gillies, S. D., King, M., Mangada, J., Greiner, D. L., and Handgretinger, R. (2005) J. Immunol 174, 6477
52. Ishikawa, F., Yasukawa, M., Lyons, B., Yoshida, S., Miyamoto, T., Yoshimoto, G., Watanabe, T., Akashi, K., Shultz, L. D., and Harada, M. (2005) Blood 106, 1565
53. Ishikawa, F., Livingston, A. G., Wingard, J. R., Nishikawa, S., and Ogawa, M. (2002) Exp Hematol 30, 488
54. Watanabe, S., Terashima, K., Ohta, S., Horibata, S., Yajima, M., Shiozawa, Y., Dewan, M. Z., Yu, Z., Ito, M., Morio, T., Shimizu, N., Honda, M., and Yamamoto, N. (2007) Blood 109, 212
55. Banchereau, J. and Steinman, R. M. (1998) Nature 392, 245
56. Wu, L. and Liu, Y. J. (2007) Immunity 26, 741
57. Palucka, A. K., Gatlin, J., Blanck, J. P., Melkus, M. W., Clayton, S., Ueno, H., Kraus, E. T., Cravens, P., Bennett, L., Padgett-Thomas, A., Marches, F., Islas-Ohlmayer, M., Garcia, J. V., and Banchereau, J. (2003) Blood 102, 3302
58. Melkus, M. W., Estes, J. D., Padgett-Thomas, A., Gatlin, J., Denton, P. W., Othieno, F. A., Wege, A. K., Haase, A. T., and Garcia, J. V. (2006) Nat Med 12, 1316
59. Mosier, D. E., Gulizia, R. J., MacIsaac, P. D., Torbett, B. E., and Levy, J. A. (1993) Science 260, 689
60. Tary-Lehmann, M., Saxon, A., and Lehmann, P. V. (1995) Immunol. Today 16, 529
61. Sun, Z., Denton, P. W., Estes, J. D., Othieno, F. A., Wei, B. L., Wege, A. K., Melkus, M. W., Padgett-Thomas, A., Zupancic, M., Haase, A. T., and Garcia, J. V. (2007) J Exp Med 204, 705
62. Ito, M., Kobayashi, K., and Nakahata, T. (2008) Curr Top Microbiol Immunol 324, 53
63. Okamoto, N., Chihara, R., Shimizu, C., Nishimoto, S., and Watanabe, T. (2007) J Clin Invest 117, 997

Part III
Targeted Immune Therapy

CD40 Stimulation and Antitumor Effects

Danice E.C. Wilkins and William J. Murphy

Abstract CD40–CD40L interactions play an important role in the generation of humoral and cell-mediated immunity. Due to the expression of CD40 on antigen presenting cells, it has become an attractive target for immunotherapy against cancer. Recent studies have focused on using CD40 stimulation as an adjuvant, and in conjunction with cytokines and other factors to elicit antitumor responses. However, due to the pleiotropic effects of CD40 stimulation, and the wide array of cell types upon which it is expressed, new studies are also focusing on the nonimmune related consequences of systemic and local CD40 stimulation. Systemic administration of immunotherapy regimens containing CD40 stimulation via soluble ligands and agonist antibodies has been associated with some toxicities, and direct stimulation of CD40 expressed on various malignancies and vascular endothelium has elucidated a possible role for CD40 in the transformation and progression of malignancies. This review focuses on the role of CD40 stimulation in the generation of innate and adaptive antitumor responses, as well as the direct effects of CD40 stimulation on tumor survival, death, and angiogenesis.

Introduction

CD40 is a 48 kDa type I transmembrane glycoprotein that belongs to the tumor necrosis factor receptor (TNFR) superfamily [1, 2], and is expressed on a variety of cell types. In humans, CD40 was first described on B cells and urinary bladder carcinomas, but it has since been identified on hematopoietic progenitors, dendritic cells (DCs), monocytes, fibroblasts, eosinophils, thymic epithelial cells and endothelial cells, and $CD8^+$ T cells [3–5]. In addition, CD40 has also been demonstrated to be expressed on several carcinomas [6].

W.J. Murphy (✉)
Department of Microbiology and Immunology 320, School of Medicine, University of Nevada, Reno, NV 89557-0320
e-mail: wmurphy@medicine.nevada.edu

J. Lustgarten et al. (eds.), *Targeted Cancer Immune Therapy*,
DOI 10.1007/978-1-4419-0170-5_13,

Among certain TNFR superfamily members, such as Fas, TNFRI, and TRAIL receptor, CD40 is unique because it lacks the intracellular death domain (DD) that the other members possess [1, 7]. Upon ligation, CD40 instead signals through the TNF receptor-associated factor (TRAF) family of adaptor proteins, specifically TRAF2, TRAF6, and TRAF3 [8], which act to further activate several signaling pathways including c-jun N-terminal kinase (JNK), mitogen activated kinases (MAPK), extracellular-regulated kinase (ERK), and most notably nuclear factor κB (NF-κB) [7, 9–11].

The ligand for CD40 is CD154 (CD40L), a trimeric type II transmembrane glycoprotein belonging to the tumor necrosis factor (TNF) superfamily [2, 12]. CD154 is predominantly found on activated $CD4^+$ T cells, where its expression is not only tightly regulated, but has also been identified on basophils, platelets, monocytes, NK cells, eosinophils, and activated B cells [1].

CD40–CD40L interactions are crucial for the development of normal innate and adaptive immune responses. CD40 is expressed predominantly on B cells and professional antigen presenting cells (APC) such as monocytes and DCs, and plays a major role in the survival, development, and activation of these cell types [4]. On APCs, CD40 functions as a costimulatory molecule. Upon the interactions between a T cell receptor (TCR) and an MHC/antigen complex presented on the surface of an APC, CD40–CD40L binding acts to activate the T cell and induce cytokine secretion by the APC. This interaction also occurs between T cells expressing CD40L and resting B cells, which express CD40, and upon ligation, become activated and enter the cell cycle [13].

CD40 is also crucial for the generation of mature B cells. It has been observed that in the absence of CD40 signaling, there is a loss of memory B cell function, the absence of germinal centers, and an inability for B cells to immunoglobulin isotype class switch [14]. In humans, a mutation in the CD40L gene leads to defective CD40 signaling and a condition known as X-linked hyper IgM syndrome. This syndrome is characterized clinically by severe susceptibility to bacterial infections, increased occurrence of carcinomas and lymphomas, and an over-abundance of IgM antibody [7, 15, 16].

CD40 and Antitumor Responses: Bridging the Gap Between Innate and Adaptive Immunity

Upon ligation of CD40, it has been found that macrophages can mediate T cell independent antitumor effects [1, 17–20]. Some groups have used CD40 stimulation as a method to activate monocytes and macrophages to induce antitumor effects, both directly and indirectly. Direct antitumor effects induced by macrophages are predominantly mediated through the release of soluble factors such as nitric oxide, INFγ, and TNFα, which can act to disrupt tumor cells and vasculature [17, 18, 21–24]. Indirect consequences of macrophage activation include the release of IFNγ, which in turn results in the further upregulation of CD40 on the macrophage

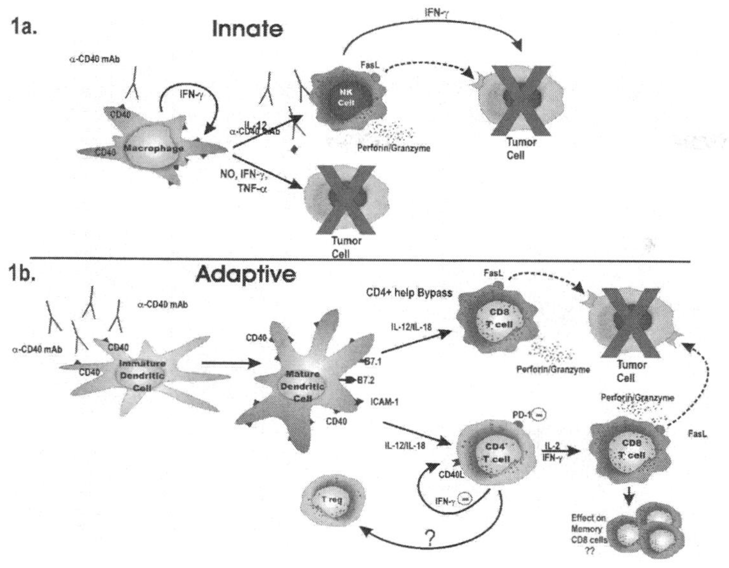

Fig. 1 Effects of CD40 stimulation on innate and adaptive antitumor responses

surface, and the secretion of IL-12, which in turn can activate natural killer cells (NK) to mediate antitumor effects (Fig. 1a) [21, 25].

Bone marrow-derived APC, primarily DCs, play a crucial role in the generation of adaptive immune responses. CD40 stimulation plays an integral role in the activation and maturation of DCs. DC maturation via CD40 ligation has been found to result in the upregulation of MHC II, additional costimulatory and adhesion molecules such as B7.1, B7.2, ICAM-1, and CD70, as well as the induction of Th1 cytokines such as IL-12 and IL-18, thus enabling them to effectively program cytotoxic T cell responses (Fig. 1b) [26–28]. DC maturation can occur through the ligation of toll-like receptors (TLRs) by microbial based ligands such as LPS, or in the absence of infection, through the ligation of CD40 on the DC surface by CD40L on activated $CD4^+$ T helper cells. The state of DC maturation at the time of DC–T cell interactions has been found to be a crucial factor for determining the nature of the T cell responses initiated.

Immature DCs have long been implicated to play a role in the generation and maintenance of central and peripheral tolerance to self-reactive T cells [29, 30]. It has been shown that stimulation of T cells with immature DCs results in the generation of tolerance to both self and exogenous antigens [31]. Steinman and Nussenzweig proposed that immature DCs circulate through the body in the steady state, processing and presenting self antigen. If they come into contact with a T cell that recognizes the presented self antigen, the immature DC will neutralize that T cell, thus maintaining peripheral tolerance [31, 32]. It has also been suggested that immature DCs play a role in the development of T regulatory cells (Tregs), and that immature DCs are capable of producing suppressive cytokines such as IL-10 and transforming growth factor β (TGFβ) [32]. It is interesting to note that, the tolerogenic states induced by immature DCs are reversible upon DC maturation via CD40 stimulation. Sotomayor et al. observed that CD40 stimulation can overcome tumor antigen-specific CD4+ T cell tolerance, and restore tumor vaccination responses [33]. In a concurrent publication, Diel et al. determined that CD40 stimulation can overcome peptide vaccine-induced CD8+ T cell tolerance [34]. Studies examining the role of DCs in the generation of Th1 antitumor responses found CD40 stimulation to be requisite for the generation of IL-12, thus illustrating the importance of CD40 signaling on DCs for the generation of Th1-Type cytokines, and subsequent cell-mediated antitumor responses [35, 36]. Stimulation of CD40 via agonist antibodies has also been found to bypass the need for CD4+ T cell help in the generation of cytotoxic T cell responses [12, 37–40]. Taken together, these studies demonstrate the necessity of DC maturation for the generation of effective cytotoxic T lymphocyte (CTL) responses, and the crucial role that CD40 stimulation plays in this process.

Anti-CD40 and Interleukin-2: Coordination of Innate and Adaptive Immunity

Many preclinical studies have adopted the use of agonist anti-CD40 antibodies to simulate the interaction between CD40 and CD40L. CD40 stimulation has been investigated for use as an adjuvant in coordination with DC vaccines and cytokine therapies to generate antigen specific T cell responses. In addition to these studies, an effective form of immunotherapy has been developed by combining CD40 stimulation via agonist antibodies, with the cytokine interleukin-2 (IL-2). As independent agents, both of these treatments have proved beneficial for the treatment of renal cell carcinoma and melanoma [41–47]; however, it has become apparent that cytokines and receptor agonist antibodies work better when used in concert with each other, rather than independently.

In previous studies, our laboratory used an agonist murine CD40 antibody, which when administered in combination with IL-2, resulted in synergistic antitumor effects in an orthotopic model of renal cell carcinoma [47]. We hypothesized that these antitumor responses were the result of the coordinated activation and maturation of APCs, namely DCs by anti-CD40, and the induction of T cell proliferation and survival by IL-2. We observed that stimulation with IL-2 or anti-CD40 alone resulted in moderate increases in survival, as well as T cell and DC proliferation, but only the combination therapy resulted in optimal antitumor responses. Studies using depleting antibodies, and knockout mice have shown that the antitumor effects generated with the combination therapy were CD8+ T cell-mediated, and were dependent on the expression of Fas ligand and interferon gamma (IFNγ) [47].

Interestingly, we later found that IFNγ, which is crucial for the development of primary antitumor effects after therapy, resulted in high levels of CD4+ T cell death. It has been previously established that stimulation through CD40 can bypass the need for CD4+ T cell help in the generation of primary CD8+ T cell responses;

however, it is widely accepted that $CD4^+$ T cell help is crucial for the generation or maintenance of secondary $CD8^+$ T cell memory responses [37, 48–52]. In our studies, we found that the IFNγ-mediated death of $CD4^+$ T cells after anti-CD40 and IL-2 immunotherapy resulted in the loss of subsequent secondary antitumor responses. It is also interesting to note that the negative effects of anti-CD40/IL-2 on $CD4^+$ T cells are not unique to this therapy, as we have also observed this phenomena in mice that received other immunotherapeutic regimens such as anti-CD40/IL-15 and CpG/IL-12 [46].

After the induction of strong immune activation, such as generated with anti-CD40/IL-2 immunotherapy, there are several inhibitory mechanisms that come into play to prevent undo damage to the host. Another observation we have made with anti-CD40/IL-2 immunotherapy is a marked expansion in $CD4^+$ $CD25^+$ $FoxP3^+$ regulatory T cells (Tregs). It is interesting to note that the cell death we observed in the conventional $CD4^+$ T cell population was largely absent from the Treg population. We found that this is due to the preferential upregulation of programmed death 1 (PD-1) on the surface of the conventional $CD4^+$ T cells, which was not seen on the Treg cell population. We hypothesized that the mechanisms of the IFNγ-mediated $CD4^+$ T cell loss after immunotherapy might be due to the upregulation of B7H-1 on the surface of various cells types, in coordination with the upregulation of PD-1 on the surface of the conventional $CD4^+$ T cells [53].

Another consequence of anti-CD40 and IL-2 immunotherapy is the conversion of $CD4^+$ and $CD8^+$ T cell populations to a memory phenotype [46]. Further studies are underway to determine the consequence of global immune activation and the conversion of T cell populations to memory. These studies will have a particular application to studies in the aged population, as they have been found to have a larger percentage of their T cells expressing a memory phenotype, and are less likely to develop new naïve T cells due to thymic involution.

In our hands and others, the combination therapy of CD40 mAb and IL-2 has also been associated with deleterious toxicities [54–56]. Due to the presence of these toxicities, as well as the ability of anti-CD40 and IL-2 therapy to expand Treg populations, alternate therapies are currently being investigated.

CD40 Signaling on Tumor Cells: Activation-Induced Cell Death and Cytokine Production

Aside from hematologic malignancies, CD40 expression has been found on carcinomas of the bladder, breast, lung, colon, ovary, cervix, prostate, kidney, and melanoma [57–63]. This expression is of interest because the healthy tissue counterparts generally do not express CD40. While CD40 stimulation has by-in-large been examined for its immunomodulatory effects, new studies are coming out that show that stimulation of CD40 expressed on carcinomas and lymphomas may have either a deleterious or advantageous effect on the cancers. Some reports have shown that CD40 stimulation can induce cell death on several types of carcinoma [64–66], whereas others have reported that constitutive signaling through CD40 can aid in tumor progression and multidrug resistance in breast carcinomas and lymphomas [67, 68]. It has also been suggested that CD40 expressed by carcinomas can lead to impaired T cell function by inducing the downregulation of CD40L expressed on activated T cells [6].

Because CD40 lacks a DD, it is unable to directly signal death pathways such as Fas-associated death domain (FADD), TNF receptor associated death domain (TRADD), and caspase-3, which lead to apoptosis of the cell [11]. However, recent studies have suggested that the apoptotic action of CD40 stimulation may be triggered by the induction of other pro-apoptotic molecules. Our lab has previously demonstrated that CD40 stimulation of aggressive histology lymphomas with a human trimeric soluble recombinant CD40L is effective in inducing apoptosis, via the induction of the pro-apoptotic protein, bax (Fig. 2b) [69]. This study corroborated what had been observed with CD40 stimulation in other aggressive B cell lymphomas, such as Burkitt's lymphomas and EBV lymphomas [70, 71]. However, in studies performed using more indolent cell lines such as follicular lymphoma, CD40 stimulation promoted tumor growth and progression [10, 69].

Data examining the effects of CD40 stimulation on solid tumors such as carcinomas of the breast, ovaries, and kidney have been even more conflicting. A paradigm shifting paper published by Baxendale et al. in 2005 demonstrated that primary human breast carcinomas express both CD40 and CD40L, and that constitutive signaling of CD40 promoted neoplastic growth and transformation in an NFκB dependent manner [67]. Other publications had demonstrated the coexpression of CD40 and CD40L on breast carcinomas, but this was the first to demonstrate that

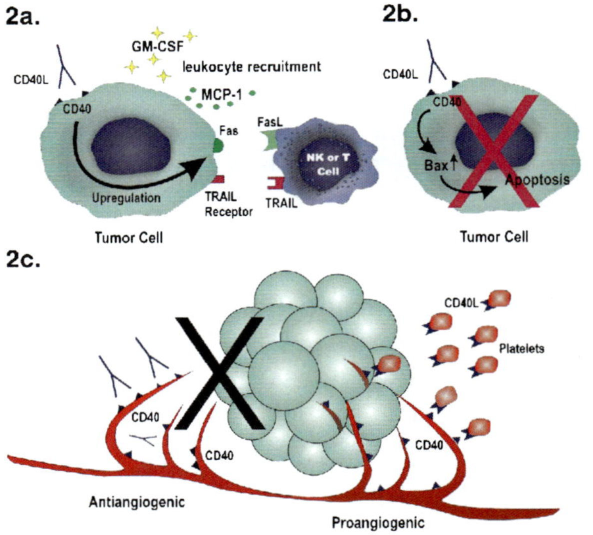

Fig. 2 Direct effects of CD40 stimulation on tumor survival, chemokine production, and vasculature

CD40 stimulation may play a role in the transformation of healthy cells into cancerous cells, and not merely function as an autocrine loop after the cells have become neoplastic [72, 73].

These reports are in striking contrast with other studies which have shown that the stimulation of breast carcinomas and other solid carcinomas with soluble CD40L can lead to growth inhibition and apoptosis, through activation-induced cell death (AICD) and the upregulation of other TNF receptor superfamily members such as Fas and TRAIL (Fig. 2a) [57, 66, 74, 75]. Similar growth inhibitory and apoptotic effects have also been observed in ovarian carcinomas after CD40 stimulation [59, 76]. It may be that the culture conditions, type of tumor, and the extent of CD40 stimulation all play a role in the outcome.

In addition to the direct inhibitory effects induced by CD40 stimulation, our group has also observed that stimulation of CD40 constitutively expressed on renal cell carcinomas results in the upregulation of chemokines such as granulocyte macrophage colony stimulating factor (GM-CSF) and monocyte chemotactic protein-1 (MCP-1), and led to an increase in leukocyte chemotaxis to the tumor site (Fig. 2a) [77]. These studies are of interest because decreases in tumor size were observed after treatment with anti-CD40, even when experiments were performed in mice lacking CD40 expression, thus negating the possibility of any CD40 stimulated immune antitumor effects.

CD40 Stimulation and Vascular Effects: Another Antitumor Pathway

In light of the pleiotropic effects of CD40 signaling on tumor cells and immune mediators, it is not surprising that CD40 stimulation can also have profound effects on endothelial cells. Coexpression of CD40 and CD40L on vascular endothelial cells and smooth muscle cells has been implicated to play a role in the development of atherosclerotic lesions, and CD40 stimulation of tumor-associated endothelial cells has been observed to induce the production of vascular endothelial growth factor (VEGF) [13, 78–80]. As such, the effects of systemic CD40 stimulation may not only trigger immune-mediated antitumor effects, but it may also lead to the production of factors and mechanisms that aid in angiogenesis and tumor progression. In a clinical study of patients with localized and metastatic disease, Romero et al. observed that high VEGF levels correlated with increased metastasis and a decrease in the presence of angiostatic chemokines and cytokines such as IP-10 and IFN-γ. The decreases in IP-10 were also associated with the downregulation of HLA class I expression by the tumor, which would conceivably make the tumor a more attractive target for NK cells, but which would also decrease the effectiveness of a T cell-mediated response [81].

The effects of CD40 stimulation on endothelial cells are becoming of more interest in light of two recent publications. Chiodoni et al. examined the role of CD40 in the generation of rat Her-2/*neu* driven breast carcinomas [82].

In their model, they utilized wildtype and CD40$^{-/-}$ mice, which both developed spontaneous breast carcinomas due to the expression of the rat Her-2/*neu* oncogene. They originally hypothesized that in the absence of CD40 signaling, they would see an acceleration in tumor growth and invasiveness due to the lack of CD40 expression on APC, and the resulting diminution of immune responses. Surprisingly, they observed that tumors grew more slowly in the CD40$^{-/-}$ mice than they did in their wildtype counterparts. They went on to postulate that CD40 expression on murine endothelial cells might be playing a role in the angiogenesis and invasiveness of the spontaneously arising tumors. Subsequent studies showed a decrease in vasculature in the tumors of CD40$^{-/-}$ mice compared with the WT controls. They further postulated that the pro-angiogenic effects were the result of CD40 signaling mediated by interactions between the CD40 receptor expressed on endothelial cells, and CD40L expressed on platelets (Fig. 2c) [82].

In contrast to this study, Hamzah et al. utilized the expression of CD40 on endothelial cells as a target for the treatment of spontaneously arising islet cell carcinomas. In a spin-off of the combination therapy reported by our group, they created a fusion protein of an anti-CD40 antibody and IL-2, which preferentially homed to the sites of tumor vasculature. The antitumor effects that resulted from treatment with the fusion protein were greater than those obtained with the unconjugated anti-CD40 antibody and IL-2 [83]. In contrast to our studies, they concluded that the antitumor effects after intratumor injection of the fusion protein were due to the disruption of the vasculature, and were not immune-mediated (Fig. 2c). It is interesting to note that they did not see a loss of antitumor effects when mice were depleted of CD4$^+$ and CD8$^+$ T cells. In fact, the abrogation of antitumor effects were seen when they treated tumors in mice whose endothelium lacked CD40 expression. In keeping with the variable expression of CD40 on transformed cells, immunohistochemistry studies in these mice also showed that CD40 expression was only upregulated on the vascular endothelium of tumors, and was not observed on normal pancreatic parenchyma and endothelium [83].

Further Considerations: Properties of Agonist CD40 Antibodies and Potential Toxicities

Based on the studies presented in this review, it is clear that there are several factors which can determine whether the outcomes of cancer immunotherapy via CD40 stimulation are advantageous to the host, or to the tumor. Among the factors that dictate the direct effects of CD40 stimulation are the aggressive or indolent nature of the tumor, the prevalence of CD40 expression on the tumor and its associated endothelium, and the strength of signaling through the CD40 receptor. The method used to mimic CD40L interactions can have a profound impact on the antitumor effects generated. Some studies have utilized cells that are virally transfected to express human CD40L [64, 68], or a soluble recombinant human CD40L which is commercially available as a source of CD40 stimulus *in vitro* [59, 66, 69, 75].

CD40L transfected cells have the benefit of presenting membrane-bound ligand to CD40, which has been shown to have significant effects on the strength of the signaling sent to the CD40 expressing cell [84]. The human CD40 ligand is also a trimer, which allows for augmented signaling capabilities [12].

Many mouse studies have used agonist antibodies as a method of CD40 stimulus both *in vitro* and *in vivo*. The application of agonist antibodies for CD40 stimulation has both advantages and draw-backs. One advantage is that *in vivo*, the ligation of antibodies to CD40 expressing tumor cells may allow for the triggering of AICD, and may affect antibody dependent cellular cytotoxicity (ADCC). For *in vitro* studies, the crosslinking of anti-CD40 antibodies by plate binding or capture antibodies is sufficient to induce apoptosis in several B cell lymphoma cell lines, as well as some human breast carcinoma lines [66]. One caveat of using monoclonal antibodies to trigger CD40 signaling is that not all CD40 agonist antibodies confer the same level of activation. The agonistic properties of the antibody used can have a profound impact on the nature of the immune and antitumor responses generated. For example, the rat anti-mouse CD40 antibody used in our studies and others (clone FGK115-B3) is a strong agonist while SGN-40, the humanized antibody currently in phase I and II clinical trials for the treatment of multiple myeloma and various hematological malignancies, is a partial agonist. As a partial agonist, SGN-40 has not been observed to induce normal B cell proliferation; however, it does result in the inhibition of proliferation, and the induction of apoptosis, and ADCC in a variety of human high-grade B-cell lymphoma and multiple myeloma cell lines [85–87]. In contrast, FGK115-B3 is a potent inducer of normal B cell proliferation, and mediates the majority of its antitumor effects through the induction of systemic antitumor immunity [88]. It is important to note that due to the differing agonistic properties of the rat and humanized antibodies, the mechanism of action differs significantly between the two.

A limiting factor for the use and efficacy of CD40 stimulation as a systemic cancer therapeutic regimen are the associated toxicities. Among the more striking features in the publication by Hamzah et al. was the surprising lack of toxicity associated with the systemic administration of the fusion protein, compared with the independent agents of anti-CD40 and IL-2 [83]. Our group and others have shown that systemic administration of agonist CD40 antibodies can result in dose limiting toxicities that include splenomegaly, the induction of pro-inflammatory cytokines such as TNFα, IFNγ, and IL-12, and the development of intestinal lesions [54–56, 83]. The intestinal effects of CD40 stimulation are such that an agonist CD40 mAb was recently used to simulate a model of wasting disease and colitis in immune deficient mice [89].

In light of the potentially severe toxicities that are generated with strong CD40 stimulation in mice, and the disparities in the agonistic properties of mouse and human antibodies, the translation of preclinical agonist antibodies such as CD40 to the clinic has been under heavy scrutiny. This scrutiny has intensified in the wake of the Northwick Park incident, in which a phase I clinical trial testing a superagonistic anti-CD28 antibody (TGN1412) resulted in the prolonged hospitalization of healthy volunteers [90–94]. Animal studies in both rodent and nonhuman primate models had demonstrated that administration of a TGN1412 resulted in the expansion of T regulatory cells, which in turn ameliorated the development of some autoimmune conditions, with minimal toxicities [93, 94]. In March of 2006, TGN1412 was administered to six healthy human volunteers as part of a first-in-human phase I clinical trial. Within hours of administration, all patients developed lymphopoenia and a cytokine storm-induced inflammatory condition, which culminated in multisystem organ failure. This study raised several questions about how and why these effects were not predicted based on the preclinical data, and what interspecies differences might account for such dramatic differential effects in humans [95–97]. Nevertheless, these studies would suggest that caution be applied when attempting to use strong agonist stimulation of CD40 due to systemic immune effects leading to toxicities.

Summary

Due to the unique role that CD40 plays in the generation of both innate and adaptive immune responses, further studies are needed into additional therapeutic combinations that might push for greater cell-mediated responses, without the generation of toxicities and suppressive mechanisms. It may be that by combining anti-CD40 treatment with other T cell targeting cytokines such as IL-15 or IL-7, it will be possible to induce T cell-mediated antitumor responses without expanding Treg populations and inducing such great toxicities. In light of the conflicting effects of CD40 stimulation on transformed cells, it will be important to balance out the tumor promoting vs. tumor inhibitory effects CD40 ligation may have when determining the best model for immunotherapy. It is likely that the immunomodulatory effects of CD40 stimulation in vivo may outweigh the tumor promoting effects produced in response to CD40 ligation on the tumor. Additional studies are needed to further elucidate the role of CD40 expression on tumor endothelial cells, and whether it provides a new target for therapy, or will aid in tumor angiogenesis and progression.

References

1. Vogel, L. A., and Noelle, R. J. (1998) Semin Immunol 10, 435
2. Dallman, C., Johnson, P. W., and Packham, G. (2003) Apoptosis 8, 45
3. Tong, A. W., and Stone, M. J. (2003) Cancer Gene Ther 10, 1
4. van Kooten, C., and Banchereau, J. (2000) J Leukoc Biol 67, 2
5. Biancone, L., Cantaluppi, V., and Camussi, G. (1999) Int J Mol Med 3, 343
6. Batrla, R., Linnebacher, M., Rudy, W., Stumm, S., Wallwiener, D., and Guckel, B. (2002) Cancer Res 62, 2052
7. Eliopoulos, A. G., and Young, L. S. (2004) Curr Opin Pharmacol 4, 360
8. Davies, C. C., Bem, D., Young, L. S., and Eliopoulos, A. G. (2005) Cell Signal 17, 729
9. Dempsey, P. W., Doyle, S. E., He, J. Q., and Cheng, G. (2003) Cytokine Growth Factor Rev 14, 193

10. van Kooten, C., and Banchereau, J. (1997) Int Arch Allergy Immunol 113, 393
11. Gaur, U., and Aggarwal, B. B. (2003) Biochem Pharmacol 66, 1403
12. Tutt, A. L., O'Brien, L., Hussain, A., Crowther, G. R., French, R. R., and Glennie, M. J. (2002) J Immunol 168, 2720
13. Grewal, I. S., and Flavell, R. A. (1998) Annu Rev Immunol 16, 111
14. Kawabe, T., Naka, T., Yoshida, K., Tanaka, T., Fujiwara, H., Suematsu, S., Yoshida, N., Kishimoto, T., and Kikutani, H. (1994) Immunity, 1, 167
15 . Callard, R. E., Armitage, R. J., Fanslow, W. C., and Spriggs, M. K. (1993) Immunol Today 14, 559
16. Hayward, A. R., Levy, J., Facchetti, F., Notarangelo, L., Ochs, H. D., Etzioni, A., Bonnefoy, J. Y., Cosyns, M., and Weinberg, A. (1997) J Immunol 158, 977
17. Lum, H. D., Buhtoiarov, I. N., Schmidt, B. E., Berke, G., Paulnock, D. M., Sondel, P. M., and Rakhmilevich, A. L. (2006) J Leukoc Biol 79, 1181
18. Lum, H. D., Buhtoiarov, I. N., Schmidt, B. E., Berke, G., Paulnock, D. M., Sondel, P. M., and Rakhmilevich, A. L. (2006) Immunology 118, 261
19. Tian, L., Noelle, R. J., and Lawrence, D. A. (1995) Eur J Immunol 25, 306
20. Rakhmilevich, A. L., Buhtoiarov, I. N., Malkovsky, M., and Sondel, P. M. (2008) Cancer Immunol Immunother 57, 1151
21. Buhtoiarov, I. N., Lum, H., Berke, G., Paulnock, D. M., Sondel, P. M., and Rakhmilevich, A. L. (2005) J Immunol 174, 6013
22. Buhtoiarov, I. N., Lum, H. D., Berke, G., Sondel, P. M., and Rakhmilevich, A. L. (2006) J Immunol 176, 309
23. Chen, G. G., Chu, Y. S., Chak, E. C., Leung, B. C., and Poon, W. S. (2002) J Neurooncol 57, 179
24. Havell, E. A., Fiers, W., and North, R. J. (1988) J Exp Med 167, 1067
25. Turner, J. G., Rakhmilevich, A. L., Burdelya, L., Neal, Z., Imboden, M., Sondel, P. M., and Yu, H. (2001) J Immunol 166, 89
26. Cella, M., Scheidegger, D., Palmer-Lehmann, K., Lane, P., Lanzavecchia, A., and Alber, G. (1996) J Exp Med 184, 747
27. French, R. R., Taraban, V. Y., Crowther, G. R., Rowley, T. F., Gray, J. C., Johnson, P. W., Tutt, A. L., Al-Shamkhani, A., and Glennie, M. J. (2007) Blood 109, 48105
28. Taraban, V. Y., Rowley, T. F., and Al-Shamkhani, A. (2004) J Immunol 173, 65426
29. Hawiger, D., Inaba, K., Dorsett, Y., Guo, M., Mahnke, K., Rivera, M., Ravetch, J. V., Steinman, R. M., and Nussenzweig, M. C. (2001) J Exp Med 194, 769
30. Garza, K. M., Chan, S. M., Suri, R., Nguyen, L. T., Odermatt, B., Schoenberger, S. P., and Ohashi, P. S. (2000) J Exp Med 191, 2021
31. Steinman, R. M., and Nussenzweig, M. C. (2002) Proc Natl Acad Sci USA 99, 3518
32. Steinman, R. M., Hawiger, D., and Nussenzweig, M. C. (2003) Annu Rev Immunol 21, 685
33. Sotomayor, E. M., Borrello, I., Tubb, E., Rattis, F. M., Bien, H., Lu, Z., Fein, S., Schoenberger, S., and Levitsky, H. I. (1999) Nat Med 5, 780
34. Diehl, L., Den Boer, A. T., van der Voort, E. I., Melief, C. J., Offringa, R., and Toes, R. E. (2000) J Mol Med 78, 3631
35. Mackey, M. F., Gunn, J. R., Maliszewsky, C., Kikutani, H., Noelle, R. J., and Barth, R. J., Jr. (1998) J Immunol 161, 2094
36. Mackey, M. F., Barth, R. J., Jr., and Noelle, R. J. (1998) J Leukoc Biol 63, 418
37. Schoenberger, S. P., Toes, R. E., van der Voort, E. I., Offringa, R., and Melief, C. J. (1998) Nature 393, 480
38. Ridge, J. P., Di Rosa, F., and Matzinger, P. (1998) Nature 393, 474
39. French, R. R., Chan, H. T., Tutt, A. L., and Glennie, M. J. (1999) Nat Med 5, 548
40. Bennett, S. R., Carbone, F. R., Karamalis, F., Flavell, R. A., Miller, J. F., and Heath, W. R. (1998) Nature 393, 478
41. Sokoloff, M. H., Daneshmand, S., and Ryan, C. W. (2005) Urol Oncol 23, 289
42. Sokoloff, M. H., deKernion, J. B., Figlin, R. A., and Belldegrun, A. (1996) CA Cancer J Clin 46, 284
43. Fyfe, G., Fisher, R. I., Rosenberg, S. A., Sznol, M., Parkinson, D. R., and Louie, A. C. (1995) J Clin Oncol 13, 688

44. Fyfe, G. A., Fisher, R. I., Rosenberg, S. A., Sznol, M., Parkinson, D. R., and Louie, A. C. (1996) J Clin Oncol 14, 2410
45. Rosenberg, S. A., Yang, J. C., Topalian, S. L., Schwartzentruber, D. J., Weber, J. S., Parkinson, D. R., Seipp, C. A., Einhorn, J. H., and White, D. E. (1994) JAMA 271, 907
46. Berner, V., Liu, H., Zhou, Q., Alderson, K. L., Sun, K., Weiss, J. M., Back, T. C., Longo, D. L., Blazar, B. R., Wiltrout, R. H., Welniak, L. A., Redelman, D., and Murphy, W. J. (2007) Nat Med 13, 354
47. Murphy, W. J., Welniak, L., Back, T., Hixon, J., Subleski, J., Seki, N., Wigginton, J. M., Wilson, S. E., Blazar, B. R., Malyguine, A. M., Sayers, T. J., and Wiltrout, R. H. (2003) J Immunol 170, 2727
48. Shedlock, D. J., and Shen, H. (2003) Science 300, 337
49. Sun, J. C., and Bevan, M. J. (2003) Science 300, 339
50. Schuurhuis, D. H., Laban, S., Toes, R. E., Ricciardi-Castagnoli, P., Kleijmeer, M. J., van der Voort, E. I., Rea, D., Offringa, R., Geuze, H. J., Melief, C. J., and Ossendorp, F. (2000) J Exp Med 192, 145
51. Janssen, E. M., Droin, N. M., Lemmens, E. E., Pinkoski, M. J., Bensinger, S. J., Ehst, B. D., Griffith, T. S., Green, D. R., and Schoenberger, S. P. (2005) Nature 434, 88
52. Janssen, E. M., Lemmens, E. E., Wolfe, T., Christen, U., von Herrath, M. G., and Schoenberger, S. P. (2003) Nature 421, 852
53. Alderson, K. L., Zhou, Q., Berner, V., Wilkins, D. E., Weiss, J. M., Blazar, B. R., Welniak, L. A., Wiltrout, R. H., Redelman, D., and Murphy, W. J. (2008) J Immunol 180, 2981
54. Gendelman, M., Halligan, N., Komorowski, R., Logan, B., Murphy, W. J., Blazar, B. R., Pritchard, K. A., Jr., and Drobyski, W. R. (2005) Blood 105, 428
55. Hixon, J. A., Anver, M. R., Blazar, B. R., Panoskaltsis-Mortari, A., Wiltrout, R. H., and Murphy, W. J. (2002) Biol Blood Marrow Transplant 8, 316
56. Hixon, J. A., Blazar, B. R., Anver, M. R., Wiltrout, R. H., and Murphy, W. J. (2001) Biol Blood Marrow Transplant 7, 136
57. Lee, J. K., Seki, N., Sayers, T. J., Subleski, J., Gruys, E. M., Murphy, W. J., and Wiltrout, R. H. (2005) Cell Immunol 235, 145
58. Sabel, M. S., Yamada, M., Kawaguchi, Y., Chen, F. A., Takita, H., and Bankert, R.B. (2000) Cancer Immunol Immunother 49, 101
59. Gallagher, N. J., Eliopoulos, A. G., Agathangelo, A., Oates, J., Crocker, J., and Young, L. S. (2002) Mol Pathol 55, 110
60. Rokhlin, O. W., Bishop, G. A., Hostager, B. S., Waldschmidt, T. J., Sidorenko, S. P., Pavloff, N., Kiefer, M. C., Umansky, S. R., Glover, R. A., and Cohen, M. B. (1997) Cancer Res 57, 1758
61. Thomas, W. D., Smith, M. J., Si, Z., and Hersey, P. (1996) Int J Cancer 68, 795
62. Ziebold, J. L., Hixon, J., Boyd, A., and Murphy, W. J. (2000) Arch Immunol Ther Exp 48, 225
63. Altenburg, A., Baldus, S. E., Smola, H., Pfister, H., and Hess, S. (1999) J Immunol 162, 4140
64. Hess, S., and Engelmann, H. (1996) J Exp Med 183, 159
65. Young, L. S., Eliopoulos, A. G., Gallagher, N. J., and Dawson, C. W. (1998) Immunol Today 19, 502
66. Hirano, A., Longo, D. L., Taub, D. D., Ferris, D. K., Young, L. S., Eliopoulos, A. G., Agathanggelou, A., Cullen, N., Macartney, J., Fanslow, W. C., and Murphy, W. J. (1999) Blood 93, 2999
67. Baxendale, A. J., Dawson, C. W., Stewart, S. E., Mudaliar, V., Reynolds, G., Gordon, J., Murray, P. G., Young, L. S., and Eliopoulos, A. G. (2005) Oncogene 24, 7913
68. Voorzanger-Rousselot, N., Alberti, L., and Blay, J. Y. (2006) BMC Cancer 6, 75
69. Szocinski, J. L., Khaled, A. R., Hixon, J., Halverson, D., Funakoshi, S., Fanslow, W. C., Boyd, A., Taub, D. D., Durum, S. K., Siegall, C. B., Longo, D. L., and Murphy, W. J. (2002) Blood 100, 217
70. Murphy, W. J., Funakoshi, S., Beckwith, M., Rushing, S. E., Conley, D. K., Armitage, R. J., Fanslow, W. C., Rager, H. C., Taub, D. D., Ruscetti, F. W. et al. (1995) Blood 86, 1946
71. Funakoshi, S., Longo, D. L., Beckwith, M., Conley, D. K., Tsarfaty, G., Tsarfaty, I., Armitage, R. J., Fanslow, W. C., Spriggs, M. K., and Murphy, W. J. (1994) Blood 83, 2787

72. Voorzanger-Rousselot, N., and Blay, J. Y. (2004) Leuk Lymphoma 45, 1239–1245
73. Tong, A. W., Papayoti, M. H., Netto, G., Armstrong, D. T., Ordonez, G., Lawson, J. M., and Stone, M. J. (2001) Clin Cancer Res 7, 691
74. Wischhusen, J., Schneider, D., Mittelbronn, M., Meyermann, R., Engelmann, H., Jung, G., Wiendl, H., and Weller, M. (2005) J Neuroimmunol 162, 28
75. Eliopoulos, A. G., Davies, C., Knox, P. G., Gallagher, N. J., Afford, S. C., Adams, D. H., and Young, L. S. (2000) Mol Cell Biol 20, 5503
76. Melichar, B., Patenia, R., Gallardo, S., Melicharova, K., Hu, W., and Freedman, R. S. (2007) Gynecol Oncol 104, 707
77. Shorts, L., Weiss, J. M., Lee, J. K., Welniak, L. A., Subleski, J., Back, T., Murphy, W. J., and Wiltrout, R. H. (2006) J Immunol 176, 6543
78. Mach, F., Schonbeck, U., Sukhova, G. K., Bourcier, T., Bonnefoy, J. Y., Pober, J. S., and Libby, P. (1997) Proc Natl Acad Sci USA 94, 1931
79. Reinders, M. E., Sho, M., Robertson, S. W., Geehan, C. S., and Briscoe, D. M. (2003) J Immunol 171, 1534
80. Melter, M., Reinders, M. E., Sho, M., Pal, S., Geehan, C., Denton, M. D., Mukhopadhyay, D., and Briscoe, D. M. (2000) Blood 96, 3801
81. Romero, J. M., Aptsiauri, N., Vazquez, F., Cozar, J. M., Canton, J., Cabrera, T., Tallada, M., Garrido, F., and Ruiz-Cabello, F. (2006) Tissue Antigens 68, 303
82. Chiodoni, C., Iezzi, M., Guiducci, C., Sangaletti, S., Alessandrini, I., Ratti, C., Tiboni, F., Musiani, P., Granger, D. N., and Colombo, M. P. (2006) J Exp Med 203, 2441
83. Hamzah, J., Nelson, D., Moldenhauer, G., Arnold, B., Hammerling, G. J., and Ganss, R. (2008) J Clin Invest 118, 1691
84. Georgopoulos, N. T., Steele, L. P., Thomson, M. J., Selby, P. J., Southgate, J., and Trejdosiewicz, L. K. (2006) Cell Death Differ 13, 1789
85. Law, C. L., Gordon, K. A., Collier, J., Klussman, K., McEarchern, J. A., Cerveny, C. G., Mixan, B. J., Lee, W. P., Lin, Z., Valdez, P., Wahl, A. F., and Grewal, I. S. (2005) Cancer Res 65, 8331
86. Francisco, J. A., Donaldson, K. L., Chace, D., Siegall, C. B., and Wahl, A. F. (2000) Cancer Res 60, 3225
87. Kelley, S. K., Gelzleichter, T., Xie, D., Lee, W. P., Darbonne, W. C., Qureshi, F., Kissler, K., Oflazoglu, E., and Grewal, I. S. (2006) Br J Pharmacol 148, 1116
88. Erickson, L. D., Durell, B. G., Vogel, L. A., O'Connor, B. P., Cascalho, M., Yasui, T., Kikutani, H., and Noelle, R. J. (2002) J Clin Invest 109, 613
89. Uhlig, H. H., McKenzie, B. S., Hue, S., Thompson, C., Joyce-Shaikh, B., Stepankova, R., Robinson, N., Buonocore, S., Tlaskalova-Hogenova, H., Cua, D. J., and Powrie, F. (2006) Immunity 25, 309
90. Suntharalingam, G., Perry, M. R., Ward, S., Brett, S. J., Castello-Cortes, A., Brunner, M. D., and Panoskaltsis, N. (2006) N Engl J Med 355, 1018
91. Muller, N., van den Brandt, J., Odoardi, F., Tischner, D., Herath, J., Flugel, A., and Reichardt, H. M. (2008) J Clin Invest 118, 1405
92. Beyersdorf, N., Hanke, T., Kerkau, T., and Hunig, T. (2005) Ann Rheum Dis 64 (Suppl 4), iv91
93. Beyersdorf, N., Gaupp, S., Balbach, K., Schmidt, J., Toyka, K. V., Lin, C. H., Hanke, T., Hunig, T., Kerkau, T., and Gold, R. (2005) J Exp Med 202, 445
94. Schmidt, J., Elflein, K., Stienekemeier, M., Rodriguez-Palmero, M., Schneider, C., Toyka, K. V., Gold, R., and Hunig, T. (2003) J Neuroimmunol 140, 143
95. Legrand, N., Cupedo, T., van Lent, A. U., Ebeli, M. J., Weijer, K., Hanke, T., and Spits, H. (2006) Blood 108, 238
96. Stebbings, R., Findlay, L., Edwards, C., Eastwood, D., Bird, C., North, D., Mistry, Y., Dilger, P., Liefooghe, E., Cludts, I., Fox, B., Tarrant, G., Robinson, J., Meager, T., Dolman, C., Thorpe, S. J., Bristow, A., Wadhwa, M., Thorpe, R., and Poole, S. (2007) J Immunol 179, 3325
97. Nguyen, D. H., Hurtado-Ziola, N., Gagneux, P., and Varki, A. (2006) Proc Natl Acad Sci USA 103, 7765

Immunocytokines: A Novel Approach to Cancer Immune Therapy

Stephen D. Gillies

Abstract The induction of a long-lived immune response to cancer has been a long-term goal of modern medicine, but to date has not been realized despite evidence that the immune system is capable of responding to tumors. Immunocytokines represent a new class of biopharmaceuticals composed of two well-known immune components – antibodies and cytokines – with the unique ability to target cytokines to the tumor microenvironment and thereby induce long-term and protective immune responses in preclinical mouse tumor models. Several immunocytokines have now reached clinical development where it is hoped that the exciting preclinical efficacy results will translate to effective therapy for cancer patients. Integration of such a treatment modality with current standard of care, as well as newly emerging targeted therapies, will be essential for the success of this approach.

Introduction

The concept of specifically targeting therapeutic substances as a form of immunotherapy is more than a century old [1]. A "magic bullet" for cancer therapy has still not been realized although several of the necessary technical components are now available including: a source of a mono-specific, tumor-targeting antibody, a means of adapting it as a drug, and finally the methods for determining the nature of the payload that would have a mechanism for fighting cancer. The first hurdle was solved by the introduction of monoclonal antibody technology in the mid 1970s [2], followed shortly thereafter by the introduction of antibody engineering in the early 1980s [3]. After it became possible to engineer potential magic bullets, many payloads have been assessed in the last two decades. These include various radioisotopes, small molecules, and toxins (all of which can and have been chemically conjugated to purified antibodies), as well as effector proteins that can be fused at the genetic

S.D. Gillies (✉)
Provenance Biopharmaceuticals Corp., 830 Winter Street, Waltham, MA 02451
e-mail: sgillies@provenancebio.com

J. Lustgarten et al. (eds.), *Targeted Cancer Immune Therapy*,
DOI 10.1007/978-1-4419-0170-5_14,

level to create antibody fusion proteins. The focus of this article is the fusion of cytokines, as the effector component, to tumor targeting antibodies to create what are now called immunocytokines [4]. The concept, in this case, is to have both a direct immune-mediated effect on the tumor cell (via innate immune cells) as well as an indirect immune response through the induction of an adaptive T cell-mediated response. This is achieved by targeting cytokines to the tumor microenvironment and thereby activating a local immune response, the nature of which is based on the cytokine and the format in which it is delivered. While the literature is filled with descriptive reports of the construction, expression and in vitro characterization of such molecules, I will focus on the more recent advances of second-generation molecules, early signs of relevant clinical activity with IL-2-based immunoctyokines and how best to position this class of drug for future success in treating cancer.

Immunocytokine Structures

The basic concept of combining a tumor targeting antibody and a cytokine opens up a vast number of possible molecular configurations based on the extensive array of genetically engineered antibody formats that have been described [5–13]. It is beyond the scope of this article to review all of these formats but they can be generally divided into two categories – small, monomeric antibody-cytokine fusions and large, dimeric antibody-cytokine fusions (Fig. 1). Ironically, this was the difference between the first immunocytokines reported by two groups in 1991 – the first based on the use of a genetically engineered Fab fragment as the antibody component [14], and the second based on an engineered cytokine fusion to the heavy chain of a whole antibody [15].

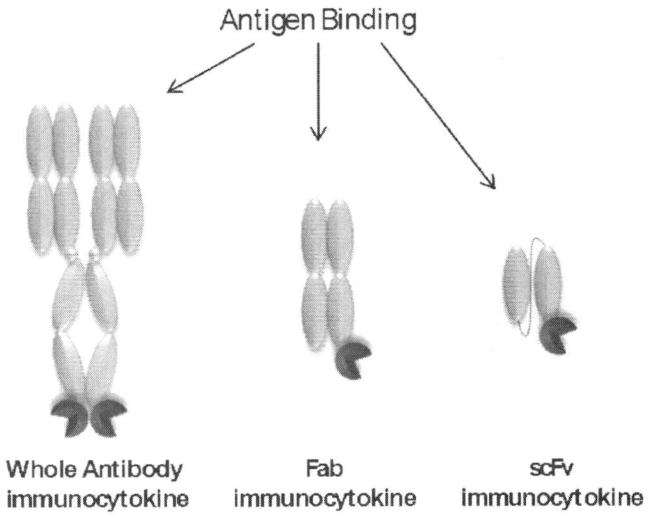

Fig. 1 Immunocytokine structures

Since that time, additional formats have been described but in all cases they differ primarily by molecular size and whether they are monomeric or covalent dimers in nature, at least with respect to the antibody component. Size is highly relevant to the pharmacokinetic behavior in vivo when the immunocytokine is small enough to be removed from the circulation through kidney filtration. One argument for small size has been to increase tumor penetration, but this is not been proven formally in either animals or in patients. Some experiments have shown increased tumor to blood ratios using small rather than large antibodies but this is not due to increased tumor penetration but rather, faster clearance from the blood pool [16]. While this is an advantage for radiologic imaging, it may be more important for tumor targeted cytokine delivery to increase the absolute amount reaching the tumor rather than the ratio. What matters most is antitumor activity and a published study comparing IL-2-based immunocytokines composed of whole antibody or with a single-chain variable Fv (scFv) binding domain, clearly showed the superiority of the former [17]. It was hypothesized that both longer circulating half-life and antibody effector functions played roles in the increased activity.

Targeting Concepts

The most obvious way to target an agent to a tumor is to use an antibody against an antigen on the tumor cell surface. Several early immunocytokines were constructed using antitumor antibodies that were available at the time including those targeting the ganglioside, GD2 [18], the epithelial antigens Lewis^{Y} [19] and EpCAM [20], the B lymphoma antigen Lym-1 [21], and Her2neu [22], to give some examples. While these have appeared to be useful targets in preclinical studies in mice, it remains to be determined what will prove to be the ideal criteria for a cell surface antigen for clinical efficacy. Some considerations include [1] the level of expression on the tumor; [2] the tumor specificity; [3] whether the antigen is shed or internalized; and [4] whether binding to the cell surface target alone contributes in some way to antitumor activity. In most cases, it is unlikely that simple antibody binding would have sufficient antitumor activity to contribute to overall efficacy, especially for monovalent immunocytokines. This is due primarily to the fact that immunocytokine dosing is limited by the biological activity of the cytokine by at least a factor of 10, and the relatively shorter circulating half-life (and thus shorter exposure) of both large and small immunocytokines. Thus, even bivalent forms would be unlikely to contribute direct antibody-mediated effects unless such processes occur at low concentrations, for example, by apoptosis induction.

A less obvious way to target cytokines to tumors is by what has been termed "tumor necrotic therapy" or TNT, pioneered by Epstein et al. [23]. In this case, antibodies specific for nucleic acids are used to target RNA and/or DNA that has been released by dying cells undergoing necrotic cell death. The idea is that this approach would bring active cytokine into the vicinity of dying tumor cells including the necrotic core and stimulate an immune response. Still another indirect approach is to target the tumor microenvironment rather than the tumor. Two groups are using antibodies against oncofetal fibronectin to deliver cytokines to the vascular bed of the tumor [24, 25]. One argument for this approach is that this region of the tumor microenvironment may be more accessible to large biomolecules than the internal part of the tumor mass, based on the finding that tumor interstitial pressures prevent effective tumor uptake of antibodies and other large proteins.

In considering which of these targeting approaches is most effective, it is necessary to consider the overall therapeutic modality one is trying to achieve and what other antibody-based mechanisms are desired to be maintained in the immunocytokine. These are discussed further below.

Immunocytokines Containing Modified IL-2

Directed mutagenesis of IL-2 has been used for many years to study which residues are responsible for receptor binding to the two polypeptide chains that make up the intermediate affinity IL-2R (β and γ), as well as the third chain (α) that, together with βγ chains, makes up the high affinity IL-2R [26, 27]. This has led investigators to try to modulate either free IL-2 or the IL-2 contained in immunocytokines to activate one or the other class of receptor selectively with the hope of separating antitumor activity and the side effects commonly associated with high dose IL-2. This is based on the fact that while most immune cells express the intermediate IL-2R, the high affinity IL-2R is quite restricted to activated T cells and a few antigen presenting cells under normal physiological conditions. Therefore, normal or even high dosing of an IL-2 molecule selective for on the high affinity receptor would have a far greater effect on the subset of activated cells than on the majority of immune cells in the circulation that are more commonly associated with IL-2 toxicity [28].

The earliest study of a reduced toxicity IL-2 was reported by Shanafelt et al. [27] based on selective elimination of binding to the β chain of IL-2 by an N88R mutation and this molecule has since been studied in both nonhuman primates, as well as in human clinical trials. Unfortunately, while early dosing demonstrated a good selectivity for IL-2R subtypes, and improved tolerability, continuous dosing appears to lead to normal IL-2 toxicity [29]. The same result was obtained using an immunocytokine (NHS-IL2LT or Selectikine) with a different mutation in the IL-2 component that eliminates binding to the β chain, D20T [30]. In the latter case, the use of intermittent dosing of 3 days, followed by 18 days without dosing (one cycle every 3 weeks), was found to be very well tolerated in mouse models. Importantly, even the first 3 days of dosing resulted in significant antitumor activity in a lung metastasis model. This is particularly interesting for the additional reason that the targeting component of this D20T mutated immunocytokine was an anti-DNA antibody (TNT targeting). The fact that it was effective in a micro-metastasis model (where tumor necrosis would not be expected) suggests that the DNA epitopes recognized by this antibody may be displayed on the surface of the individual cells of the metastatic lesions, perhaps during the early stages of apoptosis. Earlier studies of cells undergoing this process support that DNA or DNA-containing structures are detectable in both autoimmune disease and in cancer cells [31, 32]. Thus, anti-DNA antibody targeting may not only be useful for TNT approaches but also for treatment of residual disease as well.

Effector Cell Mechanisms

Since immunocytokines can be highly varied in structure, one option is to limit the therapeutic approach to the simple delivery of a cytokine to the tumor cell or microenvironment. This is true of most immunocytokine formats other than those made with whole antibodies. In this case the effector mechanism is based primarily on the biological activity of the chosen cytokine. For example, activation and proliferation of natural killer (NK) and T cells would result from the delivery of IL-2, whereas the delivery of IL-12 may have more antiangiogenic effects based on the known properties of this cytokine [33]. If one desires a more multidimensional therapeutic approach, it may be advantageous to retain the antibody effector functions found in the constant region of the Ig heavy chain. These include antibody-dependent cellular cytotoxicity (ADCC) and complement-dependent cytotoxicity (CDC), both of which are triggered by antibody binding directly to antigen on the cell surface. In the first case, bound antibody mediates a bridging between the tumor cell and an effector cell (such as an NK cell) via an Fc receptor that results in the activation of a lytic program mediated by the pore-forming protein perforin and granzyme that kills the tumor target [34]. In the second case, the binding of antibody to certain cell surface antigens results in binding of the complement system component C1q, which results in the triggering of additional complement components leading to both direct cell death and opsinization by monocytic cells [35].

The role that antibody effector function plays in antitumor activity has been tested in mouse models by several groups for both naked antibodies [36, 37] and whole antibody-based immunocytokines [38], although in the latter case, the majority of studies only tested tumor cell killing in vitro. More importantly, clinical data with the anti-CD20 antibody, Rituxan, indicate that polymorphisms of the Fc receptor associated with NK cell-mediated ADCC have a significant effect on response to therapy [39]. In this case, higher binding to FcRIII is correlated with improved clinical response to Rituxan. More recently another anti-CD20 antibody, HuMab CD20 – selected based on its increased ability to mediate CDC – appears to have significant clinical activity in patients that have relapsed after combined Rituxan and chemotherapy [40]. Thus, it appears that these antibody effector functions can and do contribute to the antitumor response in cancer patients – at least with antibodies against the CD20 target.

A recent study of an anti-CD20 IL-2-based immunocytokine indicates that the traditional antibody effector functions may not play as significant a role in antitumor activity, at least not in the SCID mouse model it was tested in [41].

In this study, DI-Leu16-IL2 was constructed as a whole antibody-IL2 immunocytokine and shown in vitro to maintain its anti-CD20 binding, as well as its ability to mediate ADCC against human B lymphoma cells. CDC activity was reduced, relative to the naked antibody, but was still present in the immunocytokine. These activities were abrogated by enzymatic deglycosylation of DI-Leu16-IL2 – a process known to destroy both ADCC and CDC activities of antibodies [42], and the resulting immunocytokine was compared with the original molecule for antitumor activity. Surprisingly, the groups of mice treated with a low dose of either immunocytokine showed the same growth delay (compared with untreated mice) as each other and roughly the same as the group treated with a much higher dose of Rituxan. A higher dose of normal DI-Leu16-IL2 completely prevented tumor progression, as was the case for the majority of mice in the group treated with the de-glycosylated immunocytokine lacking antibody effector functions. This result is quite interesting when considering the fact that the major immune effector cell in SCID mice is thought to be the NK cell – the cell type most closely associated with ADCC activity. While additional studies are needed to elucidate the antitumor mechanism(s) invoked by DI-Leu16-IL2 and the role of antibody effector activities, it is clear that they are very different from the naked anti-CD20 antibody.

Finally, another potential effector mechanism has been proposed for immunocytokines based on the multiple binding components of the antibody and the cytokine. In this case, the binding of IL-2 to IL-2 receptor (IL-2R) on effector T cells was reported to result in tumor cell killing, and that this activity was dependent on the Fas/FasL receptor system [43]. This intriguing possibility suggests an additional mechanism of antitumor activity based on the recruitment of any activated T cell expressing IL-2R and FasL and in a non-MHC-restricted or antigen-specific way – much like what has been reported for antitumor/anti-CD3 bi-specific molecules [44]. In these studies, the authors used a mono-specific antibody-IL2 fusion targeting Her2neu and showed enhancement of antitumor activity in vivo when combined with adoptively transferred, nonspecific T cells preactivated through the T cell receptor with anti-CD3 antibody. Based on these data, one could speculate that additional immune cells, capable of expressing IL-2R and FasL could mediate this same activity, e.g., NK cells and monocytes, and perhaps explain the unexpectedly high activity of de-glycosylated DI-Leu16-IL2 in SCID mice. In this case, target cell bridging would be mediated through binding of IL-2 to the IL-2R, rather than the antibody and the FcR. Furthermore, the bivalent nature of DI-Leu16-IL2 could enhance this potential bridging activity beyond what has already been described for the monovalent molecule.

The role of effector functions for immunocytokines containing cytokines other than IL-2 is less well studied. One exception is GM-CSF-based immunocytokines reported by several groups [45–47]. GM-CSF has been reported to increase ADCC mediated by neutrophils and monocytes [38] and therefore would be expected to increase the contribution of this function to overall antitumor activity. Additional immunocytokines have been described containing TNFα and TNFβ (originally called lymphotoxin), as well as IL-12 [48–50], but little has been done to assess the contribution of antibody effector activity in vivo. One reason is due to the complexity and large size of the active forms of these molecules. For example, the TNF family of cytokines naturally form trimers and bind to their cognate receptors in this configuration [51]. This has led most groups to construct TNF immunocytokines fused to scFv antibody domains lacking the Fc portion of the antibody so that trimerization would be facilitated [52, 53]. Nonetheless, the first TNF immunocytokines reported were constructed as whole antibody fusions and could be purified with full TNF bioactivity if special care was taken to avoid exposure to low pH [48]. Later studies of this immunocytokine have focused on its ability to activate a T cell response in syngeneic tumor models, and the observation that local targeting to the tumor was associated with the induction of peritumoral tertiary lymphoid tissue [54].

In summary, effector activities provided by immunocytokines are a composite of all of the biological properties contained in the fusion protein. In most cases, this is likely to be dominated by the activity of the cytokine rather than the antibody but the information obtained from often unpredictable mouse tumor models should not deter us from using all potential immunological weapons available. Therefore, one should consider leaving the antibody effector functions intact unless there is a potential safety issue of normal tissue targeting, or if inclusion of these functions has a negative impact on other important parameters such a clearance in vivo. There is precedence for this last possibility in which case FcR binding was shown to increase the clearance of an IL-2 immunocytokine [55]. Fortunately, additional changes in the molecule made it possible overcome this issue and allow the immunocytokine to retain its ADCC function [56].

Evidence for Antitumor Activity in Mouse Tumor Models

Numerous mouse tumor efficacy studies of immunocytokines have been reported by several laboratories utilizing either human tumor targets in immune compromised, SCID, mice or mouse tumor targets in syngeneic immune competent models. The details of many of these early studies can be found in several review articles [4–13]. In summary, the necessity of specific tumor targeting of these molecules is essential for antitumor activity and the immunoctyokine is generally far more effective than treatment with the antibody and cytokine components alone or in combination. In immune competent mice, cytotoxic CD8 T cells are the most important effector cells whereas in SCID mouse models, NK cells tend to mediate the cellular effector activity. An exception to this rule was reported in which the same syngeneic tumor expressing either high or low levels of class I MHC antigens was effectively treated with an IL-2 immunocytokine through two distinct mechanism. When class I molecules were expressed at normal levels, CD8 cells predominated the antitumor response, but when their expression was low, NK cells were predominant [57].

Another key result, at least with IL-2-based immunocytokines, is that an effective therapy in a syngeneic tumor model leads to immune memory and the ability of the treated animal to reject a challenge with the original tumor – even when the antibody target antigen is not expressed on the tumor cell [58, 59]. This is an important aspect of the entire therapeutic approach in which an antibody target antigen (e.g. GD2 or EpCAM) serves as a mailing address for binding the immunocytokine to at least some of the tumor cells in the host. Once the immune system is activated by the cytokine that is delivered to the tumor microenvironment, the antigens to which the cellular immune response is generated against are not necessarily derived from the targeting antigen. In fact, it is most likely that this would not be the case, since target antigens are often self molecules to which the T cell immune response is either tolerant or ignorant [60]. Instead, mutated self antigens are less likely to be tolerized and therefore capable of inducing a cellular immune response [61]. The role of the immunocytokine, in effect, is to overcome tumor-induced immune suppression that likely masks responses to these "private" antigens. Furthermore, immune escape by antigen loss or mutation is less likely to occur if immunity is directed against altered self-proteins involved in the malignant transformation process.

Early Clinical Studies of Immunocytokines

The use of mouse efficacy data for helping to guide dosing strategies in the clinic is not straightforward for immunocytokines due, in part, to limitations in mouse studies caused by the inherent immunogenicity of the specific molecules generated for human use. Not only are human immunoglobulin sequences highly immunogenic in mice, but also the fusion of a cytokine such as IL-2 or GM-CSF serves as a potent adjuvant for the generation of an anti-IC antibody response. In fact, this limited dosing regimens in immune competent mouse tumor models to the period of time prior to the generation of a high antibody titer and prevents repeat dosing cycles. Fortunately, nonhuman primates do not exhibit this same degree of immunogenicity to human immunocytokines and are very useful for predicting safe dosing regimens, including those with repeat cycles. This has provided appropriate safety information for the initiation of several phase I clinical trials.

The first trials of whole antibody immunocytokines (Table 1) were conducted with humanized molecules, hu14.18-IL2 and huKS-IL2 [62–64]. Both were administered by a 4-h infusion for 3 consecutive days followed by a second cycle of administration 4 weeks after the first dose. This regimen was chosen based on studies in nonhuman primates indicating that daily administration led to lymphopenia, but that this was followed by lymphocytosis beginning on day 4, even with continued dosing. Since emerging immune cells were expected to express increased levels of IL-2R, it seemed that additional immunocytokine given on day 4 would be consumed by this cell population and not effectively target tumor cells. The dosing interval of 4 weeks was chosen based on the time it took immune cells in nonhuman primates to return to baseline after a 3-day dosing cycle, although some later immunocytokine studies have shortened this interval to 3 weeks to be more aligned with chemotherapeutic dosing schedules.

The anti-GD2 ganglioside IC, hu14.18-IL2, was tested in both adult melanoma patients as well as in pediatric neuroblastoma patients [62, 63]. Doses were escalated after an initial starting dose of 0.5 mg/m^2 (equivalent to 1.5×10^6 units of IL-2) until

Table 1 Immunocytokines in clinical development*

Immunocytokine	Antibody target	Clinical trial	Reference
Hu14.18-IL2	GD2	Phase I melanoma	62
Hu14.18-IL2	GD2	Phase I neuroblastoma	63
Hu14.18-IL2	GD2	Phase II neuroblastoma	66
HuKS-IL2	EpCAM	Phase I hormone-refractory prostate CA	64
HuKS-IL2	EpCAM	Phase I in combination with low-dose cytoxan	Unpublished (clinicaltrials.gov)
HuKS-IL2	EpCAM	Phase II small-cell lung cancer with low-dose cytoxan	Unpublished (merckserono.com)
DI-Leu16-IL2	CD20	Phase I IST in non-Hodgkin's lymphoma	Unpublished (clinicaltrials.gov)
L19-IL2	Oncofetal fibronectin	Phase I solid tumors	67
L19-TNF	Oncofetal fibronectin	Phase I sarcoma with melphalan using isolated limb perfusion	69
BC1-IL12	Oncofetal fibronectin	Phase I in renal carcinoma and melanoma	Unpublished (antisoma.com)

*Data was obtained from publications, company websites and through public information but cannot be guaranteed to be accurate or up to date.

a maximum tolerated dose (MTD) was reached. MTDs of 7.5 and 14 mg/m^2 were reported for adult melanoma and pediatric neuroblastoma patients, respectively. This discrepancy was considered to be age-related rather than disease-related since children generally tolerate high levels of drugs than adults. Dose-limiting toxicities consisted of adverse events typically seen with IL-2. However, some patients also exhibited peripheral nerve pain (treatable with narcotics) typically observed with the naked ch14.18 antibody [65], albeit at far less intensity than seen with the antibody. This reduced intensity may be related to the shorter circulating half-life of the immunocytokine compared with the antibody [62], as well as lower CDC activity of the immunocytokine, compared with the hu14.18 antibody.

Phase I clinical testing of the anti-EpCAM immunocytokine, huKS-IL2, began with hormone-refractory prostate cancer patients and the same dosing schedule of 3 consecutive daily 4-h infusions, every 4 weeks [64]. In this case, the MTD was established as 6.4 mg/m^2. In all cases, the dose-limiting toxicities were the same as IL-2 with no additional toxicities based on targeting EpCAM. Interestingly, there were some patients in this study who had reductions in PSA or who showed periods of disease stabilization, but there did not appear to be a correlation between possible benefit and increased dose. This suggests that immunocytokines, as agonists, likely have a bell-shaped response curve (or optimal biological dose – OBD), and should not necessarily be dosed at MTD in the same manner as antagonist drugs. Determining what the OBD is for each immunocytokine presents a challenge that likely will require translational research studies for the development of appropriate immune biomarkers associated with positive clinical outcome. Such studies need to be conducted in clinical setting designed to measure efficacy rather than in settings of progressive disease that are unlikely to respond to immunological intervention.

Further testing of hu14.18-IL2 and huKS-IL2 is underway (Table 1). Most notably, hu14.18-IL2 was tested in a phase II efficacy study designed to test the relationship between tumor burden and potential response. Patients were stratified as having (1) measurable tumor burden; (2) tumor detected by sensitive radiologic (MIBG) imaging and/or microscopic detection in bone marrow; or (3) true minimal residual disease detected using specialized detection methods in bone marrow. The results, reported by the Children's Oncology Group (COG), clearly showed that patients in the intermediate tumor burden group, but not the high tumor burden group, responded to monotherapy with hu14.18-IL2, with several CRs and near CRs being reported [66]. This is not the only sign of clinical efficacy for this molecule. In the phase I adult melanoma study, several patients with no evidence of disease after surgical resection of metastatic disease were included in the dose-escalation study. Because their disease could not be assessed after treatment, this group was limited by the protocol to only two cycles of three doses, and this varied from a very low to close of 0.5 mg/m^2 to the MTD. Nonetheless, three out of five such patients receiving only this limited amount of dosing have remained disease-free for 8 to 10 years with no additional therapy. While anecdotal, this data, combined with the evidence of direct antitumor activity in the phase II neuroblastoma study clearly suggests meaningful clinical activity.

Again, the setting of reduced or minimal disease burden seems to be a factor for the success of monotherapy. Like almost all successful cancer drugs, combination therapy is needed for clinical success in patients with high tumor burden. In this regard, it should be mentioned that a refractory neuroblastoma patient with measurable disease burden, and treated in the phase I study of hu14.18-IL2, received sequential treatment with Fenretinide (a cytotoxic derivative of retinoic acid also being tested in neuroblastoma) and the immunocytokine. After two sequential cycles, a complete response was reached and has been maintained for more than 5 years. Clearly, such a result warrants further exploration in the disease setting of high unmet medical need, as well as for the general use of this combination with other IL-2-based immunocytokines. Study of the immune parameters associated with this combination therapy approach may also be generally useful for determining OBD, especially since this patient was part of a cohort receiving only a low dose of 2 mg/m^2, rather than the MTD dose used in the phase II COG study (12 mg/m^2). Future therapy of pediatric patients would be well served by protocols using rational combinations of drugs given at effective but well tolerated doses.

Less information is available with respect to the phase II study of huKS-IL2 that is currently being studied for the treatment of small cell lung cancer, a very rapidly progressing cancer that has not seen much success in past immune therapy clinical trials. This study follows a second phase I safety study in epithelial cancer patients in which 3 days of dosing was preceded by a first low dose of cyclophosphamide. Based on the results with the neuroblastoma study, just described, it seems that most patients entering such a trial would be unlikely to respond to what is essentially monotherapy, primarily due to relatively high tumor burden and a tendency for rapid progression of disease in this setting.

The anti-CD20 immunocytokine, DI-Leu16-IL2 (described earlier), has also entered phase I clinical testing in an investigator-sponsored trial. In this case, non-Hodgkin's lymphoma patients first receive the anti-CD20 antibody Rituxan to deplete peripheral B cells that could serve as a decoy for efficient tumor targeting. In addition to standard safety and pharmacokinetic analyses, this study also measures several immune parameters with the intent of establishing the OBD for use in subsequent efficacy studies.

Another group of investigators is developing a set of immunocytokines in the clinic based on targeting of the tumor vasculature using the L19 antioncofetal fibronectin protein. The first of these proteins to reach the clinic is the IL-2-based protein, L19-IL2 [67]. In this case, the immunocytokine is monomeric, in contrast to the two whole antibody immunocytokine, discussed above. With respect to antigen binding activity, this is not likely to be an issue, since the original antibody and its scFv derivative are of high affinity in this monomeric form, and apparently sufficient for tumor targeting as demonstrated in animal tumor models [68]. The smaller overall size of this construct would predict a more rapid clearance from the circulation than for the whole antibody immunocytokines. These investigators reported an MTD of 22.5 million IU of IL-2 for this phase I study. This is a bit lower than the dose of 6.4 mg/m^2 MTD reported for huKS-IL2, based on IL-2 activity units, and adjusted for body surface (roughly 30 million IU assuming an adult body surface of 1.6 m^2). Additional phase II studies are currently underway with L19-IL2 in combination with Gemcitabine in pancreatic carcinoma patients, with DTIC in melanoma patients, and as monotherapy for renal carcinoma. This group is also studying a TNF-based immunocytokine, L10-TNF, in combination with melphalan in patients with sarcoma, but administering the drug by isolated limb perfusion [69].

An IL-12-based immunocytokine has also reached phase I clinical testing. This molecule, BC1-IL12, also targets oncofetal fibronectin, but unlike L19-based immunocytokines it is constructed as a whole antibody fusion protein [70]. As such, it is expected to have a much longer circulating half-life in patients than the monomeric molecules constructed with scFvs. Preclinical testing in mouse tumor models reported potent antitumor activity against human tumors growing in immune deficient SCID mice, as well as enhanced binding to the target antigen of the immunocytokine, relative to the naked antibody.

Future Directions

The slow success of immune therapy of cancer may be due in part to the standard approach of conducting early safety studies in late-stage patients that have few other treatment options. The failure in such trials to see the standard signs of antitumor activity, typical of chemotherapeutic approaches, often reduces the interest in pursuing later stage clinical testing in appropriate patient populations. Nonetheless, there appears to be a paradigm shift based on recent findings that standard evaluation tools for measuring response to therapy (so called RECIST criteria) do not always predict overall patient benefit for immune therapies [71]. Furthermore, there is now evidence that patients that have received but have not responded well to certain immune therapies (by normal criteria), often respond surprisingly well to subsequent chemotherapy [72, 73]. While these results were obtained following cancer vaccine trials, the same might be expected following immunocytokine therapy, which at least in syngeneic mouse tumor models induces long-term memory T cell responses [74]. In fact, the nature of the immune response induced by immunocytokines may have a certain benefit over that induced by a vaccine antigen, in that the local stimulation in the tumor microenvironment activates subsets of high-avidity T cells already responding to tumor antigens but suppressed by factors secreted from the tumor. Standard vaccine antigens are by their design, shared among the general population and therefore likely to be either tolerized or capable of generating only low avidity T cells. In contrast, higher avidity T cells responding to mutated self antigens have been reported to result from the process of antigen spreading in both mouse tumor models [75] and in clinical trials [76, 77].

With these factors in mind, a future strategy for clinical development of immunocytokines should consider the clinical situation and the potential of the tumor burden in a given patient to resist or limit the effectiveness of therapy. For example, treatment of patients with minimum residual disease following standard therapies is certainly an opportunity for monotherapy, as evidenced by the recent success in neuroblastoma with hu14.18-IL2, described above. As the tumor burden increases, one needs to consider therapeutic combination partners that not only reduce that burden, but do so in a manner consistent with immune stimulatory approaches. There are several standard therapies that may on the surface appear to be immune suppressive in nature but, in fact, stimulate the innate or adaptive immune system. These include localized radiotherapy [78], several chemotherapies such as those with taxanes [79], doxorubicin [80], Gemcitabine [81], and anti-inflammatory drugs such as COX-2 inhibitors [82]. This concept has been taken even further, with studies showing that high-dose immune-ablative regimens can be used to condition patients for immune therapy [83]. In this case, an environment is created where immunotherapy is given as the immune system is reconstituting: a situation of strong lymphocyte expansion through stimulation with endogenous IL-7 and IL-15. Immune suppressive cells would also be greatly reduced in such a setting, thus providing a more favorable clinical setting of reduced tumor burden and proimmune functions such as those provided by immunocytokines.

Some experimental data combining immunocytokines with standard cancer therapies have already been reported. For example, pretreatment of tumor-bearing mice with cyclophosphamide or taxol prior to treatment with huKS-IL2 was shown to increase uptake of the immunocytokine into the tumor, and to significantly improve antitumor responses [84]. Studies with an IL-12-based immunocytokines in tumor-bearing dogs suggest that treatment prior to local radiation greatly improved antitumor responses and even long-term survival (unpublished). This does not appear to be a property unique to IL-12 immunocytokines. Recent studies with radiofrequency ablation have shown a strong combination effect with huKS-IL2 in mouse tumor models that leads to a greater number or tumor regressions and more potent long-term immune responses than either treatment alone (Johnson et al., in press). It will also be interesting to see the results of the current clinical trials with L19-IL2 that is being used in combination with Gemcitabine in pancreatic carcinoma patients.

While the approach with L19-IL2 may have been based on combining this immunocytokine with standard therapy for this indication, Gemcitabine might be an especially good drug in general to combine with IL-2-based immunocytokines. This is due to its ability to reduce the number and function of myeloid-derived suppressor cells (MDSCs), a population of immature cells capable of inhibiting antitumor T cell immune responses [81]. Therefore, combinations with Gemcitabine (perhaps at lower doses than used for cytotoxic therapy) and IL-2-based immunocytokines might be an approach for treatment of other types of cancer. This should be studied first in indications for which Gemcitabine is approved (e.g., nonsmall cell lung cancer, ovarian cancer) and if successful, expanded to additional settings. Other drugs that affect the MDSC population in a manner that could promote antitumor immunity include retinoic acids, e.g., all-trans retinoic acid (ATRA), and their derivatives [85]. It is tempting to speculate that the patient treated with alternating courses of Fenretinide and hu14.18-IL2 (see above), benefited through the combined actions of immune stimulation and MDCS suppression to mount a more effective and long-lasting immune response to their neuroblastoma.

The situation for immunocytokine therapy is not unlike that of the new targeted therapies based on selective inhibition of distinct growth and survival signaling pathways [86]. Nearly all of the successful examples of this approach require combination with chemotherapy or radiation for sufficient clinical activity for licensure. These agents include both antagonist antibodies (e.g., Herceptin, Rituxan, Erbitux, and Avastin) and small molecule kinase inhibitors (Sorafinib, Sutent, and Erlotinib). It is becoming clear that the same may be true for immune therapy, at least in patients with significant tumor burden. Not only combinations with traditional cytotoxic approaches, but also the combination of certain targeted therapies and immune therapy can be envisioned in which the targeted therapies reduce disease progression and its associated immune suppression to the extent that they can create an effective immune response. For example, many of the targeted therapies affect not only tumor growth and survival, but also tumor angiogenesis. The combination of immunocytokine treatment, and reducing angiogenesis with an αv integrin inhibitor, has been shown to have synergistic antitumor activity and to dramatically increase immune cell infiltration into tumors in multiple mouse models [87]. These results suggest that other antiangiogenic agents such as Avastin could provide similar benefits to immunocytokine therapies. Hopefully, further clinical development of immunocytokines will move in the direction of intelligent combination therapy with both standard cytotoxics as well as new targeted therapies against both tumor and supportive cell targets.

References

1. Silverstein, A. M. (1988) A History of Immunology, Jovanovich, H. B. (Ed.). Academic Press Inc., San Diego
2. Kohler, G., and Milstein, C. (1975) Nature 256, 495
3. Morrison, S. L. (1988) Science 229, 1202
4. Davis, C. B., and Gillies, S. D. (2003) Cancer Immunol Immunother 52, 297
5. Reisfeld, R. A., and Gillies, S. D. (1996) J Clin Lab Anal 10, 160
6. Reisfeld, R. A., and Gillies, S. D. (1996) Curr Top Microbiol Immunol 213, 27
7. Reisfeld, R. A., Becker, J. C., and Gillies, S. D. (1997) Melanoma Res (Suppl 2), S99
8. Penichet, M. L., Harvill, E. T., and Morrison, S. L. (1997) Hum Antibodies 8, 106
9. Lode, H. N., Xiang, R., Becker, J. C., Gillies, S. D., and Reisfeld, R. A. (1998) Pharmacol Ther 80, 277
10. Penichet, M. L., and Morrison, S. L. (2001) J Immunol Methods 248, 91
11. Helguera, G., Morrison, S. L., and Penichet, M. L. (2002) Clin Immunol 105, 233
12. Dela Cruz, J. S., Huang, T. H., Penichet, M. L., and Morrison, S. L. (2004) Clin Exp Med 4, 57
13. Schrama, D., Reisfeld, R. A., and Becker, J. C. (2006) Nat Rev Drug Discov 5, 147
14. Fell, H. P., Gayle, M. A., Grosmaire, L., and Ledbetter, J. A. (1991) J Immunol 146, 2446
15. Gillies, S. D., Reilly, E. B., Lo, K. M., and Reisfeld, R. A. (1992) Proc Natl Acad Sci USA 89, 1428
16. Colcher, D., Pavlinkova, G., Beresford, G., Booth, B. J., Choudhury, A., and Batra, S. K. (1998) Q J Nucl Med 42, 225
17. Liu, S. J., Sher, Y. P., Ting, C. C., Liao, K. W., Yu, C. P., and Tao, M. H. (1998) Blood 92, 2103
18. Mujoo, K., Cheresh, D. A., Yang, H. M., and Reisfeld, R. A. (1987) Cancer Res 47, 1098
19. Hellstrom, I. Garrigues, H. J., Garrigues, U., and Hellstrom, K. E. (1990) Cancer Res 50, 2183
20. Varki, N. M., Reisfeld, R. A., and Walker, L. E. (1984) Cancer Res 44, 681
21. Epstein, A. L., Marder, R. J., Winter, J. N., Stathopoulos, E., Chen, F. M., Parker, J. W., and Taylor, C. R. (1987) Cancer Res 47, 830
22. Challita-Eid, P. M., Penichet, M. L., Shin, S. U., Poles, T., Mosammaparast, N., Mahmood, K., Slamon, D. J., Morrison, S. L., and Rosenblatt, J. D. (1998) J Immunol 160, 3419
23. Epstein, A. L., Chen, F. M., and Taylor, C. R. (1988) Cancer Res 48, 5842
24. Neri, D., Carnemolla, B., Nissim, A., Leprini, A., Querzè, G., Balza, E., Pini, A., Tarli, L., Halin, C., Neri, P., Zardi, L., and Winter, G. (1997) Nat Biotechnol 15, 1271
25. Mariani, G., Lasku, A., Balza, E., Gaggero, B., Motta, C., Di Luca, L., Dorcaratto, A., Viale, G. A., Neri, D., and Zardi, L. (1997) Cancer 80, 2378
26. Ju, G., Collins, L., Kaffka, K. L., Tsien, W. H., Chizzonite, R., Crowl, R., Bhatt, and Kilian, P. L. (1987) J Biol Chem 262, 5723
27. Shanafelt, A. B., Lin, Y., Shanafelt, M. C., Forte, C. P., Dubois-Stringfellow, N., Carter, C., Gibbons, J. A., Cheng, S. L., Delaria, K. A., Fleischer, R., Greve, J. M., Gundel, R., Harris, K., Kelly, R., Koh, B., Li, Y., Lantz, L., Mak, P., Neyer, L., Plym, M. J., Roczniak, S., Serban, D., Thrift, J., Tsuchiyama, L., Wetzel, M., Wong, M., and Zolotorev, A. (2000) Nat Biotechnol 18, 1197
28. Assier, E., Jullien, V., Lefort, J., Moreau, J. L., Di Santo, J. P., Vargaftig, B. B., Lapa e Silva, J. R., and Theze, J. (2004) J Immunol 172, 7661
29. Margolin, K., Atkins, M. B., Dutcher, J. P., Ernstoff, M. S., Smith, J. W. 2nd, Clark, J. I., Baar, J., Sosman, J., Weber, J., Lathia, C., Brunetti, J., Cihon, F., and Schwartz, B. (2007) Clin Cancer Res 13, 3312
30. Gillies, S. D., Lan, Y., Lauder, S., Brunkhorst, B., Sun, Y., and Lo, K. M. (2004) Proc Amer Assoc Cancer Res 45, 654
31. Casciola-Rosen, L. A., Anhalt, G., and Rosen, A. (1994) J Exp Med 179, 1317
32. Gorgani, N. N., Smith, B. A., Kono, D. H., and Theofilopoulos, A. N. (2002) J Immunol 169, 4745
33. Sgadari, C., Angiolillo, A. L., and Tosato, G. (1996) Blood 87, 3877

34. Wagner, C., Iking-Konert, C., Denefleh, B., Stegmaier, S., Hug, F., and Hänsch, G. M. (2004) Blood 103, 1099
35. Goldman, A. S., and Prabhakar, B. S. (1996) Baron's Medical Microbiology, 4th ed. University of Texas Medical Branch, Texas
36. Herlyn, D., Herlyn, M., Steplewski, Z., and Koprowski, H. (1985) Cell Immunol 92, 105
37. Clynes, R. A., Towers, T. L., Presta, L. G., and Ravetch, J. V. (2000) Nat Med 6, 443
38. Metelitsa, L. S., Gillies, S. D., Super, M., Shimada, H., Reynolds, C. P., and Seeger, R. C. (2002) Blood 99, 4166
39. Cartron, G., Dacheux, L., Salles, G., Solal-Celigny, P., Bardos, P., Colombat, P., and Watier, H. (2002) Blood 99, 754
40. Taylor, R. P., and Lindorfer, M. A. (2008) Curr Opin Immunol 20, 444
41. Gillies, S. D., Lan, Y., Williams, S., Carr, F., Forman, S., Raubitschek, A., and Lo, K. M. (2005) Blood 105, 3972
42. Dorai, H., Mueller, B. M., Reisfeld, R. A., and Gillies, S. D. (1991) Hybridoma 10, 211
43. Lustgarten, J., Marks, J., and Sherman, L. A. (1999) J Immunol 162, 359
44. Fanger, M. W., Morganelli, P. M., and Guyre, P. M. (1992) Crit Rev Immunol 12, 101
45. Batova, A., Kamps, A., Gillies, S. D., Reisfeld, R. A., and Yu, A. L. (1999) Clin Cancer Res 5, 4259
46. Hornick, J. L., Khawli, L. A., Hu, P., Lynch, M., Anderson, P. M., and Epstein, A. L. (1997) Blood 89, 4437
47. Dela Cruz, J. S., Trinh, K. R., Morrison, S. L., and Penichet, M. L. (2000) J Immunol 165, 5112
48. Gillies, S. D., Young, D., Lo, K. M., Foley, S. F., and Reisfeld, R. A. (1991) Hybridoma 10, 347
49. Gillies, S. D., Young, D., Lo, K. M., and Roberts, S. (1993) Bioconjug Chem 4, 230
50. Gillies, S. D., Lan, Y., Wesolowski, J. S., Qian, X., Reisfeld, R. A., Holden, S., Super, M., and Lo, K. M. (1998) J Immunol 160, 6195
51. Smith, R. A., and Baglioni, C. (1987) J Biol Chem 262, 6951
52. Yang, J., Moyana, T., and Xiang, J. (1995) Mol Immunol 32, 873
53. Bauer, S., Adrian, N., Fischer, E., Kleber, S., Stenner, F., Wadle, A., Fadle, N., Zoellner, A., Bernhardt, R., Knuth, A., Old, L. J., and Renner, C. (2006) J Immunol 177, 2423
54. Schrama, D., thor Straten, P., Fischer, W. H., McLellan, A. D., Bröcker, E. B., Reisfeld, R. A., and Becker J. C. (2001) Immunity 14, 111
55. Gillies, S. D., Lan, Y., Lo, K. M., Super, M., and Wesolowski, J. (1999) Cancer Res 59, 2159
56. Gillies, S. D., Lo, K. M., Burger, C., Lan, Y., Dahl, T., and Wong, W. K. (2002) Clin Cancer Res 8, 210
57. Imboden, M., Murphy, K. R., Rakhmilevich, A. L., Neal, Z. C., Xiang, R., Reisfeld, R. A., Gillies, S. D., and Sondel, P. M. (2001) Cancer Res 61, 1500
58. Becker, J. C., Varki, N., Gillies, S. D., Furukawa, K., and Reisfeld, R. A. (1996) Proc Natl Acad Sci USA 93, 7826
59. thor Straten, P., Guldberg, P., Schrama, D., Andersen, M. H., Moerch, U., Seremet, T., Siedel, C., Reisfeld, R. A., and Becker, J. C. (2001) Eur J Immunol 31, 250
60. Gajewski, T. F., Meng, Y., Blank, C., Brown, I., Kacha, A., Kline, J., and Harlin, H. (2006) Immunol Rev 213, 131
61. Kmieciak, M., Morales, J. K., Morales, J., Bolesta, E., Grimes, M., and Manjili, M. H. (2008) Cancer Immunol Immunother 57, 1391
62. King, D. M., Albertini, M. R., Schalch, H., Hank, J. A., Gan, J., Surfus, J., Mahvi, D., Schiller, J. H., Warner, T., Kim, K., Eickhoff, J., Kendra, K., Reisfeld, R., Gillies, S. D., and Sondel, P. (2004) J Clin Oncol 22, 4463
63. Osenga, K. L., Hank, J. A., Albertini, M. R., Gan, J., Sternberg, A. G., Eickhoff, J., Seeger, R. C., Matthay, K. K., Reynolds, C. P., Twist, C., Krailo, M., Adamson, P. C., Reisfeld, R. A., Gillies, S. D., and Sondel, P. M. (2006) Clin Cancer Res 12, 1750
64. Ko, Y. J., Bubley, G. J., Weber, R., Redfern, C., Gold, D. P., Finke, L., Kovar, A., Dahl, T., and Gillies, S. D. (2004) J Immunother 27, 232
65. Saleh, M. N., Khazaeli, M. B., Wheeler, R. H., Allen, L., Tilden, A. B., Grizzle, W., Reisfeld, R. A., Yu, A. L., Gillies, S. D., and LoBuglio, A. F. (1992) Hum Antibodies Hybridomas 3, 19

66. Shusterman, S., London, W. B., Gillies, S. D., Hank, J. A.,Voss, S., Seeger, R., Hecht, T., Reisfeld, R. A., Maris, J. M., and Sondel, P. M. (2008) J Clin Oncol 26, abstract 3002
67. Curigliano, G., Spitaleri, G., De Pas, T., Noberasco, C., Giovannoni, L., Menssen, H., Zardi, L., Milani, A., Neri, D., and de Braud, F. (2007) J Clin Oncol 25, 3057
68. Wagner, K., Schulz, P., Scholz, A., Wiedenmann, B., and Menrad, A. (2008) Clin Cancer Res 14, 4951
69. Philogen, S. P. A. http://www.philogen.com/philogen/pipeline.html
70. Lo, K. M., Lan, Y., Lauder, S., Zhang, J., Brunkhorst, B., Qin, G., Verma, R., Courtenay-Luck, N., and Gillies, S. D. (2006) Cancer Immunol Immunother 56, 447
71. Schlom, J., Arlen, P. M., and Gulley, J. L. (2007) Clin Cancer Res 13, 3776
72. Gribben, J. G., Ryan, D. P., Boyajian, R., Urban, R. G., Hedley, M. L., Beach, K., Nealon, P., Matulonis, U., Campos, S., Gilligan, T. D., Richardson, P. G., Marshall, B., Neuberg, D., and Nadler, L. M. (2005) Clin Cancer Res 11, 4430
73. Antonia, S. J., Mirza, N., Fricke, I., Chiappori, A., Thompson, P., Williams, N., Bepler, G., Simon, G., Janssen, W., Lee, J. H., Menander, K., Chada, S., and Gabrilovich, D. I. (2006) Clin Cancer Res 12, 878
74. Becker, J. C., Varki, N., Gillies, S. D., Furukawa, K., and Reisfeld, R. A. (1996) J Clin Invest 98, 2801
75. Chakraborty, M., Abrams, S. I., Coleman, C. N., Camphausen, K., Schlom, J., and Hodge, J. W. (2004) Cancer Res 64, 4328
76. Cavacini, L. A., Duval, M., Eder, J. P., and Posner, M. R. (2002) Clin Cancer Res 8, 368
77. Butterfield, L. H., Ribas, A., Dissette, V. B. et al. (2003) Clin Cancer Res 9, 998
78. Roses, R. E., Xu, M., Koski, G. K., and Czerniecki, B. J. (2008) Oncogene 27, 200
79. Chan, O. T. M., and Yang, L.-X. (2000) Cancer Immunol Immunother 49, 181
80. Mitchell, M. S. (1992) Semin Oncol 19, 51
81. Suzuki, E., Kapoor, V., Jassar, A. S., Kaiser, L. R., and Albelda, S. M. (2005) Clin Cancer Res 11, 6713
82. Zeytin, H. E., Patel, A. C., Rogers, C. J., Canter, D., Hursting, S. D., Schlom, J., and Greiner, J. W. (2004) Cancer Res 64, 3668
83. Wrzesinski, C., and Restifo, N. P. (2005) Curr Opin Immunol 17, 195
84. Holden, S. A., Lan, Y., Pardo, A. M., Wesolowski, J. S., and Gillies, S. D. (2001) Clin Cancer Res 7, 2862
85. Mirza, N., Fishman, M., Fricke, I., Dunn, M., Neuger, A. M., Frost, T. J., Lush, R. M., Antonia, S., and Gabrilovich, D. I. (2006) Cancer Res 66, 9299
86. Bicknell, R. (2005) Br J Cancer 92, S2–S5
87. Lode, H. N., Moehler, T., Xiang, R., Jonczyk, A., Gillies, S. D., Cheresh, D. A., and Reisfeld, R. A. (1999) Proc Natl Acad Sci USA 96, 1591

Immune Escape: Role of Indoleamine 2,3-Dioxygenase in Tumor Tolerance

Jessica B. Katz, Alexander J. Muller, Richard Metz, and George C. Prendergast

Summary Indoleamine 2,3 dioxygenase (IDO) degrades the essential amino acid tryptophan in mammals, catalyzing the initial, rate-limiting step in de novo biosynthesis of the metabolic cofactor nicotinamide adenine dinucleotide (NAD). Broad evidence implicates IDO and the tryptophan catabolic pathway in the generation of immune tolerance to foreign antigens in tissue microenvironments. In particular, recent findings have established that IDO is overexpressed in both tumor cells and antigen-presenting cells in tumor-draining lymph nodes where it promotes the establishment of peripheral immune tolerance to tumor antigens. In the normal physiologic state, IDO is important in creating an environment that limits damage to tissues due to an overactive immune system. However, by fostering immune suppression, IDO can facilitate the survival and growth of tumor cells expressing unique antigens that would otherwise be recognized normally as foreign. In preclinical studies, small-molecule inhibitors of IDO can reverse this mechanism of immune suppression, strongly leveraging the efficacy of classical cancer chemotherapeutic agents to trigger regression of tumors that are otherwise largely resistant to treatment. These results have spurred clinical translation of IDO inhibitors, the first of which entered Phase I human trials in late 2007. In this chapter, we survey work defining IDO as an important mediator of peripheral tolerance, review evidence of IDO dysregulation in cancer cells, and provide an overview of the development of IDO inhibitors as a new immunoregulatory modality to enter clinical trials for cancer treatment.

Introduction to Cancer Immunoediting: Immune Surveillance, Equilibrium, and Escape

Tumor immunity is defined as the ability of the immune system to reject a tumor. However, this ability is a double-edged sword, because tumor immunity also exerts a selective pressure on the genetically plastic cells of the tumor, facilitating the

J.B. Katz, A.J. Muller, R. Metz, and G.C. Prendergast (✉)
Lankenau Institute for Medical Research, Department of Pathology, Anatomy and Cell Biology, Jefferson Medical School, Thomas Jefferson University, Philadelphia, PA, USA
e-mail: PrendergastG@mlhs.org

J. Lustgarten et al. (eds.), *Targeted Cancer Immune Therapy*,
DOI 10.1007/978-1-4419-0170-5_15, © Springer Science+Business Media, LLC 2009

evolution of immune resistant variants. This phenomenon is similar to the situation in which antibiotics select for bacterial resistance or chemotherapy selects for tumor resistance. The mechanisms of tumoral immune resistance can either be passive, such as loss of antigenicity, or active, such as establishment of tolerance. Ultimately, this selection process can lead to immune escape, which is vital for tumor outgrowth, invasion, and metastasis [1]. Active suppression of antitumor immune responses may be especially relevant to malignant disease and therapeutic failure. In recent years, many of the pathways and the cellular crosstalk involved in establishing immunoregulatory networks that favor the generation of immune tolerance and escape in the tumor microenvironment have become subjects of intense investigation.

In 1863, Rudolf Virchow, the father of cellular pathology, observed that leukocyte infiltration of tumors occurred quite commonly, leading him to suggest a functional relationship between inflammatory infiltrates and malignant growth. The potential of cancer immunotherapy was first documented by William Coley in 1890, when he realized that surgery had been much more effective in curing cancer before the use of antiseptics when infection was a normal side effect of surgery. On this basis, Coley hypothesized that infections helped patients to recover from their cancer because it stimulated the immune system. To test this, he treated patients by injecting various bacterial products (toxins) directly into patients with inoperable tumors. Despite reports of positive responses, some dramatic [2, 3], these observations were not widely developed and with the advent of radiation therapy Coley's toxins fell out of favor. Nevertheless, on this basis, a theory of cancer immune surveillance did emerge, whereby the immune system protects the host against tumor formation based on the detection of "foreign" tumor antigens, formed initially by Paul Ehrlich in the early twentieth century and enunciated again by Lewis Thomas and Macfarlane Burnet in the 1950s [1]. However, the general concept of cancer immunosurveillance was largely discredited among cancer researchers when studies carried out on partially immunodeficient "nude" mice in the 1960s and 1970s provided arguments against the theory. This remained the prevailing attitude until the late 1990s and early 2000s when carcinogenesis experiments revisiting this question were conducted in transgenic mice that had precisely-defined defects in innate and/or adaptive immunity. Indeed, these more rigorous studies strongly supported the idea that, in fact, immunodeficient mice are more prone to spontaneous and carcinogen-induced tumors than their immunocompetent counterparts [4]. Thus, cancer immunosuppression moved again into the limelight, this time as a component of Robert Schreiber's three-stage immunoediting model, where immunosurveillance that initially drives tumor cell elimination also imposes a selective pressure that can facilitate the evolution of equilibrium (dormancy) and perhaps ultimately immune escape of the tumor.

As elegantly described by Schreiber and Smyth and their colleagues [5, 6], immunoediting starts when precancerous lesions are detected as a result of genetic mutations that not only initiate cancer but also activate the immune system [7]. The first stage of immunoediting involves the response of the immune system against the nascent tumor (immune surveillance). At this stage there is no clinical evidence of disease, as a result of effective eradication of tumor cells by the immune system. However, as a result of the selective pressure applied by immunosurveillance, a second stage may begin in which a small number of tumor cells evolve the capability to gain some resistance to immune-mediating killing and/or colonize sites in a hospitable tissue microenvironment, which provides partial protection against the immune system. At this stage, tumor cells may continue to divide but the immune system would mainly continue to hold the tumor at bay (immune equilibrium). Key players in tilting the immune system from an antagonistic to supportive (suppressive) role in cancer are shown in Fig. 1.

At the stage of immune equilibrium, tumors may be dormant and occult, existing at a subclinical level where detection may be incidental. A recent study offers the

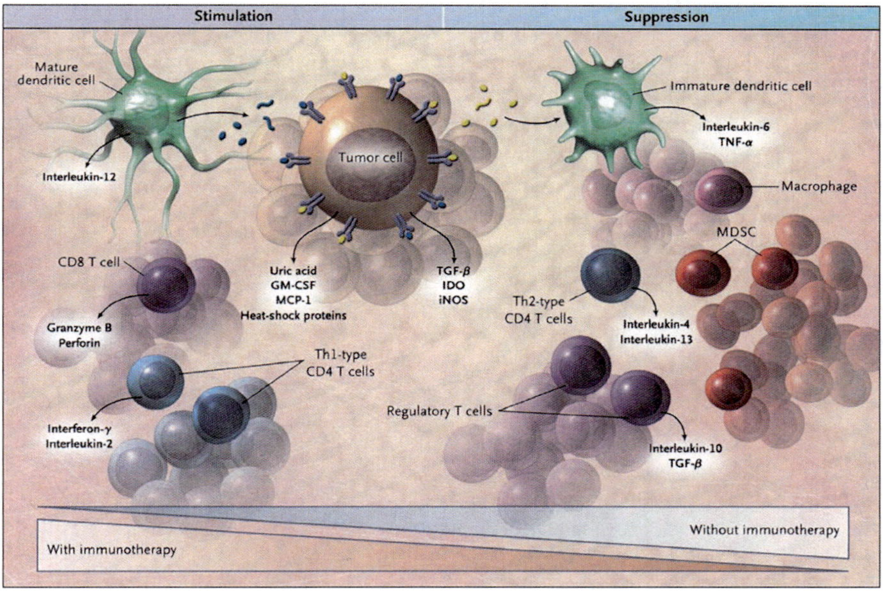

Fig. 1 Immune stimulation vs. immune suppression by the tumor. *Left side*, immune stimulation. Tumor antigens and other secreted proteins attract mature dendritic cells (DCs) that absorb the antigens and move to the tumor-draining lymph node. At that site, the DCs stimulate Th1-type helper T cells to produce interferon-γ (IFN-γ) and expand cytotoxic T cells that can destroy the tumor cells with granzyme B and perforin. *Right side*, immune suppression. Tumors can tip the balance toward immune suppression by expressing TGF-β, IDO, iNOS and other molecules that promote maturation of immature DCs that secrete IL-6 and TNF-α and stimulate Th2-type helper T cells that secrete IL-4 and IL-13, all of which help restrict anti-tumor immunity. Supportive cells recruited by these processes include macrophages, myeloid-derived suppressor cells (MDSC), and T regulatory cells. At diagnosis, immune suppression dominates. Thus, immunotherapies that restore immune balance are needed for effective antitumor strategies. GM-CSF, granulocyte-macrophage colony-stimulating factor; IDO, indolamine-2,3-dioxygenase; iNOS, inducible nitric oxide synthase; MCP-1, monocyte chemotactic protein 1; TGF-β transforming growth factor-β. Figure is copied with permission from Finn, O. J. (2008) N Engl J Med 358, 2404

first direct in vivo support for the existence of occult microtumors corresponding to the immune equilibrium stage, which never manifest as overt disease unless T cell immunity is compromised [8]. Clinical evidence from organ transplant patients also supports the idea that dormant lesions unlinked to viral or bacterial infections can exist in immune equilibrium for many years, only emerging as frank cancer under conditions of immune suppression in the organ recipient [9].

The third and final stage of immunoediting, termed immune escape, is reached when the tumor has evolved a state in which it can effectively evade, suppress, and overcome the immune system at multiple levels. At this point, the lesion progresses to become clinically apparent. Viewed from this perspective, gaining a greater understanding of how immune escape evolves is critical to understanding cancer pathophysiology at a clinical level, because immune escape mechanisms may distinguish preclinical dormant lesions from clinically relevant disease. As shown in Fig. 2, immune escape is a distinct hallmark of cancer, which along with other cell-intrinsic and cell-extrinsic traits is crucial for cancer development [10]. Developing effective methods to attack the underpining mechanisms of tumoral immune escape could offer the prospect of managing cancer like an infection, that is, either by eliminating it like an acute infection, or managing it like holding a chronic infection at bay, with the aim of prolonging overall progression-free survival.

The role of immune surveillance in controlling tumorigenicity has support in epidemiologic studies of immunosuppressed transplant patients. It is well established that immunosuppressed patients are at increased risk for virally-induced tumors based on early follow-up studies of immunosuppressed transplant recipients.

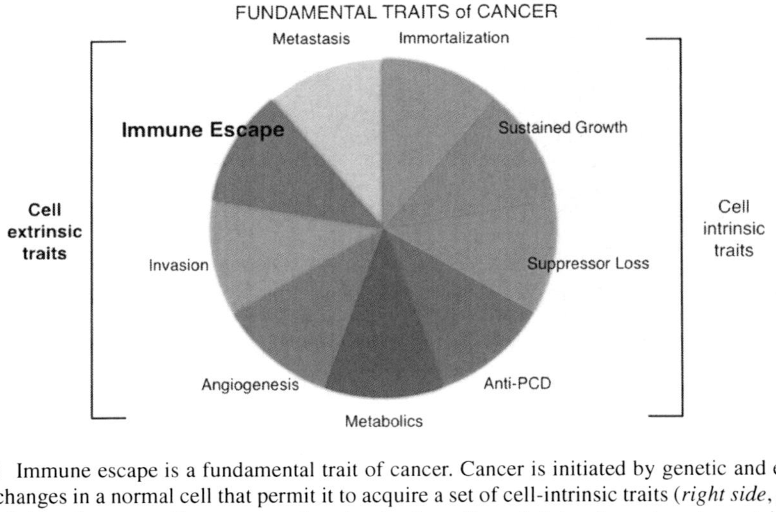

Fig. 2 Immune escape is a fundamental trait of cancer. Cancer is initiated by genetic and epigenetic changes in a normal cell that permit it to acquire a set of cell-intrinsic traits (*right side, grey*). For an initiated cancer cell to progress from benign to malignant status, it must master restrictions in its microenvironment. To do so it must acquire a set of cell-extrinsic traits that include immune escape (*left side, color*). Figure is copied with permission from Prendergast, G. C. (2008) Oncogene 27, 3889

Individuals with primary immunodeficiencies likewise have a significantly higher relative risk for developing cancer [11, 12]. On the basis of long-term studies, it appears that some of this higher risk was due to the development of tumors of viral origin. In transplant registries, there was a high incidence of non-Hodgkin's lymphoma, Kaposi's sarcoma, and carcinomas of the genitourinary and anogenital regions. Many of these malignancies are linked to viral infections (Epstein-Barr virus, human herpesvirus 8, and human papilloma virus), and they occur with increased frequency in acquired immuno deficiency syndrome patients. The increased incidence of virally induced tumors in immunocompromised patients represents one line of evidence for cancer immune surveillance [13–19].

There is accumulating evidence that the immune system can protect against the development of tumors of nonviral origin as well [3, 11]. Transgenic mouse models have offered particularly convincing evidence that immune escape is a crucial feature of tumorigenesis, for example, based on the increased incidence of solid tumors in knockout mice for the central immunoregulatory genes interferon-γ (IFN-γ), Stat1, and Rag2. Mouse studies reveal a dynamic interplay in the interaction of genetically plastic tumor cells with both the innate and adaptive immune systems. Early in tumor development, proinflammatory effects of immune cells may promote eradication, but by providing a selective pressure for the development of evasive tactics by early stage tumor cells, such as the aberrant cytokine production, immune cells may reinforce a supportive tumor microenvironment later in progression. Thus, inflammatory conditions in the tumor microenvironment may become altered such that the immune response to tumor antigens is ultimately subverted [20]. For example, Th1 polarization in the inflammatory response that promotes the development of cytotoxic T cells may be blunted in established neoplasia, while Th2 polarization associated with humoral immunity may be favored [21].

The dual nature of tumoral immune surveillance is apparent at the level of immune cytokines. Tumor necrosis factor (TNF) is important in natural killer cell and CD8 lymphocyte-mediated killing of tumor cells, but tumor-promoting effects of TNF are also well described [22]. This duality reflects the coevolution of "smouldering" inflammatory states with immune escape [23], and may explain recent clinical observations that might be considered mutually contradictory. A role for TNF in immune surveillance may explain recent clinical observations that might be considered mutually opposing. On the one hand, patients treated with anti-TNF monoclonal antibodies for various rheumatologic conditions are at increased risk for malignancy, especially lymphomas and lung cancer [24]. TNF overexpression has been reported in other human tumors where it portends a poorer prognosis [25, 26]. On the basis of such observations, anti-TNF monoclonal antibodies have entered phase II clinical trials for breast [27], ovarian [28], and renal cell carcinoma [29]. On the other hand, patients treated with anti-TNF monoclonal antibodies for various rheumatologic conditions are at increased risk for malignancy, especially lymphomas and lung cancer [24], and complete resolution of an advanced nonsmall cell lung cancer was observed in a patient with Crohn's disease after suspending therapy of the anti-TNF antibody adalimumab [30]. Studies in genetic knockout mice further illustrate the dual nature of TNF in cancer. When evaluated on a chemical carcinogenesis protocol, mice lacking TNF have an increased susceptibility to papilloma formation but a reduced susceptibility for progression of these benign lesions to frank carcinoma [31]. Thus, immune cytokines such as TNF are likely to have more than one role in immunoediting at different stages of disease. If so, contextually defined combinations of cytokines, played like notes on a musical instrument, will determine whether or not immune activation or immune escape occurs in the tumor microenvironment.

In the last decade, there have been significant advances in understanding how tumors evolve the capacity to escape the immune system [20, 32]. Although most immunotherapeutic strategies to date have focused on stimulating or supplementing immune effector cells, such approaches may be thwarted by dominant immune escape mechanisms involving active suppression networks fostered by the tumor or by stromal cells under the influence of the tumor. One implication of these advances is that disrupting these mechanisms of immune suppression may relieve suppression and permit the restoration of antitumor immunity. Enticingly, these immune suppressive networks offer new targets for therapeutic intervention with small molecular compounds instead of biological agents, which can be more expensive, more difficult to deliver, and may have decreasing efficacy over time [33]. In particular, small molecule inhibitors of indoleamine 2,3 dioxygenase (IDO), discussed in more detail below, offer one innovative and promising strategy for the therapeutic correction of immune escape.

Indoleamine 2,3-Dioxygenase

IDO is a tryptophan catabolizing enzyme (IDO; EC 1.13.11.42) encoded by the *INDO* gene at human chromosome 8p12. Tryptophan degradation by IDO is the initial step of the kynurenine pathway, the de novo biosynthetic route for nicotinamide adenine dinucleotide (NAD) [34–36]. In a seminal 1998 study, David Munn and Andrew Mellor and their colleagues at the Medical College of Georgia reported that IDO activity was crucial to prevent allogeneic fetal rejection due to maternal T cell immunity in mice [37]. Subsequent studies have much more broadly extended an immunosuppressive role for IDO [38], for example, in supporting a variety of chronic infections including viral, parasitic, and bacterial infections such as HIV, malaria, hepatitis C, *Toxoplasma gondii*, and chlamydia [39–42].

A relationship between cancer and elevated tryptophan catabolism was first recognized in the 1950s from analysis of the urine of bladder cancer patients [43]. Additional studies demonstrated similar findings of elevated urinary tryptophan metabolites in breast cancer, prostate cancer, Hodgkins lymphoma, and leukemia [44–47]. The determination that this relationship could not be attributed to the hepatic enzyme tryptophan dioxygenase (TDO2; EC 1.13.11.11) led, in part, to the isolation of the IDO enzyme from rabbit intestine [48].

The isolation of IDO, originally called D-tryptophan pyrrolase, was reported in 1963 [49, 50]. TDO2 is expressed in the liver, while IDO is expressed ubiquitously and at much higher levels in lung, gut, epididymis, and thymus. Likewise, these enzymes have different inducers. IDO is inducible by virus, lipopolysaccharide, and interferons, while TDO2 is inducible by tryptophan, tyrosine, histidine, glucocorticoids, and kynurenine [51]. TDO2 functions as a homotetramer of 320 kDa whereas IDO functions as a monomeric enzyme of 41 kDa. They are antigenically dissimilar and share little homology by amino acid sequence [52]. TDO2 has greater substrate stringency for tryptophan, while IDO can cleave other indole-containing compounds, including serotonin, tryptamine, and 5-hydroxytryptophan.

Crystallographic studies of human IDO reveal a two-domain structure of alpha-helical domains with a centrally located heme group [53]. IDO activity is dependent on the heme moiety and an electron donor. The heme moiety of IDO provides a superoxide anion to donate oxygen to tryptophan. To achieve full in vitro activity, flavin or tetrahydrobiopterin cofactors are required as reductants in the reaction, suggesting a related requirement in vivo. The cofactor binding site is separate from the substrate-binding site [54], implying the potential for allosteric regulation and possibly opportunities for developing noncompetitive as well as competitive enzyme inhibitors for IDO.

Studies of the human *INDO* gene have revealed genetic variability that may contribute to differences in IDO activity between individuals. *INDO* comprises 10 exons spanning ~15 kb at chromosome 8p12 that encodes a 403 amino acid polypeptide [55, 56]. To identify genetic variants, Arefayene and colleagues [57] sequenced 96 samples of DNA from the Coriell DNA repository, identifying 16 IDO variants including two nonsynonymous single nucleotide polymorphisms (SNPs) in coding exons 1 and 3. In evaluating the functional effects of each alteration, by expressing variant proteins in COS-7 and HEK293 cells, a complete loss of catalytic activity occurred in the exon 3 variant. This finding documented a naturally occurring polymorphism leading to a nonfunctional allele of the *INDO* gene in human populations.

IDO in Human Cancer and Immune Disorders

IDO activation represents one mechanism by which tumor cells can escape the immune system. The survival benefit of this mechanism to a tumor cell is balanced by the cost of depriving itself of an essential amino acid. Tryptophan catabolites are elevated in the urine of cancer patients, and this effect is reversed upon cytoreductive surgery [46]. IDO overexpression in human tumors explains this phenomenon [58].

Several studies have suggested that IDO overexpression is associated with poor prognosis. In a small study of serous ovarian cancers, overexpression of IDO mRNA in surgically resected tumor specimens from patients with stage IIIc disease was positively associated with paclitaxel resistance, a first line chemotherapeutic agent in ovarian cancer. Additionally, the pattern of IDO staining in tumor sections correlated inversely with patient survival with stage III and IV serous-type ovarian cancer [59]. For sporadic (n = 12), focal (n = 3), and diffusely (n = 2) staining tumors, the 50% survival of patients was 41, 17, and 11 months, respectively. Patients whose tumors did not stain for IDO exhibited 100% 5-year survival (n = 7), reportedly irrespective of the patients' stages at diagnosis [59]. In a study of colorectal cancer, IDO enzyme levels were examined by immunohistochemisty in 143 patients [60]. High IDO expression was documented in 39.2% (56/143) cases with the remaining 60.8% (87/143) cases exhibiting lower levels. High IDO expression was associated with a significant reduction of CD3+ infiltrating T cells when compared with tissue samples expressing low IDO. Furthermore, IDO-high immunoreactivity significantly correlated with the frequency of liver metastases. Seventy-one percent of patients with low IDO-expressing primary tumors were free of metastasis, while only 50% of patients with high-expressing primary tumors were free of metastasis. Kaplan-Meier survival analysis showed the crossing of survival curves at 45 months, and therefore they could not show any survival advantage. However, high IDO expression emerged as an independent prognostic variable. Interestingly, the same group had observed elevated IDO in inflammatory bowel disease, a condition that is associated with a significant increase in the risk of colon cancer [61]. In a study of liver cancer, immunohistochemical analysis revealed IDO overexpression in 35.5% of 138 liver tumor resections with weak staining of the remaining 64.5% cases. Again, high IDO expression was correlated significantly with metastatic disease, and IDO was an independent prognostic indicator for poor outcome [62].

Studies of IDO in lung cancer and melanoma also suggest that IDO is overexpressed in tumor stromal cells and tumor-draining lymph nodes. In a small study of nonsmall cell lung cancer (NSCLC), IDO overexpression was observed in tumor-infiltrating eosinophils, and the level of the IDO-positive eosinophil infiltrate was associated with poor survival [63]. In melanoma patients, IDO-positive dendritic cells in tumor-draining lymph nodes was correlated with poor prognosis, and moreover, their presence in sentinel nodes was noted before overt metastasis was discovered [64, 65].

IDO enzymatic activity has been evaluated in acute myeloid leukemia (AML). An evaluation of serum kynurenine/tryptophan ratio (Kyn/Trp) in patients revealed higher levels than in healthy people, suggesting higher IDO activity associated with the cancer [66]. Patients with higher Kyn/Trp ratios also showed lower survival. Recently, it was reported that AML blast cells also overexpress IDO and this is sufficient to convert cocultured $CD25^{low}$ T cells into CD25+ T regulatory cells [67]. These observations suggest IDO as a therapeutic target in AML.

Positive correlations have been reported between IDO expression and accumulation of T regulatory cells that blunt antigen-dependent immune responses. In a small study of pancreatic ductal adenocarcinoma (PDA), upregulation of IDO in metastatic cells was correlated with an increase in FoxP3+ T regulatory cells (Tregs) in the primary tumor and tumor-draining lymph nodes, which exhibited metastases [68]. IDO expression was detected in all tumors (n = 17) that had lymph node metastases and the intensity of immunohistochemical staining was stronger in metastatic foci than primary tumors, suggesting that IDO may help tumor cells evade immune detection during distant spread in PDA. In cases of CIN-3 cervical intraepithelial neoplasia, this association was seen in the uterine cervix where marked expression in microinvasive cancer cells was observed. Interestingly, both FoxP3+CD25+ Tregs and cancer cells that were immunohistochemically positive for IDO expression were colocalized predominantly at the invasive border of the tumor [69]. No significant differences were reported in the relative proportion of Tregs cells in the stroma vs. epithelium of nonmetastatic or metastatic cancers, compared with primary lesions; however, there was a significant increase in the proportion of Tregs in tumor-draining lymph nodes that harbored metastastic tumor cells. Although no correlation was reported in this study between IDO expression, Treg level, and patient prognosis, it seemed that cancer progression occurred with IDO expression at the invasive edge of tumor. Unlike epithelial ovarian or colorectal adenocarcinoma, cervical cancer is most often virally induced, suggesting there may be some pathway variablitity in immune responses to different types of antigens.

It should be noted that some counterexamples in the literature exist regarding the purported link between Treg-mediated immune suppression and poor prognosis. In Hodgkin's lymphoma (HL), an increase in Tregs was reported to be associated with good prognosis [70]. Likewise, in head and neck cancers, a good correlation was found between increased Tregs and locoregional control [71]. These two studies did not evaluate IDO status; however, in one study of liver cancer, the recurrence-free survival rate was reported to be higher in IDO-positive cases. [72]. Similarly, IDO expression in vascular endothelial cells in a study of renal cell carcinomas was found to be correlated with improved long-term survival [73]. In this study, the tumor cells did not constitutively express IDO, leading the investigators to theorize that IDO expression in endothelial cells might have a nonimmune role in limiting the influx of tryptophan from the blood to the tumor or in generating tumor-toxic metabolites, either of which might contribute to survival by restricting tumor growth. It will be important to extend all of these observations into larger and better clinically defined studies to determine both the nature as well as the germane context where IDO may act as a driver of immune escape and malignant progression.

Emerging data on the role of IDO in autoimmune disorders conveys a similarly complex picture regarding its role in disease pathology. Synovial fluid (SF) of RA patients contains large numbers autoreactive T cells expressing high levels of CD45RO (found in effector and memory T cells). Adoptive transfer of synovial infiltrating T cells derived from RA patients causes inflammatory arthritis in SCID mice. Partial elimination or inhibition of T cells by immunosuppressive drugs or anti-T cell antibodies ameliorates the disease. Counterintuitively, RA patient-derived SF DC expressed high levels of IDO while those from healthy donors did not [74]. IFN-γ, TNF, and other cytokines in the SF of RA patients increased the activity of tryptophanyl-tRNA-synthetase (TTS) in synovial T cells. Additionally, IDO was found to be expressed only in the DCs from RA patient SF, not in SF from normal controls [74]. The authors hypothesized that increased TTS activity promoted resistance to IDO-mediated tryptophan deprivation in RA patient-derived SF T cells, thereby making them difficult to restrain. Additionally, the IDO-secreting

RA dendritic cells could stimulate allogenic T cell proliferation, but the proliferation was greatly enhanced in the presence of 1MT [74]. This finding suggested that synovial DCs of RA patients express functional IDO that is able to catabolize tryptophan and inhibit T cell proliferation. However, the synovial T cells from RA patients could resist the effect of IDO due to the increased TTS activity, which enhanced the reservoir of tryptophan-tRNA available for protein synthesis. Although IFN-γ induces IDO in DCs, it also upregulates TTS in T cells in the RA SF microenvironment. Thus, it appeared that IDO could not suppress the autoreactive T cells in RA, because TTS increases the intracellular tryptophan reservoir in T cells and thereby counters the immunosuppressive effect of IDO. Overall, these findings suggested that IDO dysregulation may drive autoreactivity or immunosuppression, depending on the contribution of the local microenvironment.

IDO2: A Second Tryptophan Catabolic Enzyme

A recent new twist in the IDO field is the discovery of a second related gene identified as *IDO2* or *INDOL1* [75–77]. Blast searches of the publicly available human genome database for IDO-related sequences led to identification of the larger *IDO2* gene immediately downstream of the IDO-encoding *INDO* gene at human chromosome 8p12. This region had previously included an anonymous designator LOC169355, which referred to an incomplete gene fragment, but it turned out that this region of the human gene had been misannotated in the database. The human and mouse *IDO2* genes span 11 exons in an ~74 kb genomic region, encoding highly conserved IDO2 proteins of 420 and 405 amino acids, respectively. Tissue expression of *IDO2* is much narrower than *INDO*, confined mainly to liver, placenta, and antigen-presenting immune cells. Although the IDO and IDO2 proteins do not share a high degree of homology (43% identity), amino acids determined by crystallographic and mutagenesis studies to be critical for the catalytic activity of IDO are all conserved in the IDO2 protein. Tryptophan catabolic activity of IDO2 was confirmed by expression of recombinant proteins [78].

In characterizing the human *IDO2* gene, Metz and colleagues identified two SNPs that nearly abolish tryptophan catabolic activity yet occur commonly in human populations [78]. Y359X generates a premature stop codon. R248W is structurally analogous to the key conserved R231 residue, which is critical for enzymatic activity in human IDO. Both of these genetic polymorphisms are widely represented in human populations, with as many as 50% of individuals of European or Asian descent and 25% of individuals of African descent inferred to lack functional *IDO2* alleles [78]. The frequent presence of these SNPs suggests that there may be some evolutionary benefits in human populations to attenuating IDO2 activities, perhaps reflecting competing selective pressures to maintain immunological responsiveness and tolerance in an optimal balance in a complex environment of pathogenic and symbiotic microorganisms. Further, as discussed further below, this variation may have significant bearing on the interpretation of clinical responses to IDO inhibitors that may inhibit IDO2 as well or better than IDO itself [77].

Cellular Pathways of Tryptophan Catabolism Signaling Regulating T Cell Immunity

Studies of IDO have revealed that depletion of tryptophan and production of tryptophan catabolites such as kynurenine both contribute to suppressing effector T cell function [79–81]. At present, while there is little insight into how catabolites may act, some information exists on how tryptophan depletion may mediate IDO function, as summarized in Fig. 3. By depleting microenvironmental levels of tryptophan, IDO activity can trigger local induction of GCN2, a kinase stimulated by uncharged tRNA at the ribosome that initiates an integrated stress response by phosphorylating the central translation initiation factor eIF2α [81]. In T cells, the resulting cell growth arrest alters expression of the T cell receptor zeta chain and prevents antigen-dependent activation, thereby promoting anergy and the production of a regulatory T cell phenotype [82, 83]. Kynurenine contributes to suppressing T effector cells by sensitizing them to apoptosis [79]. T cells to appear relatively more sensitive to these effects of tryptophan catabolism, selectively focuses the effects of IDO activation on the immune system. Activation of either IDO or IDO2 triggers eIF2α phosphorylation and induction of LIP, an inhibitory isoform of the immunoregulatory transcription factor NF-IL6 (also known as CEBP-β), by shifting the translational start site to a downstream initiation codon [77]. In this manner, induction of LIP antagonizes NF-IL6 and causes the transcriptional upregulation of downstream target genes encoding IL-6, IL-10, and TGF-β [23], three immunoregulatory cytokines that support "smouldering" inflammation and immune suppression in the tumor microenvironment.

Although both IDO and IDO2 induce the GCN-eIF2α-LIP pathway, there are differences in how this pathway is switched off after its induction. In vitro experiments indicate that restoring tryptophan after depletion quickly abolishes the LIP response if IDO induced it, but not if IDO2 did [84]. Thus, after IDO2 induction, LIP expression is maintained in a tryptophan-independent manner, indicating a stable effect of tryptophan catabolism signaling via IDO2. Although the significance of this distinction is yet to be evaluated in vivo, one implication is that IDO2 might differ from IDO in its ability to transmit a stable immune regulatory signal. LIP-mediated signaling initiated by IDO2 could alter distal immunity, since the signal could persist in microenvironments where tryptophan levels are normal. Alternately, IDO2 might produce a stable differentiation signal. In any case, the discovery that IDO and IDO2 elevate LIP reveals a likely mechanism for immune regulation by tryptophan catabolism through modulation of NF-IL6/CEBPβ activity [78].

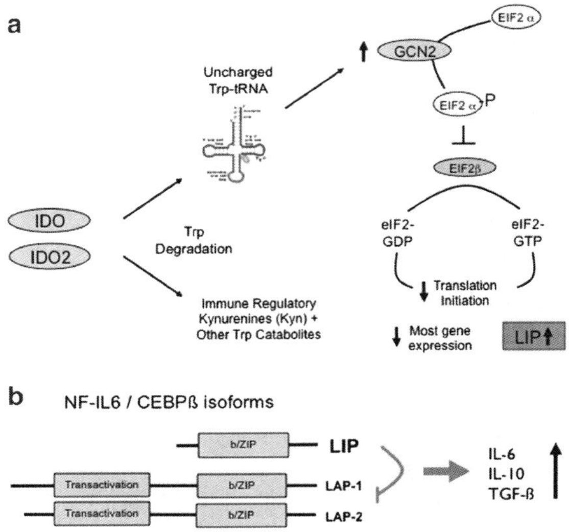

Fig. 3 Tryptophan catabolism signaling pathway triggered by IDO and IDO2. (**a**) Tryptophan starvation to LIP activation. Tryptophan catabolism generates kynurenine and other products that modulate T cell immunity and starve a microenvironment for tryptophan. In T cells starvation triggers GCN2, a stress kinase that responds to amino acid deprivation by phosphorylating the translation initiation factor eIF2α. This event blocks translation initiation from most mRNAs with the exception of certain factors such as LIP that are involved in mediating stress responses. (**b**) LIP is a dominant negative isoform of the immune regulatory b/ZIP transcription factor NF-IL6, also known as CEBP-β. LIP is an alternately translated isoform of the transcription factor NF-IL6/ CEBPβ implicated in differentiation, proliferation and immunity. Starvation switches NF-IL6 expression from LAP isoforms to LIP isoform through use of a downstream translation start site in the mRNA. LIP encodes only a b/ZIP dimerization domain, so it functions as a "natural" dominant inhibitory molecule that disrupts NF-IL6 function by competing with LAP isoforms for binding to target gene promoters. NF-IL6 target genes include the immune suppressive cytokines IL-6, IL-10, and TGF-β which are upregulated as a result of LIP induction. Both IDO and IDO2 switch on LIP, but restoring tryptophan after its depletion only switches LIP off in the case of IDO, offering a possible mechanism for IDO2 to propagate immune suppression away from a local tumor microenvironment

With the emergence of its immunosuppressive role, IDO has become recognized as a tumor supporting enzyme. This is in striking contrast to the initial theories of the role of IDO in cancer. The early discovery that the *INDO* gene is strongly induced at the transcriptional level by interferon-γ (IFN-γ) prompted an initial reinterpretation of longstanding clinical observations that tryptophan catabolites are elevated in urine from cancer patients [43, 44, 46]. The hypothesis was that IDO driven by IFN-γ caused the elevation of tryptophan catabolites in cancer patients [85]. IFN-γ was known to have tumor-suppressing properties, so it was proposed that IDO mediated these properties in part by starving tumor cells for tryptophan [86]. Later, with the discovery of its immunosuppressive properties discussed later, it became apparent that the deleterious effects of tryptophan depletion on the tumor might be more than counterbalanced by the benefit that immune escape could provide in supporting tumor survival. IFN-γ promotes formation of an immune stimulatory Th1 response. In addition to supporting the major histocompatibility complex (MHC) class II antigen-processing pathway in antigen-presenting cells, IFN-γ inhibits expression of IL-4, which is key to production of a Th2 response. Moreover, IFN-γ can blunt angiogenesis by inhibiting the synthesis of basic fibroblast growth factor (bFGF), IL-8, and collagenase IV and by limiting endothelial cell migration. The antitumor properties ascribed to IFN-γ secretion by activated T cells would seem to be at odds with its ability to potent induce *INDO* transcription in APCs that suppress T cell activation, prompting the idea that IDO may normally participate in a negative feedback mechanism on IFN-γ signaling. In the tumor microenvironment, IDO activity may lead to an impairment of antigen-dependent T cell activation, thereby contributing to pathologic immune tolerance to tumor associated antigens. In this sense, IDO can be considered prooncogenic.

As noted earlier, IFN-γ is a major inducer of IDO in many cells, particularly in antigen-presenting cells such as DCs [87–90]. Transcriptional induction of the *INDO* gene is mediated through Jak1 and Stat 1 [91]. Stat 1 acts through direct binding of GAS sites within the *INDO* promoter as well as indirectly through induction of interferon regulatory factor 1 (IRF-1), which binds the *INDO* promoter at two interferon-stimulated response element (ISRE) sites [91–95]. The immunoregulatory transcription factor NF-κB also contributes to *INDO* induction. In particular, IFN-γ and TNF, which signal through NF-κB, can act synergistically to induce expression of IRF-1 and IDO [96].

Studies indicate that IDO is integrated in a complex milieu of factors that promote immune tolerance. One important regulator of its expression may be the proinflammatory prostaglandin E2 (PGE2), which is frequently elevated during cancer progression as a result of activation of cyclooxygenase 2 (COX-2). IDO is induced by PGE2, consistent with the role of COX-2 in promoting immune suppression. COX-2 is an inducible enzyme, becoming abundant in activated macrophages and other cells at sites of inflammation. Interestingly, while PGE2 is employed widely as an in vitro maturation factor for DCs, treatment of these cells with PGE2 has been reported to elevate IDO expression approximately 100-fold [97]. Although it remains unresolved whether such preparations actually compromise the desired immunostimulatory activity of DCs used for cancer vaccines, it has been reported in a small melanoma vaccination trial [98] that the DC maturation cocktail, which included PGE2, induced IDO in the treated DCs and that IDO-expressing cells continued to be observed in situ at the DC injection site where accumulation of FOXp3+ cells, indicative of regulatory T cells, was also evident. The concept that IDO is downstream of COX-2 is further supported by evidence that induction of IDO activity can be blocked in vitro by COX-2 inhibitors, such as aspirin, indomethacin, and phenylbutazone, but not by antiinflammatory agents that do not affect prostaglandin [99]. The relationship between PGE-2 and IDO is clearly complex insofar as IDO activity can also affect the ratio of prostaglandin synthesis [100].

Other important immune regulatory agents that can influence IDO activity are nitric oxide (NO) and transforming growth factor-β (TGF-β). IDO and inducible nitric oxide synthase (iNOS) appear to be mutually antagonistic in DC-based studies [41, 101]. The production of NO by iNOS prevents the IFN-γ-induced expression of IDO [102], interferes directly with its enzymatic activity [102–104], and promotes its proteolytic degradation [105]. NO can directly inactivate IDO by binding directly to the heme iron, which under lowered pH conditions induces iron-His bond rupture and the formation of a 5C NO-bound derivative that is associated with protein conformational changes that may be sufficient to target the protein for ubiquitination and proteosomal degradation [106]. In the nonobese diabetic (NOD) mouse model, in vivo evidence suggests that IFN-γ signaling is impaired as the result of nitration of the downstream Stat1 transcription factor by peroxynitrate, which is derived from NO and superoxide. This impairment can be overcome by CTLA-4-Ig treatment, which, by promoting PTEN activity, relieves the negative regulation that phosphorylated Akt imposes on Fox03a-mediated transcription of superoxide dismutase (SOD2), which degrades peroxynitrate [107]. Through this complex route, the blockade to activation of IDO gene expression, to which iNOS contributes through peroxynitrate-mediated nitration of Stat1, is relieved.

There are two implications of this mechanism. First, NO agonists would be expected to reverse the immunosuppression at the level of DCs in cancer, which should benefit treatment. Second, small-molecule inhibitors of Akt developed as anticancer therapeutics may heighten immunosuppression by phenocoyping the effect of CTLA-4-Ig on IDO expression. Therapeutic evaluation of Akt inhibitors as potential anticancer agents should therefore balance consideration of their potentially useful proapoptotic effects on tumor cells against their possible proinvasive and immunosuppressive liabilities.

TGF-β may also antagonize IFN-γ-mediated induction of IDO expression of fibroblasts [108]. This finding appears to run counter to the immunosuppressive activity ascribed to TGF-β but is consistent with its ability to antagonize positively regulated targets of IFN-γ. The balance between the effects of TGF-β and IFN-γ signaling on IDO expression in different cells of tumor and peripheral microenvironments provides a complex mechanism for local control of IDO activity. Overall it seems clear that IDO is tied into many important immunoregulatory pathways in a complex network involving signaling overlaps and feedback loops.

Dendritic Cells and Immune Tolerance Mediated by IDO

DCs play a central role in defending against invaders. As "professional" antigen-presenting cells, they are numerous in organs frequently exposed to antigens, such as skin, lungs, and the digestive tract. They migrate to lymphoid organs where they present antigens to T cells to activate an immune response. Contrariwise, DCs can also be efficient at inducing tolerance and at controlling autoimmunity. A network of cytokine signaling determines whether a DC becomes tolerogenic or stimulatory. Immature DCs are tolerogenic by default until external inputs promote differentiation. They produce protolerogenic cytokines such as IL-10 and vascular endothelial growth factor. Mature tolerogenic DC subgroups also exist, although it is unclear whether they arise through alternative differentiation or as distinct lineages. These mature tolerogenic DCs can promote Th2 polarization and expand the regulatory T cell (Treg) population [109, 110]. Tumors can play a key role in determining the type of response that tumor-associated DCs will elicit [111, 112].

B7 costimulatory molecules, which are expressed on DCs, are implicated in supporting Treg homeostasis as both CD28-null and B7–1/B7–2 double null mice have markedly reduced populations of Tregs [113]. Likewise, when constitutively expressed, endogenous B7 potently limits T cell activation and maintains self-tolerance by sustaining Tregs [114, 115]. Furthermore, naïve $CD4^+CD25^-$ T cells transferred into congenic mice are converted in vivo into $CD4^+CD25^+$ Tregs only if the recipient mice express B7 costimulatory molecules [116].

Accumulating evidence indicates that $CD4^+CD25^+$ Tregs play an indispensable role in maintaining negative control over pathologic as well as physiologic immune responses [117–119]. The removal of Tregs not only elicits autoimmune diseases but also enhances responses to nonself antigens, including xenogenic proteins and allografts [120]. In mice, the absence of Tregs leads to gestational failure due to immunologic rejection [121]. Conversely, adoptive transfer of pregnancy-induced Tregs can protect against fetal rejection in abortion-prone mice [122]. The role of Tregs in maintaining chronic infections has also been studied [123]. $CD4^+CD25^+$ Tregs from persons recovered from hepatitis C virus (HCV) infection and from healthy blood donors exhibited significantly less suppressor activity than those patients with chronic HCV infection [124], while chronic HIV infection affected the tissue distribution of Tregs with a direct correlation evident between FoxP3 levels and viral load [125]. Treatment of SIV-infected macaques with CTLA-4 blockade was associated with a decrease in viral levels in the lymph nodes as well as in levels of immunosuppressive molecules such as IDO and TGFβ, which correlated with a concomitant increase in $CD4^+$ and $CD8^+$ T cell effector function [126].

Several studies have evidenced an intriguing link between B7 and CTLA-4 on DCs and T cells with the production of IDO-dependent tolerance [127–129]. CTLA-4 is a major signaling molecule for Tregs, and IDO has been implicated to be an important downstream effector for CTLA-4-mediated immune tolerance. The first in vivo evidence for this implication was the observation that administering CTLA-4-Ig in a diabetic mouse model suppressed the immune rejection of pancreatic islet allografts, an effect that was reversible by concurrent treatment with the IDO inhibitor 1MT [107, 130]. These findings also suggested that CTLA-4-Ig-mediated tolerance occurs through a heterodox mechanism of "reverse" signaling through B7 molecules on APCs, leading to IFN-γ autocrine signaling and IDO induction. Other work has confirmed that systemic administration of CTLA-4-Ig results in IDO upregulation in DC subsets. Systemic CTLA-4-Ig can also block clonal expansion and cytotoxic T lymphocyte (CTL) activity of H-2Kb-specific T cells from T cell receptor (TCR) transgenic mice adoptively transferred into H-2Kb hosts. This effect of CTLA-4-Ig was abrogated by treatment with 1MT or by using IDO-null knockout mice as hosts [131]. The latter control is particularly informative, because it provides a strong argument that IDO is an essential target for mediating the effects of 1MT [132]. Tregs that constitutively express CTLA-4 on their surface have likewise been shown to promote IDO activity in DCs through a CTLA-4-dependent mechanism [127].

Data indicating that IDO mediates the biological effects of CTLA-4 ligation support the idea that CTLA-4 inhibits immune activation, whether by preventing CD28 binding to B7 ligand, inducing immunosuppressive cytokines, or directly interfering with CD28-mediated and/or TCR-mediated signaling. [133]. The different mechanisms need not be mutually exclusive; however, considering that loss of IDO activity, either pharmacologically or genetically, does not completely phenocopy genetic loss of CTLA-4. The B7–1/B7–2-CD28/CTLA-4 pathway includes two B7 family members, B7–1 and B7–2 that have dual specificity for the stimulatory receptor CD28 and the inhibitory receptor CTLA-4. CTLA-4 is the higher-affinity receptor for B7–1 and B7–2. CD28 is constitutively expressed on the surface of T cells whereas CTLA-4 expression is rapidly upregulated following T cell activation. CTLA4 can dampen proliferation and guard against autoimmunity, perhaps most clearly illustrated by the phenotype of CTLA4-deficient mice. Waterhouse and colleagues [134] and Tivol and colleagues [135] showed that these mice died by 3–4 weeks of birth as a result of massive lymphoadenopathy, tissue infiltration, and destruction of multiple organs. The observed lymphoproliferation was later reported to be mediated by the costimulation dependent activation of CD4+ T cells [135]. The fatal lymphoproliferative disease that develops in CTLA-$4^{-/-}$ mice secondary to uncontrolled B7–1/B7–2 costimulation underscores the importance of CTLA-4 as a negative regulator of T cell responses.

CTLA-4 has a crucial role in regulating peripheral T cell tolerance, but IDO-null knockout mice have not been observed to exhibit spontaneous autoimmune disease. Nevertheless, in vivo blockade of CTLA-4 clearly augments antitumour immunity and exacerbates autoimmune responses [133, 136]. These observations suggest that IDO is not required for homeostatic maintenance of central or peripheral tolerance to self antigens. In contrast, acquired tolerance may be defective in IDO-null mice, such that IDO induction might play a role in the acquisition of tolerance to neoantigens [109]. This idea is appealing, since acquiring tolerance to neoantigens is critical to maintain pregnancy and to permit progression of early neoplastic lesions that present tumor antigens.

Much published work on the role of IDO in DCs has come from investigating the tolerogenic mechanisms elicited by CD11c+CD8α+ DCs during challenges with self and tumor antigens. One model that has been used for immune tolerance experiments is a delayed type hypersensitivity (DTH) skin test model, in which mice receiving peptide-pulsed DCs were assayed for MHC class I-restricted reactivity by challenging with peptide in the footpad. Fractionated CD8α-myeloid DCs presented with tumor/self peptide were actively immunogenic but could be effectively inhibited by reintroduction of a small percentage of CD8α+ lymphoid DCs. The Th1-associated cytokines IL-12 and IFN-γ were found to work at cross purposes in this system, with tolerogenic suppression by the CD8α+ cells relieved by pretreatment of the CD8α^- DCs with IL-12 before mixing with CD8α+ lymphoid DCs. Inhibition was reestablished by exposure of the CD8α^+ population to IFN-γ prior to mixing with the IL-12 treated CD8α-myeloid DCs [137, 138]. Addition of the IDO inhibitory compound 1MT suppressed the ability of IFN-γ to overcome the adjuvant effect of IL-12. Induction of IDO activity by IFN-γ in CD8α+ DCs, which exhibit a significant basal level of IDO expression, has been shown to be regulated both at the level of expression as well as in the posttranslational period [82]. Interestingly, in the CD8α− population, both the basal and induced levels of IDO expression appear to be comparable with the CD8α+ DC IDO levels, but IDO activity remained suppressed in response to IFN-γ. Responses to engagement of cell surface molecules on DCs were found to play a key role in determining whether DC activity would be immunogenic or tolerogenic. Engagement of CD40 with agonistic antibody blocked IFN-γ-mediated induction of IDO activity in otherwise protolerogenic CD8α+ DCs and induced these cells to actively prime rather than suppress CTL responses to self/tumor peptide I the DTH model [139]. The agonistic CTLA-4-Ig receptor/antibody fusion protein had an opposite effect as otherwise proimmunogenic CD8α-DCs treated with CTLA-4-Ig-induced IDO activity and were rendered tolerogenic [140]. Together, these findings highlight the functional plasticity of these different DC subsets.

Like CTLA-4-Ig, CD28-Ig binds B7 molecules except with variable effects of promoting immunogenicity [141] or tolerance [142] depending on the animal receiving the antibody. DCs treated with CD28-Ig exhibited early and sustained production of IL-6 that was not induced by CTLA-4-Ig. IL-6 upregulates SOCS3, which inhibits the Stat-dependent IFN-γ signaling required for IDO signaling; consistent with these signaling connections, silencing of SOCS3 expression in DCs caused CD28-Ig to elicit a CTLA-4-Ig-like tolerogenic response [143, 144]. Gene expression profiling in CD8α+ DCs has revealed that the *Tyrobp*-encoded DAP12 protein, which is controlled by IFN-γ and activates NK cells via negative transcriptional regulation imposed by IRF-8, is important for posttranslational suppression of IDO activity. CD8α+ DCs from transgenic mice overexpressing the DAP12 protein exhibited impaired tolerogenic function, while CD8α+ DCs lacking DAP12 protein exhibited increased IDO-dependent tolergenic activity [145]. These observations suggest that DAP12 is a modifier of IDO activity.

In addition to DCs, other immune cells that may utilize IDO for immunosuppression include macrophages, granulocytes, and neutrophils. The first indications of IDO involvement in the suppression of T cell activation were obtained from in vitro studies of macrophages exposed to colony-stimulating factor 1 (CSF-1), which induced IDO activity in the context of a mixed lymphocyte reaction. Expression of CSF-1 in tumors has been implicated in polarizing macrophages toward an M2 suppressor phenotypes [146]. Studies in Stat6 knockout mice support a role for both myeloid-derived suppressor cells (MDSCs) and tumor-associated macrophages (TAMs) in tumor metastasis. Stat6 knockout mice are resistant to metastasis produced by isogenic tumor grafts of the highly metastatic breast cancer cell line 4T1. The resistance observed in these animals has been linked to diminished MDSC induction coupled with a reduction in M2 TAMs. In CD-1 knockout mice, which lack IL-13-producing NKT cells, polarization toward an M2 phenotype is no longer suppported after implantation of 4T1 cells, and resulting production of cytotoxic M1 macrophages is associated with rejection of 4T1 tumors [147]. In addition, when cultured in the presence of CSF-1, macrophages display expression of IDO [148], which also suppresses effector T cell responses. The production of TGF-β and IL-10 by TAMs would also perpetuate polarization toward a protolerogenic state [146].

Precisely how IDO-mediated tryptophan catabolism elicits immune tolerance remains uncertain given evidence for different but not necessarily mutually exclusive mechanisms of action. Some studies in DCs have indicated that induction of IDO activity, triggered by exposure to either IFN-γ or CTLA-4-Ig, may be necessary for acquiring rather than directly eliciting the suppressor phenotype [138, 145]. The former possibility is consistent with the finding that DC maturation, in response to TNF or lipopolysaccharide (LPS) treatment, is suppressed by 1MT along with expression of the CCR5 and CXCR4, which mediate tumor migration and infiltration [149]. Most attention, however, has focused on the direct suppression of T cells by IDO-mediated tryptophan catabolism. The first studies examining how IDO suppresses T cell immunity proposed the core concept that starving T cells of tryptophan limits their ability to be activated by appropriately presented antigen due to a block in cell division required for activation [148]. However, other studies have shown that the catabolites produced by the IDO pathway can trigger preferential T cell apoptosis [79], and in vitro experiments meant to demonstrate which of these two mechanisms is more relevant to immunological suppression have produced contradictory results [150].

Recent in vivo data likewise seem incongruent. There is genetic evidence that signaling through the GCN2 kinase pathway, which responds to environmental depletion of tryptophan, elicits arrest in T cells. T cells from GCN2-null mice are no longer responsive to IDO-expressing DCs. IDO-mediated induction of growth arrest and anergy in responding T cells is signaled by stress signals mediated through the GCN2 kinase pathway [83]. Contrariwise, systemic treatment of mice with the IDO catabolic mimetic 3,4-DAA has been reported to ameliorate symptoms in a mouse model of multiple sclerosis. In this study 3,4-DAA interfered with IFN-γ-induced Stat1 signaling in a microglial cell line and suppressed the activation of APCs in vivo, but no data on its effects on T cells independent of APCs were presented. One possible explanation consistent with these two in vivo reports is that depletion of tryptophan might have a direct effect in suppressing T cell activation, while the accumulation of tryptophan catabolites might act indirectly to further impair T cell activation by suppressing immunogenic APCs. Fallarino and colleagues [80] reported that IDO-expressing DCs can suppress CD8+ T cell activity in mice and can also convert naïve CD4+ T cells to Foxp3+ Tregs. These effects required tryptophan depletion plus exposure to tryptophan catabolites and were mediated through GCN2 kinase. Not only did this finding address some of the confusion surrounding the physiologic mechanism of IDO-mediated immune suppression, but it is also intriguing given the relationship that was established between CTLA-4+ Tregs and their ability to induce IDO-mediated immune suppression through responsive DCs. This finding suggested that there may be a circular feed-forward mechanism in which tolerogenic DCs recruit the development of additional Tregs, which in turn recruit more toleragenic DCs through the action of IDO.

IDO as a Target for Therapeutic Intervention

Immune therapy has been evaluated extensively in a variety of cancers, including melanoma, chronic myelogenous leukemia, non-Hodgkin's lymphoma, hairy cell leukemia, AIDS-related Kaposi's sarcoma, bladder cancer (intravesicular), and renal cell cancer. Interest in immune therapy for melanoma developed because of known spontaneous remissions in patients with advanced disease and subsequent studies that showed that it was highly immunogenic [151]. In 1992, IL-2 was approved for use in metastatic melanoma, and in 1995, IFN-γ2b became the first immune therapy approved for adjuvant treatment in regionally advanced disease. Unfortunately, since that time, these agents have exhibited limited success, and several peptide vaccine trials have likewise failed to show benefit using various melanoma-associated antigens. Canvaxin is one melanoma vaccine that contained more than 20 specific antigens. However, a randomized prospective clinical trial of Canvaxin (CancerVax Corp., Carlsbad, CA) [152] in stage III/IV melanoma patients showed overall survival was 9% (stage III) and 5% (stage IV), worse than using Bacillus Calmette-Guerin antigen [151]. Thus, it was suggested that Canvaxin may actually reinforce immune suppression in these patients. Similarly, many other types of cancer vaccines have failed to improve overall survival, probably because of the major impediments to a successful immunotherapy regimen caused by tumor-induced immune suppression. At present, a better understanding of the immune system-tumor interface is encouraging the development of new strategies and targets to overcome tolerance. Recently, IDO ranked highly among new targets considered most promising for therapeutic intervention by an NCI workshop [153].

One appealing aspect of IDO as a target to enhance in vivo immune responses is that it appears to be nonessential for DC maturation. As noted earlier, IDO-null mice do not exhibit any evidence of spontaneous autoimmunity or illness. Faudeur and colleagues demonstrated that there was normal development and function of dendritic cells from IDO-null mice under conditions that mimicked in vivo conditions, such as low adherence plates and in the presence of Flt-3, despite prior demonstrations of differences in development of dendritic cell subpopulations in vitro under standard conditions [154]. Even under conditions where wild-type and IDO-null mice were challenged subcutaneously with promastigotes of *Leishmania major*, there were no differences in subpopulations of dendritic cells between wild-type and IDO-null mice. These observations support the notion that interfering with IDO will not grossly impair DC maturation.

Importantly, several studies offer sound preclinical evidence that IDO inhibition with 1MT or other small molecule inhibitors can exert potent antitumor effects. Initial evidence emerged in 2002 that 1MT could slow the growth of mouse lung carcinoma cells engrafted in a syngeneic host [155]. Similar results were obtained a part of an investigation to assess the ramifications of IDO overexpression that was detected in a wide range of human tumors [58]. In this study, ectopic overexpression of IDO in an established histiocytic tumor cell line was sufficient to promote tumor formation in animals preimmunized against a specific tumor antigen, and 1MT partially suppressed tumor outgrowth in this context. In 2005, a breakthrough was achieved regarding the potential use of IDO inhibitors to leverage the effectiveness of chemotherapy in the treatment of established tumors [156]. In the MMTV-*Neu*/HER2 transgenic mouse model of breast cancer, 1MT retarded the growth of autochthonous mammary tumors to some degree but did not elicit tumor regression when used alone, confirming that IDO inhibition may have limited antitumor efficacy as a monotherapy as had previously been observed in transplantable tumor models. In contrast, when delivered in combination with a variety of cytotoxic chemotherapeutic agents, 1MT elicited significant regression of MMTV-*Neu*/HER2 tumors, which respond poorly to most chemotherapeutic agents [156]. There was no increase in side-effects noted in mice receiving both agents, suggesting that the synergistic response seen was not due to an increase in the effective dose of the chemotherapeutic agent alone. Similar effects were produced by administration of methyl-thiohydantoin tryptophan (MTH-trp), another bioactive small molecule inhibitor of IDO identified as part of this study. Immunodepletion of CD4+ or CD8+ T cells before treatment abolished antitumor efficacy [156]. These findings confirmed that the antitumor properties conferred by IDO inhibition were elicited by a T cell-mediated pathway.

From a clinical standpoint, combining an immunomodulatory agent such as 1MT with conventional chemotherapeutic agents represents a logical and readily translatable strategy. With regard to 1MT, however, apparently contradictory evidence emerged as to which of the two stereoisomers of 1MT, D or L, was most effective. Most studies in the literature have used the racemic mixture of 1MT, which is composed of L and D stereoisomers. Although the amino acid tryptophan occurs naturally in the form of the L stereoisomer, yet, in some biological systems D-1MT seemed to be the more active form of 1MT. Hou and colleagues used recombinant human IDO in a cell-free assay system to test the ability of L-1MT and D-1MT to inhibit kynurenine production [157]. Notably, they found that L-1MT functioned as a competitive inhibitor ($K_i = 19\ \mu M$) whereas D-1MT displayed little activity ($K_i >$ $100\ \mu M$). In a cell-based assay, in which the endogenous IDO enzyme in HeLa cells was activated with IFN-γ, a pattern of inhibition similar to that of the cell-free recombinant enzyme was observed. In contrast, when primary human monocyte-derived DCs were used as IDO-expressing cells, D-1MT was at least as effective as L-1MT for IDO inhibition [157]. Using T cell proliferation in allo-mixed lymphocyte reactions (MLRs) stimulated by IDO+ monocyte-derived dendritic cells, D-1MT was also superior to either L-1MT or the racemic D, L mixture. Lastly, D-1MT was more potent as an antitumor agent when used in combination with chemotherapy in both the MMTV-Neu "oncomouse" and 4T1 graft mouse models of breast cancer [157]. The effect of D-1MT could be genetically linked to IDO as an essential drug target, on the basis of evidence that D-1MT was completely inactive in IDO-null mice used as hosts to engraft the 4T1 breast tumor cells (which do not express IDO).

The dichotomy between L-1MT's superior activity as a biochemical inhibitor of IDO and D-1MT's superior in vivo activity as an antitumor compound does not appear to be attributable to a difference in pharmacological properties between the two isomers, suggesting other explanations such as (1) in vivo racemization of the D to L isoform, (2) in vivo differences in IDO in DCs rendering it susceptible to D-1MT, or (3) in vivo involvement of another target of D-1MT that IDO requires for immunosuppression. Metz and colleagues corroborated the latter explanation with the striking finding that IDO2 is preferentially inhibited by D-1MT [77]. In contrast, L-1MT did not inhibit IDO2, but MTH-trp inhibited IDO and IDO2 equally well [77]. Together these results identified IDO2 as a relevant target for biochemical inhibition by D-1MT, possibly explaining its well-documented antitumor effects. IDO is more widely expressed, while IDO2 is expressed mainly in antigen-presenting DCs where driving tryptophan catabolism is clearly established as an immune tolerance mechanism. Given the advancement of D-1MT into clinical trials, these recent findings make IDO2 a compelling subject for further study.

As targets for drug development, IDO and IDO2 offer a number of appealing features. These enzymes are single-chain cytosolic catalytic enzymes with a well-defined biochemistry. One of the other known tryptophan catabolizing enzymes on the kynurenine pathway, TDO2, is structurally distinct from IDO and IDO2 and has a more restricted pattern of expression and substrate specificity such that it is generally unaffected by IDO inhibitory compounds, ameliorating off-target issues. A growing number of lead inhibitors of IDO and IDO2 exist that can serve as useful tools for validation and mechanism studies [158–162]. One interesting advance from drug discovery efforts to date has been the identification of the natural product brassinin as an IDO inhibitor [163, 164], a phytoalexin-type compound found in cruciferous vegetables that is known to have chemopreventative activity in breast and colon cancer mouse models [165, 166]. The design of potent inhibitors can be assisted by an understanding of the three-dimensional structure of an enzyme's active and catalytic sites, and a high resolution X-ray crystal structure of IDO bound to a simple inhibitor has been solved recently [53]. Given the intriguing features of IDO as an immune modulator in cancer and other diseases, future efforts to identify IDO inhibitors may accelerate quickly. Encouraging this effort is the fact that IDO-null mice are viable and healthy, which portends that an IDO inhibitor may not have serious side-effects [167] (although it will be important to know whether genetic ablation of IDO2 produces similarly benign effects). Given the challenges faced by many molecular targeted therapeutics in pharmacodynamic clinical testing, it is attractive to consider the prospects that the evaluation of IDO inhibitors might be possible through simple determinations of tryptophan and kynurenine in blood serum. Lastly, from a cost-of-goods standpoint, small molecule inhibitors of IDO may offer practical advantages over biological or cell-based alternatives to therapeutically modulate T cell immunity.

Concluding Comments

Conceptualization regarding the physiological role of IDO has evolved from its being a metabolic, tryptophan catabolizing enzyme into a recognized immune regulator and an important player in immunosurveillance. While IDO conceivably has a beneficial role in dampening down inflammation and reducing collateral damage that may occur in settings of marked inflammation, its place in human diseases, particularly in infectious disease and oncology, is rapidly becoming more fully described. There is now extensive evidence that IDO is overexpressed in tumors and tumor-draining lymph nodes and that its expression contributes significantly to immune escape. Certainly the evidence of cooperation between the IDO inhibitor 1MT and traditional chemotherapeutic agents in animal models creates a new and enticing way to design treatments for human tumors. Multimodality treatments can be rationalized with surgery, chemotherapy, radiation, and immunotherapy. To date, preclinical validation of IDO inhibitors supports the assertion that they may offer great promise in combination with cytotoxic drugs, but their potential to increase the response to active immunotherapeutic agents, such as cancer vaccines and Toll receptor-like (TLR) ligands, is clearly another avenue to consider. In late 2007, D-1MT entered into Phase I clinical trials. Whatever the outcome of its clinical evaluation, one would expect interest in the IDO pathway for therapeutic targets to continue to grow.

References

1. Burnet, M. (1957) Br Med J 1, 841
2. Nauts, H. C., Fowler, G. A., and Bogatko, F. H. (1953). Acta Med Scand Suppl 276, 1
3. McCarthy, E. (2006) Iowa Orthop J 26, 154
4. Dunn, G. P., Koebel, C. M., and Schreiber, R. D. (2006) Nat Rev Immunol 6, 836
5. Dunn, G. P., Old, L. J., and Schreiber, R. D. (2004) Immunity 21, 137
6. Smyth, M. J., Dunn, G. P., and Schreiber, R. D. (2006) Adv Immunol 90, 1
7. Gasser, S., and Raulet, D. H. (2006) Cancer Res 66, 3959
8. Koebel, C. M., Vermi, W., Swann, J. B., Zerafa, N., Rodig, S. J., Old, L. J., Smyth, M. J., and Schreiber, R. D. (2007) Nature 450, 903
9. MacKie, R. M., Reid, R., and Junor, B. (2003) N Engl J Med 348, 567
10. Prendergast, G. C. (2008) Oncogene 27, 3889
11. Gatti, R. A., and Good, R. A. (1971) Cancer 28, 89
12. Gutierrez, C., Guo, Z. S., Burhans, W., De Pamphilis, M. L., Farrell-Towt, J., and Ju, G. (1988) Science 240, 1202
13. Penn, I. (1999) Transplant Proc 31, 1260
14. Brown, M. R., Noffsinger, A., First, M. R., Penn, I., and Husseinzadeh, N. (2000) Gynecol Oncol 79, 220
15. Penn, I. (2000) Drug Saf 23, 101
16. Penn, I. (2000) Adv Ren Replace Ther 7, 147
17. Penn, I. (1998) Clin Transpl 147
18. Penn, I. (1997) Transplantation 64, 669
19. Penn, I. (1997) Arch Dermatol 133, 221
20. Zou, W. (2005) Nat Rev Cancer 5, 263
21. Balkwill, F., Charles, K. A., and Mantovani, A. (2005) Cancer Cell 7, 211
22. Balkwill, F. (2006) Cancer Metastasis Rev 25, 409
23. Prendergast, G. C. (2008) Oncogene 27, 3889
24. Bongartz, T., Sutton, A. J., Sweeting, M. J., Buchan, I., Matteson, E. L., and Montori, V. (2006) JAMA 295, 2275

25. Kulbe, H., Thompson, R., Wilson, J. L., Robinson, S., Hagemann, T., Fatah, R., Gould, D., Ayhan, A., and Balkwill, F. (2007) Cancer Res 67, 585
26. Szlosarek, P. W., and Balkwill, F. R. (2003) Lancet Oncol 4, 565
27. Madhusudan, S., Foster, M., Muthuramalingam, S. R., Braybrooke, J. P., Wilner, S., Kaur, K., Han, C., Hoare, S., Balkwill, F., Talbot, D. C., Ganesan, T. S., and Harris, A. L. (2004) Clin Cancer Res 10, 6528
28. Madhusudan, S., Muthuramalingam, S. R., Braybrooke, J. P., Wilner, S., Kaur, K., Han, C., Hoare, S., Balkwill, F., and Ganesan, T. S. (2005) J Clin Oncol 23, 5950
29. Harrison, M. L., Obermueller, E., Maisey, N. R., Hoare, S., Edmonds, K., Li, N. F., Chao, D., Hall, K., Lee, C., Timotheadou, E., Charles, K., Ahern, R., King, D. M., Eisen, T., Corringham, R., DeWitte, M., Balkwill, F., and Gore, M. (2007) J Clin Oncol 25, 4542
30. Lees, C. W., Ironside, J., Wallace, W. A. H., and Satsangi, J. (2008) N Engl J Med 359, 320
31. Moore, R. J., Owens, D. M., Stamp, G., Arnott, C., Burke, F., East, N., Holdsworth, H., Turner, L., Rollins, B., Pasparakis, M., Kollias, G., and Balkwill, F. (1999) Nat Med 5, 828
32. Kim, R., Emi, M., Tanabe, K., and Arihiro, K. (2006) Cancer Res 66, 5527
33. Muller, A. J., and Scherle, P. A. (2006) Nat Rev Cancer 6, 613
34. Sono, M., Roach, M. P., Coulter, E. D., and Dawson, J. H. (1996) Chem Rev 96, 2841
35. Sono, M., Taniguchi, T., Watanabe, Y., and Hayaishi, O. (1980) J Biol Chem 255, 1339
36. Botting, N. P. (1995) Chem Soc Rev 24, 401
37. Munn, D. H., Zhou, M., Attwood, J. T., Bondarev, I., Conway, S. J., B. Marshall, C. Brown, and A. L. Mellor. (1998) Science 281, 1191
38. Finn, O. (2008) N Engl J Med 25, 2704
39. Hansen, A. M., Ball, H. J., Mitchell, A. J., Miu, J., Takikawa, O., and Hunt, N. H. (2004) Int J Parasitol 34, 1309
40. Thomas, S. M., Garrity, L. F., Brandt, C. R., Schobert, C. S., Feng, G. S., Taylor, M. W., Carlin, J. M., and Byrne, G. I. (1993) J Immunol 150, 5529
41. Fujigaki, S., Saito, K., Takemura, M., Maekawa, N., Yamada, Y., Wada, H., and Seishima, M. (2002) Infect Immun 70, 779
42. Larrea, E., Riezu-Boj, J. I., Gil-Guerrero, L., Casares, N., Aldabe, R., Sarobe, P., Civeira, M. P., Heeney, J. L., Rollier, C., Verstrepen, B., Wakita, T., Borras-Cuesta, F., Lasarte, J. J., and Prieto, J. (2007) J Virol 81, 3662
43. Boyland, E., and Williams, D. C. (1955) Process Biochem 60, v
44. Ambanelli, U., and Rubino, A. (1962) Haematol Lat 5, 49
45. Ivanova, V. D. (1964) Acta Unio Int Contra Cancrum 20, 1085
46. Rose, D. P. (1967) Lancet 1, 239
47. Wolf, H., Madsen, P. O., and Price, J. M. (1968) J Urol 100, 537
48. Gailani, S., Murphy, G., Kenny, G., Nussbaum, A., and Silvernail, P. (1973) Cancer Res 33, 1071
49. Higuchi, K., and O. Hayaishi. 1967. Enzymic formation of D-kynurenine from D-tryptophan. *Arch. Biochem. Biophys.* 120:397–403.
50. Higuchi, K., Kuno, S., and Hayaishi, O. (1963) Federation Proc 22, 243 (abstr)
51. Taylor, M. W., and Feng, G. S. (1991) FASEB J 5, 2516
52. Watanabe, Y., Yoshida, R., Sono, M., and Hayaishi, O. (1981) J Histochem Cytochem 29, 623
53. Watanabe, Y., Yoshida, R., Sono, M., and Hayaishi, O. (1981) J Histochem Cytochem 29, 623
54. Sono, M. (1989) Biochemistry 28, 5400
55. Kadoya, A., Tone, S., Maeda, H., Minatogawa, Y., and Kido, R. (1992) Biochem Biophys Res Commun 189, 530
56. Najfeld, V., Menninger, J., Muhleman, D., Comings, D. E., and Gupta, S. L. (1993) Cytogenet Cell Genet 64, 231
57. Arefayene, M., Philips, S., Cao, D., Mamidipalli, S., Flockhart, D. A., Wilkes, D. S., Skaar, T. C (2009) Pharmacogenet Genomics 19, 464

58. Uyttenhove, C., Pilotte, L., Theate, I., Stroobant, V., Colau, D., Parmentier, N., Boon, T., and Van Den Eynde, B. J. (2003) Nat Med 9, 1269
59. Okamoto, A., Nikaido, T., Ochiai, K., Takakura, S., Saito, M., Aoki, Y., Ishii, N., Yanaihara, N., Yamada, K., Takikawa, O., Kawaguchi, R., Isonishi, S., Tanaka, T., and Urashima, M. (2005) Clin Cancer Res 11, 6030
60. Brandacher, G., Perathoner, A., Ladurner, R., Schneeberger, S., Obrist, P., Winkler, C., Werner, E. R., Werner-Felmayer, G., Weiss, H. G., Gobel, G., Margreiter, R., Konigsrainer, A., Fuchs, D., and Amberger, A. (2006) Clin Cancer Res 12, 1144
61. Wolf, A. M., Wolf, D., Rumpold, H., Moschen, A. R., Kaser, A., Obrist, P., Fuchs, D., Brandacher, G., Winkler, C., Geboes, K., Rutgeerts, P., and Tilg, H. (2004) Clin Immunol 113, 47
62. Pan, K., Wang, H., Chen, M.S., Zhang, H.K., Weng, D.S., Zhou, J., Huang, W., Li, J.J., Song, H.F., Xia, J.C. (2008). J Cancer Res Clin 134, 1247
63. Astigiano, S., Morandi, B., Costa, R., Mastracci, L., D'Agostino, A., Ratto, G. B., Melioli, G., and Frumento, G. (2005) Neoplasia 7, 390
64. Astigiano, S., Morandi, B., Costa, R., Mastracci, L., D'Agostino, A., Ratto, G. B., Melioli, G., and Frumento, G. (2005) Neoplasia 7, 390
65. Munn, D. H., Sharma, M. D., Hou, D., Baban, B., Lee, J. R., Antonia, S. J., Messina, J. L., Chandler, P., Koni, P. A., and Mellor, A. L. (2004) J Clin Invest 114, 280
66. Corm, S., Berthon, C., Imbenotte, M., Biggio, V., Lhermitte, M., Dupont, C., Briche, I., and Quesnel, B. (2009) Leukemia Res 33, 490
67. Curti, A., Pandolfi, S., Valzasina, B., Aluigi, M., Isidori, A., Ferri, E., Salvestrini, V., Bonanno, G., Rutella, S., Durelli, I., Horenstein, A. L., Fiore, F., Massaia, M., Colombo, M. P., Baccarani, M., and Lemoli, R. M. (2007) Blood 109, 2871
68. Witkiewicz, A., Williams, T. K., Cozzitorto, J., Durkan, B., Showalter, S. L., Yeo, C. J., and Brody, J. R. (2008) J Am Coll Surg 206, 849
69. Nakamura, T., Shima, T., Saeki, A., Hidaka, T., Nakashima, A., Takikawa, O., and Saito, S. (2007) Cancer Sci 98, 874
70. Alvaro, T., Lejeune, M., Salvado, M. T., Bosch, R., Garcia, J. F., Jaen, J., Banham, A. H., Roncador, G., Montalban, C., and Piris, M. A. (2005) Clin Cancer Res 11, 1467
71. Badoual, C., Hans, S., Rodriguez, J., Peyrard, S., Klein, C., Agueznay Nel, H., Mosseri, V., Laccourreye, O., Bruneval, P., Fridman, W. H., Brasnu, D. F., and Tartour, E. (2006) Clin Cancer Res 12, 465
72. Ishio, T., Goto, S., Tahara, K., Tone, S., Kawano, K., and Kitano, S. (2004) J Gastroenterol Hepatol 19, 319
73. Ishio, T., Goto, S., Tahara, K., Tone, S., Kawano, K., and Kitano, S. (2004) J Gastroenterol Hepatol 19, 319
74. Zhu, L., Ji, F., Wang, Y., Zhang, Y., Liu, Q., Zhang, J. Z., Matsushima, K., Cao, Q., and Zhang, Y. (2006) J Immunol 177, 8226
75. Ball, H. J., Sanchez-Perez, A., Weiser, S., Austin, C. J., Astelbauer, F., Miu, J., McQuillan, J. A., Stocker, R., Jermiin, L. S., and Hunt, N. H. (2007) Gene 396, 203
76. Murray, M. F. (2007) Curr Drug Metab 8, 197
77. Metz, R., Duhadaway, J. B., Kamasani, U., Laury-Kleintop, L., Muller, A. J., and Prendergast, G. C. (2007) Cancer Res 67, 7082
78. Muller, A. J., Metz, R., and Prendergast G. C. (in press)
79. Fallarino, F., Grohmann, U., Vacca, C., Bianchi, R., Orabona, C., Spreca, A., Fioretti, M. C., and Puccetti, P. (2002) Cell Death Differ 9, 1069
80. Fallarino, F., Grohmann, U., You, S., McGrath, B. C., Cavener, D. R., Vacca, C., Orabona, C., Bianchi, R., Belladonna, M. L., Volpi, C., Santamaria, P., Fioretti, M. C., and Puccetti, P. (2006) J Immunol 176, 6752
81. Munn, D. H., Sharma, M. D., Baban, B., Harding, H. P., Zhang, Y., Ron, D., and Mellor, A. L. (2005) Immunity 22, 633
82. Fallarino, F., Vacca, C., Orabona, C., Belladonna, M. L., Bianchi, R., Marshall, B., Keskin, D. B., Mellor, A. L., Fioretti, M. C., Grohmann, U., and Puccetti, P. (2002) Int Immunol 14, 65

83. Munn, D. H., Sharma, M. D., Baban, B., Harding, H. P., Zhang, Y., Ron, D., and Mellor, A. L. (2005) Immunity 22, 633
84. Metz, R., DuHadaway, J. B., Kamasani, U., Kleintop, L. L., Muller, A. J., and Prendergast, G. C. (2008) Cancer Res 67, 7082
85. Yasui, H., Takai, K., Yoshida, R., and Hayaishi, O. (1986) Proc Natl Acad Sci USA 83, 6622
86. Ozaki, Y., Edelstein, M. P., and Duch, D. S. (1988) Proc Natl Acad Sci USA 85, 1242
87. Carlin, J. M., Borden, E. C., Sondel, P. M., and Byrne, G. I. (1987) J Immunol 139, 2414
88. Carlin, J. M., Borden, E. C., Sondel, P. M., and Byrne, G. I. (1989) J Leukoc Biol 45, 29
89. Hwu, P., Du, M. X., Lapointe, R., Do, M., Taylor, M. W., and Young, H. A. (2000) J Immunol 164, 3596
90. Takikawa, O., Tagawa, Y., Iwakura, Y., Yoshida, R., and Truscott, R. J. (1999) Adv Exp Med Biol 467, 553
91. Du, M. X., Sotero-Esteva, W. D., and Taylor, M. W. (2000) J Interferon Cytokine Res 20, 133
92. Chon, S. Y., Hassanain, H. H., and Gupta, S. L. (1996) J Biol Chem 271, 17247
93. Chon, S. Y., Hassanain, H. H., Pine, R., and Gupta, S. L. (1995) J Interferon Cytokine Res 15, 517
94. Konan, K. V., and Taylor, M. W. (1996) J Biol Chem 271, 19140
95. Robinson, C. M., Hale, P. T., and Carlin, J. M. (2005) J Interferon Cytokine Res 25, 20
96. Pine, R. (1997) Nucleic Acids Res 25, 4346
97. Braun, D., Longman, R. S., and Albert, M. L. (2005) Blood 106, 2375
98. Wobser, M., Voigt, H., Houben, R., Eggert, A. O., Freiwald, M., Kaemmerer, U., Kaempgen, E., Schrama, D., and Becker, J. C. (2007) Cancer Immunol Immunother 56, 1017
99. Sayama, S., Yoshida, R., Oku, T., Imanishi, J., Kishida, T., and Hayaishi, O. (1981) Proc Natl Acad Sci USA 78, 7327
100. Marshall, B., Keskin, D. B., and Mellor, A. L. (2001) BMC Biochem 2, 5
101. Chiarugi, A., Rovida, E., Dello Sbarba, P., and Moroni, F. (2003) J Leukoc Biol 73, 172
102. Alberati-Giani, D., Malherbe, P., Ricciardi-Castagnoli, P., Kohler, C., Denis-Donini, S., and Cesura, A. M. (1997) J Immunol 159, 419
103. Daubener, W., Posdziech, V., Hadding, U., and MacKenzie, C. R. (1999) Med Microbiol Immunol [Berl] 187, 143
104. Thomas, S. R., Mohr, D., and Stocker, R. (1994) J Biol Chem 269, 14457
105. Hucke, C., MacKenzie, C. R., Adjogble, K. D., Takikawa, O., and Daubener, W. (2004) Infect Immun 72, 2723
106. Samelson-Jones, B. J., and Yeh, S. R. (2006) Biochemistry 45, 8527
107. Fallarino, F., Bianchi, R., Orabona, C., Vacca, C., Belladonna, M. L., Fioretti, M. C., Serreze, D. V., Grohmann, U., and Puccetti, P. (2004) J Exp Med 200, 1051
108. Yuan, W., Collado-Hidalgo, A., Yufit, T., Taylor, M., and Varga, J. (1998) J Cell Physiol 177, 174
109. Mellor, A. L., Baban, B., Chandler, P., Marshall, B., Jhaver, K., Hansen, A., Koni, P. A., Iwashima, M., and Munn, D. H. (2003) J Immunol 171, 1652
110. Mellor, A. L., Chandler, P., Baban, B., Hansen, A. M., Marshall, B., Pihkala, J., Waldmann, H., Cobbold, S., Adams, E., and Munn, D. H. (2004) Int Immunol 16, 1391
111. Ghiringhelli, F., Puig, P. E., Roux, S., Parcellier, A., Schmitt, E., Solary, E., Kroemer, G., Martin, F., Chauffert, B., and Zitvogel, L. (2005) J Exp Med 202, 919
112. Liu, Y., Bi, X., Xu, S., and Xiang, J. (2005) Cancer Res 65, 4955
113. Salomon, B., Lenschow, D. J., Rhee, L., Ashourian, N., Singh, B., Sharpe, A., and Bluestone, J. A. (2000) Immunity 12, 431
114. Lohr, J., Knoechel, B., Jiang, S., Sharpe, A. H., and Abbas, A. K. (2003) Nat Immunol 4, 664
115. Lohr, J., Knoechel, B., Kahn, E. C., and Abbas, A. K. (2004) J Immunol 173, 5028
116. Liang, S., Alard, P., Zhao, Y., Parnell, S., Clark, S. L., and Kosiewicz, M. M. (2005) J Exp Med 201, 127

117. Bluestone, J. A., and Abbas, A. K. (2003) Nat Rev Immunol 3, 253
118. Piccirillo, C. A., and Shevach, E. M. (2004) Semin Immunol 16, 81
119. Sakaguchi, S. (2004) Annu Rev Immunol 22, 531
120. Wood, K. J., and Sakaguchi, S. (2003) Nat Rev Immunol 3, 199
121. Aluvihare, V. R., Kallikourdis, M., and Betz, A. G. (2004) Nat Immunol 5, 266
122. Zenclussen, A. C., Gerlof, K., Zenclussen, M. L., Sollwedel, A., Bertoja, A. Z., Ritter, T., Kotsch, K., Leber, J., and Volk, H. D. (2005) Am J Pathol 166, 811
123. Rouse, B. T., and Suvas, S. (2007) Expert Opin Biol Ther 7, 1301
124. Boettler, T., Spangenberg, H. C., Neumann-Haefelin, C., Panther, E., Urbani, S., Ferrari, C., Blum, H. E., von Weizsacker, F., and Thimme, R. (2005) J Virol 79, 7860
125. Andersson, J., Boasso, A., Nilsson, J., Zhang, R., Shire, N. J., Lindback, S., Shearer, G. M., and Chougnet, C. A. (2005) J Immunol 174, 3143
126. Hryniewicz, A., Boasso, A., Edghill-Smith, Y., Vaccari, M., Fuchs, D., Venzon, D., Nacsa, J., Betts, M. R., Tsai, W. P., Heraud, J. M., Beer, B., Blanset, D., Chougnet, C., Lowy, I., Shearer, G. M., and Franchini, G. (2006) Blood 108, 3834
127. Fallarino, F., Grohmann, U., Hwang, K. W., Orabona, C., Vacca, C., Bianchi, R., Belladonna, M. L., Fioretti, M. C., Alegre, M. L., and Puccetti, P. (2003) Nat Immunol 4, 1206
128. Grohmann, U., Orabona, C., Fallarino, F., Vacca, C., Calcinaro, F., Falorni, A., Candeloro, P., Belladonna, M. L., Bianchi, R., Fioretti, M. C., and Puccetti, P. (2002) Nat Immunol 3, 1097
129. Munn, D. H., Sharma, M. D., Lee, J. R., Jhaver, K. G., Johnson, T. S., Keskin, D. B., Marshall, B., Chandler, P., Antonia, S. J., Burgess, R., Slingluff, C. L. J. r., and A. L. Mellor. (2002) Science 297, 1867
130. Grohmann, U., Fallarino, F., and Puccetti, P. (2003) Trends Immunol 24, 242
131. Mellor, A. L., and Munn, D. H. (2003) J Immunol 170, 5809
132. Terness, P., Chuang, J. J., and Opelz, G. (2006) Trends Immunol 27, 68
133. Sharpe, A. H., and Freeman, G. J. (2002) Nat Rev Immunol 2, 116
134. Waterhouse, P., Penninger, J. M., Timms, E., Wakeham, A., Shahinian, A., Lee, K. P., Thompson, C. B., Griesser, H., and Mak, T. W. (1995) Science 270, 985
135. Tivol, E. A., Borriello, F., Schweitzer, A. N., Lynch, W. P., Bluestone, J. A., and Sharpe, A. H. (1995) Immunity 3, 541
136. Karandikar, N. J., Vanderlugt, C. L., Bluestone, J. A., and Miller, S. D. (1998) J Neuroimmunol 89, 10
137. Grohmann, U., Bianchi, R., Belladonna, M. L., Vacca, C., Silla, S., Ayroldi, E., Fioretti, M. C., and Puccetti, P. (1999) J Immunol 163, 3100
138. Grohmann, U., Bianchi, R., Belladonna, M. L., Silla, S., Fallarino, F., Fioretti, M. C., and Puccetti, P. (2000) J Immunol 165, 1357
139. Grohmann, U., Fallarino, F., Silla, S., Bianchi, R., Belladonna, M. L., Vacca, C., Micheletti, A., Fioretti, M. C., and Puccetti, P. (2001) J Immunol 166, 277
140. Grohmann, U., Bianchi, R., Orabona, C., Fallarino, F., Vacca, C., Micheletti, A., Fioretti, M. C., and Puccetti, P. (2003) J Immunol 171, 2581
141. Orabona, C., Grohmann, U., Belladonna, M. L., Fallarino, F., Vacca, C., Bianchi, R., Bozza, S., Volpi, C., Salomon, B. L., Fioretti, M. C., Romani, L., and Puccetti, P. (2004) Nat Immunol 5, 1134
142. Sharpe, A. H., and Abbas, A. K. (2006) N Engl J Med 355, 973
143. Orabona, C., Puccetti, P., Vacca, C., Bicciato, S., Luchini, A., Fallarino, F., Bianchi, R., Velardi, E., Perruccio, K., Velardi, A., Bronte, V., Fioretti, M. C., and Grohmann, U. (2005) Blood 107, 2846
144. Orabona, C., Belladonna, M. L., Vacca, C., Bianchi, R., Fallarino, F., Volpi, C., Gizzi, S., Fioretti, M. C., Grohmann, U., and Puccetti, P. (2005) J Immunol 174, 6582
145. Orabona, C., Tomasello, E., Fallarino, F., Bianchi, R., Volpi, C., Bellocchio, S., Romani, L., Fioretti, M. C., Vivier, E., Puccetti, P., and Grohmann, U. (2005) Eur J Immunol 35, 3111
146. Mantovani, A., Sozzani, S., Locati, M., Allavena, P., and Sica, A. (2002) Trends Immunol 23, 549

147. Sinha, P., Clements, V., and Ostrand-Rosenberg, S. (2005) J Immunol 174, 636
148. Munn, D. H., Shafizadeh, E., Attwood, J. T., Bondarev, I., Pashine, A., and Mellor, A. L. (1999) J Exp Med 189, 1363
149. Hwang, S. L., Chung, N. P., Chan, J. K., and Lin, C. L. (2005) Cell Res 15, 167
150. Muller, A. J., Malachowski, W. P., and Prendergast, G. C. (2005) Expert Opin Ther Targets 9, 831
151. Kirkwood, J. M., Tarhini, A. A., Panelli, M. C., Moschos, S. J., Zarour, H. M., Butterfield, L. H., and Gogas, H. J. (2008) J Clin Oncol 26, 3445
152. Faries, M. B. M., Donald, L. (2005) BioDrugs 19, 247
153. Cheever, M. A. (2008) Immunol Rev 222, 357
154. de Faudeur, G., de Trez, C., Muraille, E., and Leo, O. (2008) Immunol Lett 118, 21
155. Friberg, M., Jennings, R., Alsarraj, M., Dessureault, S., Cantor, A., Extermann, M., Mellor, A. L., Munn, D. H., and Antonia, S. J. (2002) Int J Cancer 101, 151
156. Muller, A. J., Duhadaway, J. B., Donover, P. S., Sutanto-Ward, E., and Prendergast, G. C. (2005) Nat Med 11, 312
157. Hou, D. Y., Muller, A. J., Sharma, M. D., DuHadaway, J., Banerjee, T., Johnson, M., Mellor, A. L., Prendergast, G. C., and Munn, D. H. (2007) Cancer Res 67, 792
158. Banerjee, T., Duhadaway, J. B., Gaspari, P., Sutanto-Ward, E., Munn, D. H., Mellor, A. L., Malachowski, W. P., Prendergast, G. C., and Muller, A. J. (2008) Oncogene 27, 2851
159. Carr, G., Chung, M. K., Mauk, A. G., and Andersen, R. J. (2008) J Med Chem 51, 2634
160. Kumar, S., Jaller, D., Patel, B., Lalonde, J. M., Duhadaway, J. B., Malachowski, W. P., Prendergast, G. C., and Muller, A. J. (2008) J Med Chem 51, 4968
161. Kumar, S., Malachowski, W. P., DuHadaway, J. B., LaLonde, J. M., Carroll, P. J., Jaller, D., Metz, R., Prendergast, G. C., and Muller, A. J. (2008) J Med Chem 51, 1706
162. Muller, A. J., and Prendergast, G. C. (2007) Curr Cancer Drug Targets 7, 31
163. Gaspari, P., Banerjee, T., Malachowski, W. P., Muller, A. J., Prendergast, G. C., DuHadaway, J., Bennett, S., and Donovan, A. M. (2006) J Med Chem 49, 684
164. Banerjee, T., DuHadaway, J. B., Gaspari, P., Sutanto-Ward, E., Munn, D. H., Mellor, A. L., Malachowski, W. P., Prendergast, G. C., and Muller, A. J. (2008) Oncogene 27, 2851
165. Park, E. J., and Pezzuto, J. M. (2002) Cancer Metastasis Rev 21, 231
166. Mehta, R. G., Liu, J., Constantinou, A., Thomas, C. F., Hawthorne, M., You, M., Gerhuser, C., Pezzuto, J. M., Moon, R. C., and Moriarty, R. M. (1995) Carcinogenesis 16, 399
167. Baban, B., Chandler, P., McCool, D., Marshall, B., Munn, D. H., and Mellor, A. L. (2004) J Reprod Immunol 61, 67

Adoptive Transfer of T-Bodies: Toward an Effective Cancer Immunotherapy

Dinorah Friedmann-Morvinski and Zelig Eshhar

Abstract Adoptive immunotherapy is a valid treatment for cancer and has been widely practiced in the clinic using antitumor antibodies. Application of the cellular arm of the immune response, although more efficient, has not yet found its way for cancer treatment. The main cause for this lag is scarcity of tumor specific T cells and difficulty to obtain such functional cells from cancer patients. The "T-body" approach that we have pioneered has been designed to provide answers to these issues. T-bodies are T cells expressing a chimeric receptor composed of an antibody derived antigen recognizing unit in the form of single chain domain linked through extracellular hinge and transmembrane stretches to the cytoplasmic domains of costimulatory and stimulatory molecules. As such the engineered T-body's design takes advantage and combine the specificity and availability of antitumor antibodies with the efficient effector function of T cells. In practice, T-bodies can be prepared from peripheral blood of any cancer patient, engineered ex-vivo to express the chimeric receptor gene on their surface and reinfused back to the patient where it should migrate and accumulate at the tumor site, will undergo specific activation by the tumor antigen and cause selective elimination of the cancer. In this chapter, we describe the preparation of optimal chimeric constructs and ways to safely introduce the chimeric receptor genes to T cells. Most of the research was performed so far in animal models where it showed impressive effects, including complete responses to a large range of cancers. On the basis of this proof of concept many T-bodies have been prepared to human cancers, several of which are being tested for safety in phase I clinical trials.

Z. Eshhar (✉)
Department of Immunology, The Weizmann Institute of Science, Rehovot 76100, Israel
e-mail: zelig.eshhar@weizmann.ac.il

J. Lustgarten et al. (eds.), *Targeted Cancer Immune Therapy*,
DOI 10.1007/978-1-4419-0170-5_16,

Introduction

Cancer patients usually mount a poor, if at all, immune response against their own tumors because of the following reasons: (1) low or absent expression of tumor-specific antigens; (2) expression of antigens that are shared with normal cells at certain developmental stages, so that the immune system becomes self-tolerant or anergic; (3) escape from immune attack by down-regulation of surface expression of MHC molecules; (4) defective pathways of antigen processing and presentation; (5) absence of appropriate costimulation to deliver a complete activation stimulus to effector T-cells; (6) the presence of inhibitory molecules actively secreted by the tumor microenvironment (such as interlukin-10 and transforming growth factor-β) [1]; and (7) the expansion of naturally occurring or tumor-induced T cells with regulatory activity [2, 3]. Several approaches have been attempted to enable the immune eradication of tumor cells. These include various methodologies to augment, nonspecifically or specifically, the host immune response and treatment with specific antitumor antibodies. Nonspecific treatments, such as the use of lymphokine-activated killer (LAK) cells, are not effective in all types of cancer. The requirement for the coinjection of large amounts of IL-2 causes severe side effects, which often require the cessation of treatment. The use of antibodies in passive immunotherapy is often of limited efficacy both because of the difficulty in identifying true tumor-specific antigens, poor tumor penetration, and the short half-life of the antibodies.

A promising method developed for the immunotherapy of cancer that has proven beneficial for certain myeloma patients [4] is to remove lymphocytes from tumors, expand them ex vivo in the presence of lymphokines, and reinfuse these cells into the patient. Treatment of cancer by the infusion of such autologous tumor infiltrating lymphocytes (TIL) is patient-specific, but is inefficient because of the difficulty in obtaining sufficient numbers of functional TIL from each myeloma patient. Moreover, for many histological types of cancer, the T cell receptor (TCR)/HLA-peptide tumor target are not known. To overcome these limitations Rosenberg and colleagues have succeeded recently to confer antitumor specificity on the patient's T cells by transducting them with cDNA encoding the α and β TCR chains specific to a given HLA-peptide [5, 6]. Such manipulation has produced clinical responses in some patients; however, due to the rarity of tumor-specific T cells against the antigen found in these tumors, this approach cannot provide a general solution to most cancers. In contrast, many monoclonal antibodies have been described that bind tumor-associated antigens shared by tumors of similar histology (e.g., anti-HER2(anti-erbB2) antibodies), which are being used for the treatment of a broad spectrum of patients regardless of their HLA haplotype [7]. However, although beneficial in the treatment of vascularized, blood borne tumors (e.g., lymphomas), most clinical attempts using antibodies or immunotoxins made of such antibodies have not fulfilled expectations in the treatment of solid tumors mainly because such tumors are not sufficiently accessible to antibodies.

To take advantage of the availability of antitumor antibodies and the efficient tissue rejection of T cells, our group has pioneered the "T-body" approach, a novel

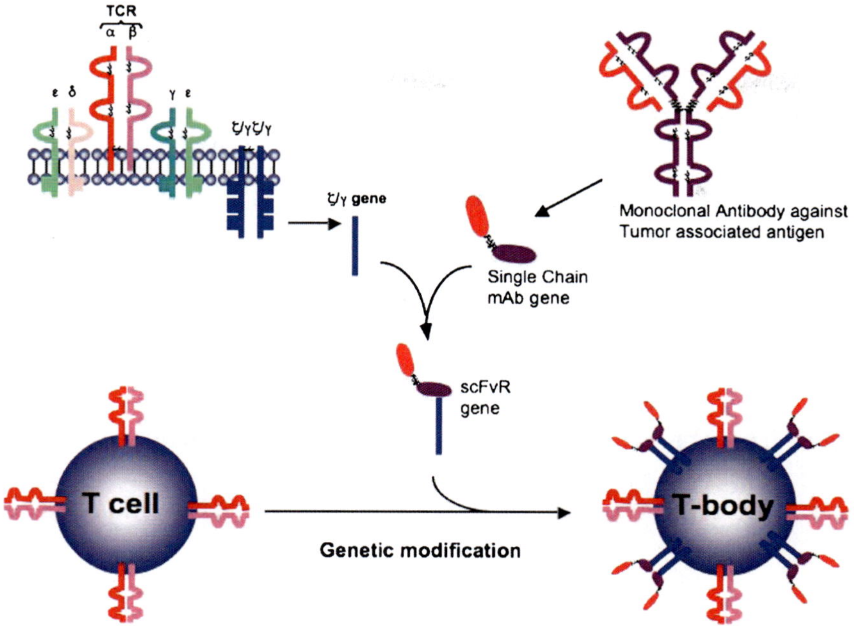

Fig. 1 General design and composition of the scFv-based chimeric receptor

approach for adoptive cancer therapy. We have joined these two approaches of adoptive immunotherapy and immunotoxin therapy to genetically engineer an improved immunocytolysin, which is an antibody recognition unit in the form of single chain variable (scFv) region attached to a cytotoxic T cell signaling molecule (Fig. 1). The first configuration of an antibody-based chimeric receptor (CR) composed of the two TCRs α and β chains in which each pair of TCR Vα and Vβ domains was replaced with a pair of V_H and V_L derived from a given antibody. These two genes were then cotransfected into T cell-lines and were found to confer to them antibody specificity [8]. This first CR design demonstrated that T cells can be activated and kill their target in an MHC nonrestricted and independent manner (for review see [9]).

In our second generation of CR, rather than using two CR chains, we developed the single chain configuration of the CR to obtain a receptor molecule that would be useful for cancer therapy. In this configuration, a single chain Fv (scFv) of an antibody is linked through an extracellular linker to transmembrane and cytoplasmic domains of lymphocyte triggering moieties such as the TCR/CD3 complex-associated ζ chain, or Fc receptor γ chain [10]. To space the scFV recognition unit from the cell surface and to allow flexibility, a hinge domain of various molecules of the immunoglobulin gene family have been added to link the scFv with the transmembrane part of the intracellular stimulatory chains (see scheme in Fig. 1). This single chain configuration, which combines antibody recognition and T cell signaling in a single continuous protein, is composed of modular structural and functional domains that are simple to manipulate, and can be readily expressed in human lymphocytes using retroviral-based vectors [11].

Today, redirection of the specificity of effector lymphocytes using single-chain CR is becoming a feasible option for adoptive cancer therapy. Many groups have adapted the "T-body" approach to endow T cells with various specificities and functions, increasing the applicability of this type of treatment [9, 12, 13]. Here we shall focus on the potential application of the CR approach for cancer therapy and will discuss the various challenges of this approach in hopes to realize its potential.

Use of Engineered T Cells for Cancer Immunotherapy

To enhance a desirable function of T cell following to their adoptive transfer, they can be engineered by means of gene transfer, for example:

1. To increase the reactivity of T cells to weak or poorly presented antigens, such as those expressed by tumor cells, usage of scFv of higher affinity could be selected
2. To favor survival of T cells even in a hostile tumor microenvironment, T cells can be equipped with antiapoptotic stimulating activity such as adding costimulatory domains to the CR
3. To provide a mechanism whereby unwanted proliferation or activity of modified T cells can be controlled, a suicide gene that will activate ectopic supply of regulatory agents could be inserted

Optimization of the Chimeric Receptor Function

To serve as a cancer-specific therapeutic agent able to eliminate the large mass of cells in solid tumors, the T-body receptor must optimally discriminate the tumor from healthy tissue. Following its systemic administration to the patient, the T-body should migrate to the tumor site, interact with the tumor cell, undergo activation, and execute its effector function, culminating in cancer elimination. Optimal performance of this series of events is dependent on predefined, intrinsic properties of the transfected T cell that are triggered and regulated by the chimeric receptor, and are dependent on its composition. The process of tumor rejection, similar to tissue rejection, is a complex one that requires both CD8 and CD4 cells that can mediate direct target cell killing and induce a local inflammatory response. Optimization of the CR activity can be achieved by modifying several features of the extracellular recognition unit, the scFv and by the activation and costimulatory sequences in its intracellular domain.

Optimal Recognition of Tumor Antigens

Apparently, a single chimeric receptor that interacts with its target antigen at high enough affinity can trigger the activation of both CD8 and CD4 T cells in which it is expressed. Nevertheless, for certain applications and specific targets, fine-tuning of the CR recognition can be achieved by the selection of scFv whose binding to the desired target antigen on the cancer cells will be optimal. Most of the cancer antigens toward which therapeutic antibodies are directed today are also expressed to some extent on healthy tissue. What makes these tumor-associated antigens (TAA) targets for the T-body approach is either quantitative (i.e., over expression on the tumor vs. the healthy tissue (e.g., erbB2)), mode of exposure (i.e., antigens that change their topological expression in the tumor in a way that make them exposed to T-cells (e.g., MUC-1 that is apical in healthy tissue and becomes exposed on all surfaces in adenocarcinomas), antigens that appear in embryonic tissues and disappear in the adult (e.g., CEA), and finally antigens that are expressed on the surface of malignant cells as well as on regenerating healthy tissues (such as hematopoietic cells which are being destroyed as well as their malignant cells by anti-CD20 antibodies). Another issue is the secretion or shading of tumor antigens into the body fluids of patients in concentrations that may block the binding of the scFv to their desired targets. Collectively, all these variables led to the realization that the strength of binding of the scFv to its target antigen (affinity) and the level of expression of cell bound or free TAA as well as this of the CR on the effector cell (avidity) are very important to the outcome of the interaction between the tumor target cell and the redirected effector T cell. Several studies have been carried out to find out the rules that govern this crucial issue using either defined chemical antigens [14] or TAA [15]. By-and-large, these data have taught us that there is a dynamic equilibrium between the affinity of the antibody-based chimeric receptor and the density of the target antigen on the tumor cell. There is a quite a broad range of avidities where a fruitful (i.e., cancer killing) situation will occur. However in the extremities, i.e., at low levels of target antigen, higher avidity interactions are required and for a low density of CR on the effector cell surface, higher levels of antigen is needed for efficient stimulation.

In practical terms, this information teaches us that T-bodies made of scFv of too high affinity is neither required nor beneficial: the resulting T-bodies will kill also healthy T-cells having low level of the TAA and will be also more vulnerable to inhibition by lower doses of circulating antigen. In addition, since the actual target cell killing is performed by recycling CTL, high affinity interactions will keep the CR occupied with the dead or dying target cell and will make the rejection process less efficient, by modifying several features of the scFv mainly the activation and costimulatory sequences in its intracellular domain.

Combining Costimulatory and Stimulatory Signals

For optimal and sustained function of T cells, their development into memory cells and their reactivation, especially by targets lacking the ligands for costimulatory molecules (which are missing on many tumor cells and assist their escape of the immune attack), an added costimulatory signal is advantageous. It has been shown that CR that lack the capacity to provide costimulatory signaling cannot activate resting or naïve lymphocytes, such as T cells derived from genetically modified stem-cells or from CR transgenic mice [16]. It is also well established that, in the absence of costimulatory signaling by CD28, resting T lymphocytes typically undergo anergy or apoptosis [17].

These obstacles have been resolved by constructing CR in which the scFv is linked to the intracellular part of CD28 or other costimulatory molecules such as OX40 (CD134), CD40L, PD-1, or 4-1BB (CD137) [18, 19]. The effect of these costimulatory domains in the context of the CR was compared in unstimulated human CD4 and CD8 T cells and was found that cytokine release and killing activity in response to target cells was dramatically enhanced by all the costimulatory sequences relative to the CR that did not contain any costimulatory signaling moieties. No practical advantage was demonstrated by ICOS, OX40, or 4-1BB over the CD28-based tripartite CR (TPCR). We designed a novel TPCR composed of a scFv recognition moiety, fused to the nonligand binding part of the extracellular and the entire transmembrane and intracellular domains of the CD28 costimulatory molecule, together with the intracellular domain of FcRγ (scFv-CD28-γ). Human PBL transduced with such a CR gene demonstrate specific stimulation of IL-2 production and target cell killing [11]. Many studies, from different groups, have demonstrated that out of the costimulatory domains, CD28 performed most effectively in various experimental settings [13, 20–24] to enhance tumor rejection in mouse models using human and murine T cells [25–28]. To prove the ultimate requirement of CD28 for antigen-specific activation and development of mature naïve T cells, we have recently generated several lines of transgenic mice expressing CR under the control of T cell-specific regulatory sequences. Unprimed, naïve T lymphocytes from mice transgenic for scFv-CD28-γ TPCR undergo high levels of proliferation, IL-2 secretion, and rescue from apoptosis following stimulation by plastic-bound cognate antigen [29]. The rescue from apoptosis by CD28 in the context of T cells stimulation through the antigen-specific CR is an important factor in the persistence of the T-bodies in the patient where there is the risk of antigen induced cell death in the absence of B7 on the surface of the tumor target cell. Additional advantage is the recent finding that CD28 costimulation overcomes transforming growth factor (TGF)-β-mediated repression of proliferation of redirected human $CD4^+$ and $CD8^+$ T cells in an anti-tumor cell attack [30]. TGF-β is known for its immunosuppressive activity that is produced by regulatory T cells and some tumors. Along this line is the finding that the inclusion of CD28 to the CR enhances chimeric T cell resistance to Treg [31].

As to the use of 4-1BB signaling domain in the context of the CR, it was found to elicit potent cytotoxicity against acute lymphoblastic leukemia cells in vitro [32].

Another interesting costimulatory molecule is CD27. Engagement of CD27 can also augment TCR-induced T cell proliferation and is required for the generation and maintenance of memory T cells in vivo [33, 34]. The administration of soluble

CD27 ligand, CD70, augmented in vivo $CD8^+$ T cell responses to viral infection and tumor challenge by increasing the expansion and maintenance of the antigen-specific T cell population, indicating that CD27 expression is not only a marker of less-differentiated T cells, but also functionally crucial for optimal immune responses [35]. In the clinics, after adoptive transfer, the frequency of TILs expressing CD27 gradually increased and was associated with the long-term maintenance of stable numbers of tumor-specific T cells in responding patients [36]. Altogether, these results predict that T cells that express CD27 selectively persist in vivo, giving rise to a stable population of memory CD8 + T cells [36, 37].

Although the performance of CD28 appears quite satisfactory both in vitro and in vivo, the inclusion of additional or alternative moieties, or combinations of costimulatory domains have been recently suggested to sustain and optimize the anticancer effect of T-bodies in vivo. The group of Sadelain has shown that primary human T cells expressing CD80 and 4-1BB ligand (4-1BBL) vigorously respond to tumor cells lacking costimulatory ligands and provoke potent rejection of large, systemic tumors in immunodeficient mice. In addition to showing costimulation of bystander T cells (transcostimulation), we show the effect of CD80 and 4-1BBL binding to their respective receptors in the immunological synapse of isolated single cells (autocostimulation) [38].T cell-encoded CD80 and 4-1BBL induce auto and transcostimulation, resulting in potent tumor rejection.

Another recent study that demonstrated the advantages of fused costimulatory domains derived from CD28 and OX40 intracellular domains used MUC-1 specific CR. Interestingly, this TPCR targeting a complex glycoprotein on the cell surface of many adenocarcinomas, needed to be extended from the cell surface by an extended hinge linker made of IgD-derived hinge [39].

Signaling Domains

In contrast to the costimulatory moieties, only a few stimulatory domains have been used in the TPCR context. The original studies used both the CD3ζ and FcRγ subunits [10] and one group used the CD3ε domain [40]. All these domains signal through the immune T cell activation motifs (ITAM) that contain a tyrosine, which undergoes phosphorylation as a result of the interaction of the TCR with antigen presenting cells. The phosphorylated ITAM facilitates docking of down stream kinases (such as ZAP70 and Syk) that are involved in signal transduction. FcRγ and CD3ε contain a single ITAM, while CD3ζ contains three such motifs. No comprehensive comparison has been done so far to identify the most active domain in the context of the CR. We prefer the FcRγ, based on early studies showing that phosphorylation of the first ITAM of the CD3ζ leads to anergy [41]. Despite the lack of consensus, we have tried to bypass signaling through the ITAM that is often impaired in T lymphocytes of tumor-bearing patients [42]. In a series of studies, we found that using the Syk cytoplasmic phosphotyrosine kinase as the signaling domain of the CR instead of an ITAM-containing signaling chain can efficiently induce T cell activation [43].

Increasing the Survival and Efficacy of the T-Bodies

Although it seems counter-intuitive that the efficacy of adoptive transfer T-body-based tumor immunotherapy can be improved by the removal of the host's immune system, several mechanisms might underlie the augmented efficacy of tumor-reactive T cells in the lymphopaenic environment. These factors include the elimination of immunosuppressive cells such as $CD4^+$ $CD25^+$ regulatory T (Treg) cells, the depletion of endogenous cells that compete for activating/growth cytokines, and the increased function and availability of natural or artificial antigen-presenting cells (APCs).

Elimination of Immunosuppressive Cells

Naturally occurring regulatory T cells are emerging as key regulators of immune responses to self-tissues and infectious agents as well as suppressors of antitumor responses. The discovery that $CD4^+$ $CD25^+$ Tregs expressed the transcription factor forkhead box P3 (Foxp3) gave credence to the notion that regulatory T cells represented a distinct T cell lineage [44–47]. Mouse Treg cells also express the glucocorticoid-induced tumor-necrosis factor (TNF)-receptor-related-protein (GITR) and cytotoxic T-lymphocyte-associated antigen 4 (CTLA-4) [48]. However, exclusive molecular signatures for human Treg cells do not currently exist because activation of $CD4^+$ T cells can also result in upregulation of Foxp3 expression [49]. Experiments using mice lacking Treg cells, owing to specific gene defects, as well as the "add-back" of these cells, have convincingly shown that they suppress the antitumor activities of adoptive transferred tumor-reactive T cells [50].

At present, no conclusive data link the in vivo function of Treg cell and the progression of cancer. Nevertheless, the suppressive effects of Treg cells might contribute to the poor clinical outcome reported in patients with cancer who receive immunotherapy in nonlymphodepleting settings. Selective elimination of Treg cells might further improve the efficacy of adoptively transferred T-bodies in the lymphodepleting setting, because Treg cell proliferation can be increased by the lymphopaenic environment and the presence of exogenous IL-2 [51, 52]. Although Treg depletion was demonstrated useful in murine system prior to antitumor treatment (active vaccination or adoptive cell transfer) [50, 53] none of these means have been practiced or approved in clinical setting. So far, the lymphodepletion protocols, given before the adoptive transfer of genetically engineered T cells (two days of cyclophosphamide (60 mg/kg) and 5 days of fludarabine (25 mg/m^2) [5]) are sufficient to eliminate Treg. Another approach is to render the T-bodies insensitive to the suppressive effects of the Treg cytokines TGF-β and IL-10. This can be achieved by coexpression, concomitantly to the TPCR, of siRNA's to these cytokine receptors or their down stream molecules (e.g., Smad for TGF-β [54] and STAT-3 and or Jak for IL-10 [55].

Minimizing the Competition for Homeostatic Cytokines

Transfer of small amounts of antigen-specific T cells into a lymphopaenic host results in the expansion and activation of the transferred T cell population, a process that is known as homeostatic proliferation [56–58]. Although host-mediated inhibition of the proliferation of adoptively transferred T cells might involve direct cellular contact, competition might also exist between transferred and host T cells for a limited amount of the cytokines that are required to support $CD8^+$ T cell homeostasis, such competition is known as the "cytokine sink" effect [59].

The importance of the availability of these cytokines has been shown in experiments in which mice deficient for IL-7 or IL-15 showed impaired homeostatic maintenance and proliferation of memory T cell population [60, 61]. Conversely, transgenic mice overexpressing IL-7 or IL-15 have increased numbers of the memory T cell population [60, 61].

IL-2 is a T cell growth factor that is commonly used to promote the expansion and function of tumor-specific T cells populations in vitro and in vivo [62]. Perhaps more importantly, IL-2 is essential for the maintenance of peripheral self-tolerance [63]. Recently it has been shown that IL-2 is important for Treg suppressive function [64]. Therefore, removal of Treg cells by lymphodepletion might result in increased antitumor reactivity of adoptively transferred T cells, not only by the elimination of direct cellular inhibition but also through increased availability of IL-2.

Improved Availability of APC and Their Function

Systemic chemotherapy and total body irradiation have both been used prior to adoptive transfer to deplete the lymphoid (including Treg) compartment of the host and make a niche for the transferred cells. Although lymphodepletion can reduce the absolute number of APCs in vivo, it can also promote their transition to an activated state [65, 66]. Activation of dendritic cells (DCs) after chemotherapy or radiotherapy might be triggered by translocation of bacterial products, such as lipopolysaccharide (LPS) and other Toll-like receptor (TRL) agonists, into the blood following damage to the integrity of mucosal barriers [67]. The production of proinflammatory cytokines such as TNF, IL-1, and IL-4 by host cells might also be involved in mediating DC maturation [65, 67–70]. In addition, lymphodepletion can also favor the transferred tumor-reactive T-bodies through decreased competition at the surface of antigen-bearing APCs. Although the effect of lymphodepletion is not as clear as in the case of Treg elimination and generation of cytokine sinks, ablation might ultimately increase the antitumor reactivity of the transferred T cells by increasing the activation and availability of APCs.

Optimizing the Safety of the Transferred T-Bodies

To enhance the safety of adoptive T-body immunotherapy, genetic strategies have been developed that enable the specific elimination of the transferred T cells and thereby control undesired T cell activity. The most common strategy relies on the inclusion of a suicide gene, which should permit elimination of genetically modified T cells upon treatment with a drug. The modification of lymphocytes with a suicide gene was first evaluated as a means of preventing graft-versus-host disease (GVHD) in patients treated with donor lymphocyte transfusions following allogeneic stem cell transplantation. The most extensively studied system is the HSV-tk suicide gene. Expression in T cells of HSV-tk confers sensitivity to the prodrug ganciclovir providing an effective means to delete the transferred cells [71]. One problem with this system is that gene product of the suicide gene is highly immunogenic and may induce immune-mediated rejection of the transduced cells. Less immunogenic suicide and selection marker genes, preferable of human origin, may reduce the immunological inactivation of genetically modified donor lymphocytes.

Another example is the use of endogenous proapoptotic molecules such as the inducible caspase-9 (iCasp-9) suicide gene. This proapoptotic gene product is activated after exposure to a small chemical inducer of dimerization (CID, AP20187), which is an analog of FK506 that has been safely tested in a phase I study [72].

Transduction of Human T Cells: Generation of T-Bodies Toward Clinical Applications

T Cell Differentiation State

Emerging findings from both mouse studies and clinical trials indicated that intrinsic properties related to the differentiation state of adoptively transferred T cell populations are crucial to the success of the T-body-based approaches.

In a study conducted by Gattinoni et al. [73] using the pmel-1 transgenic mice, the $CD8^+$ T cells that acquired terminal effector properties and had increased antitumor activity in vitro were found to be less effective at triggering tumor regression in vivo. Terminally differentiated $CD8^+$ T cells were nearly 100-fold less effective in vivo on a per-cell basis that T cells at an early stage of differentiation. Other groups, using different mouse tumor models reported similar findings [74, 75]. Once the $CD8^+$ T cells become differentiated the resulting phenotypic and functional changes makes them less "fit" to mediate antitumor responses and less able to benefit from the activating triggers in the lymphopaenic host. For example, less-differentiated, central-memory-like T cells have a higher proliferative potential, are less prone to apoptosis than more differentiated cells, and have a response better to homeostatic cytokines, because they express receptors such as the IL-7 receptor α-chain (IL-7Rα).

The same situation was observed in the clinic where T cell clones used for therapy were highly avid and showed potent tumor-specific responses in vitro, but they did not persist after infusion, indicating that they were in a state of terminal differentiation [76, 77].

Expanding the Modified T Cell Populations

So far, the only vector approved for clinical trials using cancer patients' T cells are retrovectors [78]. To genetically modify the T cells to become T-bodies, the cells need to be activated with CD3 and CD28-specific antibodies for retroviral transduction and then expanded before reinfusion into the patient, usually in the presence of IL-2 (Fig. 2). This procedure already results in the differentiation of $CD8^+$ T cells to an intermediate and late effector state. Limiting the in vitro expansion phase to a short duration might markedly improve the "quality" of the transferred T-bodies. The question remains, however, whether this improved "quality" or "fitness" can compensate for the reduced number of cells generated soon after activation. IL-2 has been shown to be an effective T cell growth factor but has undesirable effects, including the ability to decrease the expression of lymph-node homing molecules (e.g., CD62L) and to promote the terminal differentiation of T cells, predisposing

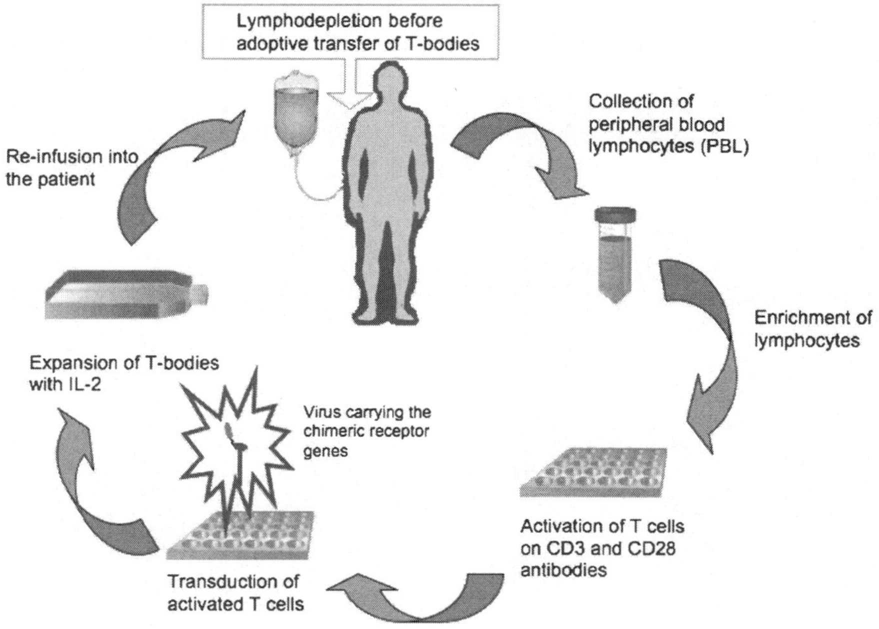

Fig. 2 The process of preparation of T-bodies for clinical application

them to activation-induced cell death [73, 79]. Other cytokines that signal through a receptor that contains γ chain, such as IL-15, IL-7, and IL-21 support the growth of T cells and have a less detrimental effect on differentiation and antitumor effect in vivo [59].

Summary and Conclusions

Genetic engineering is a powerful strategy to design tumor-associated antigen-specific T cells for immunotherapy of cancer. We have at our disposal a repertoire of diverse antitumor antibodies some of which are humanized or of human origin which have been proven safe in the clinic. We have in hand chimeric receptor configurations that delivers combined stimulatory and costimulatory signals to fully activate the effector function of T cells. These chimeric receptors can be quite efficiently, stably, and safely expressed in CD8, CD4, and NK cells, which in turn can be propagated to large quantities of functional cells. We learned how to maintain the functional properties of these cells for prolonged periods by preconditioning the patients and the use of homeostatic lymphokines to maintain the delivered cells long enough to allow them to reach their tumor target and completely eliminate it. Preclinical and clinical studies have identified multiple mechanisms contributing to successful adoptive immunotherapies, including host-related factors, as well as the phenotypic and functional characteristics of the T-bodies used for transfer.

Taken together, experiments in animal models have provided a quite substantial proof of concept that the T-body approach that expands the spectrum of diseases to which adoptive cellular immunotherapy is ready to be applied to the clinic. Several phase I and phase II clinical trials are on going or in advanced phase toward their applications in patients of a wide spectrum of cancers. We hope these trials will prove safe and pave the way for further trials that will establish the T-body approach as valid treatment for cancer therapy.

References

1. Jutel, M., Akdis, M., Blaser, K., and Akdis, C. A. (2006) Allergy 61, 796
2. Wang, R. F. (2006) Semin Cancer Biol 16, 106
3. Zou, W., (2006) Nat Rev Immunol 6, 295
4. Dudley, M. E., and Rosenberg, S. A. (2007) Semin Oncol 34, 524
5. Morgan, R. A., Dudley, M. E., Wunderlich, J. R., Hughes, M. S., Yang, J. C., Sherry, R. M., Royal, R. E., Topalian, S. L., Kammula, U. S., Restifo, N. P., Zheng, Z., Nahvi, A., de Vries, C. R., Rogers-Freezer, L. J., Mavroukakis, S. A., and Rosenberg, S. A. (2006) Science 314, 126
6. Rosenberg, S. A., Restifo, N. P., Yang, J. C., Morgan, R. A., and Dudley, M. E. (2008) Nat Rev Cancer 8, 299
7. Heimann, D. M., and Weiner, L. M. (2007) Surg Oncol Clin N Am 16, 775
8. Gross, G., Waks, T., and Eshhar, Z. (1989) Proc Natl Acad Sci USA 86, 10024
9. Gross, G., and Eshhar, Z. (1992) Faseb J 6, 3370

10. Eshhar, Z., Waks, T., Gross, G., and Schindler, D. G. (1993) Proc Natl Acad Sci USA 90, 720
11. Eshhar, Z., Waks, T., Bendavid, A., and Schindler, D. G. (2001) J Immunol Methods 248, 67
12. Baxevanis, C. N., and Papamichail, M. (2004) Cancer Immunol Immunother 53, 893
13. Willemsen, R. A., Debets, R., Chames, P., and Bolhuis, R. L. (2003) Hum Immunol 64, 56
14. Alvarez-Vallina, L., Agha-Mohammadi, S., Hawkins, R. E., and Russell, S. J. (1997) J Immunol 159, 5889
15. Chmielewski, M., Hombach, A., Heuser, C., Adams, G. P., and Abken, H. (2004) J Immunol 173, 7647
16. Brocker, T., and Karjalainen, K. (1995) J Exp Med 181, 1653
17. Boussiotis, V. A., Freeman, G. J., Gribben, J. G., and Nadler, L. M. (1995) Res Immunol 146, 140
18. Finney, H. M., Akbar, A. N., and Lawson, A. D. (2004) J Immunol 172, 104
19. Finney, H. M., Lawson, A. D., Bebbington, C. R., and Weir, A. N. (1998) J Immunol 161, 2791
20. Gong, M. C., Latouche, J. B., Krause, A., Heston, W. D., Bander, N. H., and Sadelain, M. (1999) Neoplasia 1, 123
21. Haynes, N. M., Trapani, J. A., Teng, M. W., Jackson, J. T., Cerruti, L., Jane, S. M., Kershaw, M. H., Smyth, M. J., and Darcy, P. K. (2002) J Immunol 169, 5780
22. Hombach, A., Wieczarkowiecz, A., Marquardt, T., Heuser, C., Usai, L., Pohl, C., Seliger, B., and Abken, H. (2001) J Immunol 167, 6123
23. Kowolik, C. M., Topp, M. S., Gonzalez, S., Pfeiffer, T., Olivares, S., Gonzalez, N., Smith, D. D., Forman, S. J., Jensen, M. C., and Cooper, L. J. (2006) Cancer Res 66, 10995
24. Maher, J., Brentjens, R. J., Gunset, G., Riviere, I., and Sadelain, M. (2002) Nat Biotechnol 20, 70
25. Gade, T. P., Hassen, W., Santos, E., Gunset, G., Saudemont, A., Gong, M. C., Brentjens, R., Zhong, X. S., Stephan, M., Stefanski, J., Lyddane, C., Osborne, J. R., Buchanan, I. M., Hall, S. J., Heston, W. D., Riviere, I., Larson, S. M., Koutcher, J. A., and Sadelain, M. (2005) Cancer Res 65, 9080
26. Pinthus, J. H., Waks, T., Kaufman-Francis, K., Schindler, D. G., Harmelin, A., Kanety, H., Ramon, J., and Eshhar, Z. (2003) Cancer Res 63, 2470
27. Vera, J., Savoldo, B., Vigouroux, S., Biagi, E., Pule, M., Rossig, C., Wu, J., Heslop, H. E., Rooney, C. M., Brenner, M. K., and Dotti, G. (2006) Blood 108, 3890
28. Westwood, J. A., Smyth, M. J., Teng, M. W., Moeller, M., Trapani, J. A., Scott, A. M., Smyth, F. E., Cartwright, G. A., Power, B. E., Honemann, D., Prince, H. M., Darcy, P. K., and Kershaw, M. H. (2005) Proc Natl Acad Sci USA 102, 19051
29. Friedmann-Morvinski, D., Bendavid, A., Waks, T., Schindler, D., and Eshhar, Z. (2005) Blood 105, 3087
30. Koehler, H., Kofler, D., Hombach, A., and Abken, H. (2007) Cancer Res 67, 2265
31. Loskog, A., Giandomenico, V., Rossig, C., Pule, M., Dotti, G., and Brenner, M. K. (2006) Leukemia 20, 1819
32. Imai, C., Mihara, K., Andreansky, M., Nicholson, I. C., Pui, C. H., Geiger, T. L., and Campana, D. (2004) Leukemia 18, 676
33. Hendriks, J., Gravestein, L. A., Tesselaar, K., van Lier, R. A., Schumacher, T. N., and Borst, J. (2000) Nat Immunol 1, 433
34. Hendriks, J., Xiao, Y., and Borst, J. (2003) J Exp Med 198, 1369
35. Arens, R., Schepers, K., Nolte, M. A., van Oosterwijk, M. F., van Lier, R. A., Schumacher, T. N., and van Oers, M. H. (2004) J Exp Med 199, 1595
36. Powell, D. J., Jr., Dudley, M. E., Robbins, P. F., and Rosenberg, S. A. (2005) Blood 105, 241
37. Ochsenbein, A. F., Riddell, S. R., Brown, M., Corey, L., Baerlocher, G. M., Lansdorp, P. M., and Greenberg, P. D. (2004) J Exp Med 200, 1407
38. Stephan, M. T., Ponomarev, V., Brentjens, R. J., Chang, A. H., Dobrenkov, K. V., Heller, G., and Sadelain, M. (2007) Nat Med 13, 1440
39. Wilkie, S., Picco, G., Foster, J., Davies, D. M., Julien, S., Cooper, L., Arif, S., Mather, S. J., Taylor-Papadimitriou, J., Burchell, J. M., and Maher, J. (2008) J Immunol 180, 4901

40. Schaft, N., Lankiewicz, B., Drexhage, J., Berrevoets, C., Moss, D. J., Levitsky, V., Bonneville, M., Lee, S. P., McMichael, A. J., Gratama, J. W., Bolhuis, R. L., Willemsen, R., and Debets, R. (2006) Int Immunol 18, 591
41. Kersh, E. N., Kersh, G. J., and Allen, P. M. (1999) J Exp Med 190, 1627
42. Mizoguchi, H., O'Shea, J. J., Longo, D. L., Loeffler, C. M., McVicar, D. W., and Ochoa, A. C. (1992) Science 258, 1795
43. Fehling, H. J., Krotkova, A., Saint-Ruf, C., and von Boehmer, H. (1995) Nature 375, 795
44. Fontenot, J. D., Gavin, M. A., and Rudensky, A. Y. (2003) Nat Immunol 4, 330
45. Fontenot, J. D., Rasmussen, J. P., Williams, L. M., Dooley, J. L., Farr, A. G., and Rudensky, A. Y. (2005) Immunity 22, 329
46. Hori, S., Nomura, T., and Sakaguchi, S. (2003) Science 299, 1057
47. Khattri, R., Cox, T., Yasayko, S. A., and Ramsdell, F. (2003) Nat Immunol 4, 337
48. Sakaguchi, S. (2005) Nat Immunol 6, 345
49. Walker, M. R., Kasprowicz, D. J., Gersuk, V. H., Benard, A., Van Landeghen, M., Buckner, J. H., and Ziegler, S. F. (2003) J Clin Invest 112, 1437
50. Antony, P. A., Piccirillo, C. A., Akpinarli, A., Finkelstein, S. E., Speiss, P. J., Surman, D. R., Palmer, D. C., Chan, C. C., Klebanoff, C. A., Overwijk, W. W., Rosenberg, S. A., and Restifo, N. P. (2005) J Immunol 174, 2591
51. Ahmadzadeh, M., and Rosenberg, S. A. (2006) Blood 107, 2409
52. Zhang, H., Chua, K. S., Guimond, M., Kapoor, V., Brown, M. V., Fleisher, T. A., Long, L. M., Bernstein, D., Hill, B. J., Douek, D. C., Berzofsky, J. A., Carter, C. S., Read, E. J., Helman, L. J., and Mackall, C. L. (2005) Nat Med 11, 1238
53. Grauer, O. M., Sutmuller, R. P., van Maren, W., Jacobs, J. F., Bennink, E., Toonen, L. W., Nierkens, S., and Adema, G. J. (2008) Int J Cancer 122, 1794
54. Itoh, S., and ten Dijke, P. (2007) Curr Opin Cell Biol 19, 176
55. Pestka, S., Krause, C. D., Sarkar, D., Walter, M. R., Shi, Y., and Fisher, P. B. (2004) Annu Rev Immunol 22, 929
56. Cho, B. K., Rao, V. P., Ge, Q., Eisen, H. N., and Chen, J. (2000) J Exp Med 192, 549
57. Ernst, B., Lee, D. S., Chang, J. M., Sprent, J., and Surh, C. D. (1999) Immunity 11, 173
58. Goldrath, A. W., Bogatzki, L. Y., and Bevan, M. J. (2000) J Exp Med 192, 557
59. Gattinoni, L., Powell, D. J., Jr., Rosenberg, S. A., and Restifo, N. P. (2006) Nat Rev Immunol 6, 383
60. Kieper, W. C., Tan, J. T., Bondi-Boyd, B., Gapin, L., Sprent, J., Ceredig, R., and Surh, C. D. (2002) J Exp Med 195, 1533
61. Marks-Konczalik, J., Dubois, S., Losi, J. M., Sabzevari, H., Yamada, N., Feigenbaum, L., Waldmann, T. A., and Tagaya, Y. (2000) Proc Natl Acad Sci USA 97, 11445
62. Dudley, M. E., and Rosenberg, S. A. (2003) Nat Rev Cancer 3, 666
63. Furtado, G. C., Curotto de Lafaille, M. A., Kutchukhidze, N., and Lafaille, J. J. (2002) J Exp Med 196, 851
64. Kohm, A. P., McMahon, J. S., Podojil, J. R., Begolka, W. S., DeGutes, M., Kasprowicz, D. J., Ziegler, S. F., and Miller, S. D. (2006) J Immunol 176, 3301
65. Brown, S., Konopa, J., Zhou, D., and Thompson, J. (2004) Bone Marrow Transplant 33, 359
66. Zhang, Y., Louboutin, J. P., Zhu, J., Rivera, A. J., and Emerson, S. G. (2002) J Clin Invest 109, 1335
67. Hill, G. R., Crawford, J. M., Cooke, K. R., Brinson, Y. S., Pan, L., and Ferrara, J. L. (1997) Blood 90, 3204
68. Rigby, S. M., Rouse, T., and Field, E. H. (2003) Blood 101, 2024
69. Sherman, M. L., Datta, R., Hallahan, D. E., Weichselbaum, R. R., and Kufe, D. W. (1991) J Clin Invest 87, 1794
70. Xun, C. Q., Thompson, J. S., Jennings, C. D., Brown, S. A., and Widmer, M. B. (1994) Blood 83, 2360
71. Bonini, C., Ferrari, G., Verzeletti, S., Servida, P., Zappone, E., Ruggieri, L., Ponzoni, M., Rossini, S., Mavilio, F., Traversari, C., and Bordignon, C. (1997) Science 276, 1719

72. Quintarelli, C., Vera, J. F., Savoldo, B., Giordano Attianese, G. M., Pule, M., Foster, A. E., Heslop, H. E., Rooney, C. M., Brenner, M. K., and Dotti, G. (2007) Blood 110, 2793
73. Gattinoni, L., Klebanoff, C. A., Palmer, D. C., Wrzesinski, C., Kerstann, K., Yu, Z., Finkelstein, S. E., Theoret, M. R., Rosenberg, S. A., and Restifo, N. P. (2005) J Clin Invest 115, 1616
74. Chen, B. J., Cui, X., Sempowski, G. D., Liu, C., and Chao, N. J. (2004) Blood 103, 1534
75. Wang, L. X., Huang, W. X., Graor, H., Cohen, P. A., Kim, J. A., Shu, S., and Plautz, G. E. (2004) J Transl Med 2, 41
76. Dudley, M. E., Wunderlich, J. R., Yang, J. C., Hwu, P., Schwartzentruber, D. J., Topalian, S. L., Sherry, R. M., Marincola, F. M., Leitman, S. F., Seipp, C. A., Rogers-Freezer, L., Morton, K. E., Nahvi, A., Mavroukakis, S. A., White, D. E., and Rosenberg, S. A. (2002) J Immunother 25, 243
77. Yee, C., Thompson, J. A., Byrd, D., Riddell, S. R., Roche, P., Celis, E., and Greenberg, P. D. (2002) Proc Natl Acad Sci USA 99, 16168
78. Lamers, C. H., van Elzakker, P., Langeveld, S. C., Sleijfer, S., and Gratama, J. W. (2006) Cytotherapy 8, 542
79. Refaeli, Y., Van Parijs, L., London, C. A., Tschopp, J., and Abbas, A. K. (1998) Immunity 8, 615

Targeting Toll-Like Receptor for the Induction of Immune and Antitumor Responses

Joseph Lustgarten, Dominique Hoelzinger, Maria Adelaida Duque, Shannon Smith, and Noweeda Mirza

Abstract A very unique and important feature of TLR (toll-like receptor) agonists is their ability to modulate TLR on the cells of the innate immune system resulting in changes that will induce effective and efficient adaptive immune responses. Therefore, stimulation of TLR pathways through their respective ligands presents a potentially attractive approach to activate adaptive anticancer immune responses. In this chapter, we summarize the effect of targeting some of the TLR for the induction of antitumor responses. Although the use of TLR agonists as future vaccine adjuvants seems very promising, we also need to proceed with caution and long term studies will be critical in assessing the propensity of chronic therapy to trigger autoimmune conditions or promote tumor growth.

Introduction

The immune system can be divided into innate and adaptive components. The innate immune response is the first line of defense against infectious diseases [1], while the adaptive immune response represents specific resistance, weak at first, then developing into a long-term memory response [2]. More importantly, adaptive responses are initiated when T and B cells recognize foreign molecules expressed on antigen presenting cell (APC) [3]. The major difference between the innate and adaptive immune systems lies in the mechanism of the recognition of antigens. In the adaptive immune response, T and B cell responses recognize the antigen through the T and B cell receptors, respectively, which have the capacity to recognize almost any antigenic structure. Additionally, each T or B cell expresses a unique receptor that can bind any antigen regardless of its origin. The innate response is largely mediated by white blood cells such as neutrophils, monocytes, macrophages (MΦ), and dendritic cells (DCs).

J. Lustgarten (✉)
Cancer Center Scottsdale, Mayo Clinic Arizona, 13400 East Shea Boulevard Scottsdale, AZ 85259
e-mail: lustgarten.joseph@mayo.edu

J. Lustgarten et al. (eds.), *Targeted Cancer Immune Therapy*,
DOI 10.1007/978-1-4419-0170-5_17,

In contrast to the adaptive immune response, the innate immune response relies on the recognition of the antigen by receptors that recognize specific structures found exclusively in microbial pathogens termed pathogen-associated molecular patterns (PAMPs) [4]. The recognition of PAMPs by the innate immune system can regulate the induction of adaptive immune responses [5]. For example, DCs respond to some microbial product by taking up the antigen. Concurrently, DCs synthesize a wide variety of inflammatory mediators and cytokines amplifying the immune response and, additionally, they can process and present antigens resulting in the activation of T and B cell responses and the establishment of protective immunity. Therefore, a number of microbial products are thought to function as effective adjuvants due to effects on APCs, which in turn, can influence the activation of an adaptive immune response.

More than a decade ago, Janeway postulated that regulation of PAMPs recognition must be controlled by receptors with a specificity for microbial products, thereby linking innate recognition of nonself with the induction of adaptive immunity [6]. Recent studies have demonstrated that recognition of PAMPs by APCs is mediated by a Toll-like receptor (TLR) family [7, 8]. There are currently more than ten known TLR family members capable of sensing bacterial wall components, such as LPS (TLR2/4), lipoteichoic acids (TLR2/4), CpG-DNA (TLR9), flagellin (TLR5), as well as other microbial products [9]. A wide variety of TLRs are expressed in immature or mature DCs, MΦ, and monocytes; and these receptors control the activation of those APCs [10]. Recognition of PAMPs by TLRs initiates a signaling pathway that leads to activation of NF-kB transcription factors and members of the MAP kinase family [11]. All TLRs share a common intracellular domain that is similar to the IL-1 receptors. The signal is mediated through the adaptor protein MyD88 [12]. The TLRs signaling triggers maturation and activation of APCs that includes upregulation of MHC and costimulatory molecules, and secretion of proinflammatory cytokines and chemokines [13, 14]. This maturation of APCs significantly increases their ability to prime naive T cells. In this way, TLRs link the recognition of pathogens with induction of adaptive immune responses. In this chapter, we will review the effects of targeting some of the TLR in activating and inducing an antitumor immune responses.

TLR4

The toll-like receptor 4 (TLR4) was the first human TLR to be cloned [15]. TLR4 was originally described on immune sentinel cells such as DCs, myeloid-derived dendritic cells (MDSCs), and B cells. Its function in APCs, such as DCs, is to initiate cell activation, in order to repel a potential infection of Gram-negative bacteria. Constitutive activation of TLR4 resulted in IL-1, IL-8, IL-12 TNF-α, IFN-γ, and B7.1 expression, suggesting its function as a mediator of TH1 proinflammatory responses. Since its discovery, it has been established that TLR4 predominantly recognizes and binds to bacterial lipopolysaccharides (LPS), triggering antimicrobial host defenses through the innate immune system. LPS signaling occurs through extracellular LPS binding anchoring proteins such as coreceptor MD-2 (also known as lymphocyte protein 96), CD14, and LPS binding protein [16]. Ligand binding leads to receptor oligomerization and clasical TLR downstream signaling that results in MAP kinase and NFkB activation [16].

Initial studies with LPS for the induction of antitumor responses were very successful in mouse tumor models in the 1980s, but it did not translate well to human clinical trials due to its high toxicity in humans [17]. Less toxic LPS derivatives such as MLA [18], aminoalkyl glucosamidine-4-phosphates (APGs) [19], and Corixa-675 have been developed; however, to date, only MLA has been used in a large number of patients as an allergy vaccine adjuvant. Lee et al. [20] using TLR4 wild-type mice (C3H/HeN) and $TLR4^{-/-}$ mice (C3H/HeJ) bearing syngeneic K1735 melanoma showed that *S. choleraesuis* infection significantly reduced tumor volume in a TLR4-dependent fashion. Decreases in tumor volume through *S. choleraesuis* infection in the presence of TRL4 correlated with increased presence of immune effector cells, such as $CD4^+$ and $CD8^+$ T cells, neutrophils and macrophages and secretion of high levels of IFN-γ. *Mycobacterium bovis* bacillus Calmette-Guerin (BCG) has historically been used as an immune adjuvant. Preparations of BCG cell-wall skeleton (BCG-CWS) activate both TLR2 and TLR4. Unlike the response to LPS, the BCG-driven TLR4 activation results in an atypical response defined by very low type 1 IFN induction [21]. Intravesical administration of BCG preparations has been successfully used as bladder cancer therapy for two decades [22, 23], but has been restricted to high grade tumor due to toxic side effects [24]. Most recently BCG therapy was shown to be a successful monotherapy in bladder cancer as a mechanism to prevent tumor recurrence [25, 26]. OK-432, derived from *Streptococcus pyogenes*, has been shown to have antitumor activity in mice and in human head and neck cancer [27], though this unrefined preparation could also be triggering TLR9 [28]. OK-PSA, an OK-432 derivative, has also been reported to activate TLR4 and showed efficacy in tumor bearing TLR4 mouse models [29, 30]. These results demonstrate the ability of targeting TLR4 to induce and activate antitumor responses.

Tumors can generate endogenous TLR4 ligands, which bind to and activate DCs. Tumors subjected to anthracycline-based chemotherapeutic drugs, or radiation exposure, undergo apoptosis (7). During this programmed cell death process, intracellular proteins such as heat-shock proteins and high-mobility-group-box 1 (HMG1) are released to the extra-cellular milieu. We are coming to an understanding that these proteins are immunogenic, binding to TLR4 present on DCs and eliciting a signaling cascade that involves MyD88 [31]. TLR4 expression by DCs is essential for efficient tumor-antigen presentation derived from dying tumor cells [31]. Amongst all the potential endogenous TLR4 ligands, HMG1 is the only one that regulates processing and presentation of tumor antigens derived from dying tumor cells [31, 32]. This process is thought to be due to the inhibition of lysosomal destruction of endocytosed tumor antigens through preventing the fusion between endosomes and lysozomes [33]. These findings support the usage of TLR4 agonists in support of antitumor therapy, even outside the scope of antitumor vaccines. However, there is a note of caution: breast cancer patients with mutated TLR4 (loss of function) alleles have a heightened risk of metastatic recurrence than control patients [31]. This indicates that therapies which include TLR4 activation should not be used in patients with inactive TLR4 receptors. Heat-shock protein 70 (HSP70) is also a tumor-derived TLR4 ligand. In a murine model of ovarian cancer, Chang et al. [34] showed that HSP70 produced by ovarian tumor cells generates an antigen-specific $CD8^+$ T cell immune response. This antitumor response was quenched in $CD40^{-/-}$ mice and $TLR4^{-/-}$ mice, suggesting that both CD40 and TLR4 mediate an inflammatory response through HSP70 resulting in an immune response against the tumor cells.

In addition to being expressed in immune cells, TLR4 is also expressed in various cancers, such as colon, squamous cell, salivary gland, and bladder carcinoma. This group of cancers is of epithelial origin and it is derived from tissues that constitute the first line of pathogen defense, the mucosal lining. Although the gastrointestinal track naturally expresses low levels of TLR4 [35], chronic inflammatory diseases up-regulate TLR4 expression [35], and can lead to tumorigenesis. The most well-documented instance of inflammation leading to tumorigenesis is *Heliobacter pylori* infection of the stomach, in which TLR4 stimulation is linked to neoplastic proliferation [36]. Crohn's disease and ulcerative colitis, both inflammatory diseases of the colon, can lead to colonic tumorigenesis. Colitis-associated neoplasia is linked to TLR4 expression and activation [37]. In fact, Rapamycin, an immunosuppressant used to treat autoimmune diseases, significantly inhibits TLR4 signaling (by down-regulating its expression) and reduces colon cancer invasion [38], further linking TLR4 to colon cancer progression.

TLR4 expression and function in human lung cancer promotes secretion of immunosuppressive cytokines vascular endothelial growth factor (VEGF) and transforming growth factor β (TGFβ) [39]. LPS and TLR4 are also linked to apoptosis resistance in lung cancer cell lines [39], suggesting a role in immune escape and potential therapy resistance. Similar findings are true in mouse models. TLR4 is expressed by a variety of murine tumor cell lines and it is thought to contribute to evasion of immunosurveillance [40]. LPS stimulation of MC26 colon cancer cell line *in vitro* results in secretion of factors that enhance immunosuppression. In addition to the effect of inhibiting T cell proliferation, these factors also inhibit CTL activity. Sensitivity to CTL attack is lowered through LPS- and TLR4-dependent up-regulation of B7-H1, B7-H2, and CD40 mRNA. Blocking TLR4 signaling in MC26 tumors through siRNA and a synthetic blocking peptide increases survival in Balb/c mice inoculated with MC26 tumor cells. Increased survival was linked to increased proliferation capacity of tumor infiltrating T cells, as well as a significant increase of NK cells in the TIL population (as measured by in vitro IFN-γ secretion). LPS-dependent TLR4 signaling in prostate cancer is thought to promote tumor proliferation [41], progression, metastasis, and immune escape [42]. In human ovarian cancer cell lines, it confers chemoresistance to Paclitaxel as well as promoting tumor growth [43]. The same study evaluated the link between expression of the TLR4 signaling through MyD88 and tumor progression, and concluded that loss of MyD88 expression significantly lengthened progression free survival. Taken together, agonist-based TLR4 therapies can result in both tumor proliferation and progression. Single nucleotide polymorphisms (SNPs) in TLR4 are linked to an increased gastric [44, 45] and prostate [46] cancer risk. Presumably this increased risk is due to decreased responsiveness of TLR4 to LPS, which corresponds to a higher susceptibility to bacterial infections such as *Heliobacter pylori* [47]. One should conclude that TLR4 agonist-based immunotherapy should not be considered for patients with loss of function SNPS. Taken together these results suggest that TLR4 immunotherapy should only be considered for patients with cancers that do not respond to ligand with proliferation.

TLR3

Toll-like receptor 3 (TLR3) is a member of the TLR family proteins that recognizes natural (genomic or life cycle intermediate material of many viruses) or synthetic double stranded RNA (dsRNA) and transmits signals that lead to the production of type I interferon (IFN), cytokines and chemokines, DC maturation and apoptosis of tumor cells, among other actions [48]. In addition to TLR3, dsRNA has additional cytosolic receptors such as the dsRNA-dependent protein kinase (PKR) [49], 2′-5′ oligoadenylate synthetases [50, 51], the retinoic-acid inducible gene-I (RIG-I) [52], and melanoma differentiation-associated antigen 5 (MDA5) [53].

In humans, TLR3 is expressed in the placenta, pancreas, lung, liver, heart, brain, and colon, in nonimmune cells such as intestinal epithelial cells, fibroblasts, keratinocytes, endothelial cells and in cells of the immune system such as myeloid DCs, polymorphonuclear leukocytes, T, B, and natural killer (NK) cells. In mice, TLR3 expression has been observed in lung, brain and kidney and also in response to LPS stimulation in the heart, liver, and spleen [54]. TLR3 is also expressed on murine $CD4^+$ T cells [55], IFN-producing killer dendritic cells (IKDC) [56], bone marrow-derived DCs, and macrophages [54–58].

Two decades before the finding of the TLR3, poly (I:C) was used as a therapeutic tool against tumors. Levy et al. [59] and Bart et al. [60] showed that poly (I:C) could inhibit the tumor growth rates, depress oncogenesis, and cause the regression of some established experimental tumors. These reports suggested that the antitumor effect might be related to the capacity of poly (I:C) to stimulate IFN production. Other groups reported that poly (I:C) could stimulate both cellular and humoral immunity suggesting that this compound stimulated the immune system in a nonspecific manner [61, 62]. Later on, it was demonstrated that the inhibition of tumor growth by poly (I:C) was related with the increase of cytotoxic splenic lymphocytes [63]. With the discovery of TLR3 as receptor of poly (I:C) and natural dsRNA, some of the specific mechanisms of the immune response that are activated by this molecule through this receptor and that participate in the antitumor function have been elucidated [64]. The findings of the actions of poly (I:C) on the immune system are concentrated in specific cell populations: macrophages, DCs, NK cells, and $CD8^+$ T cells [65]. Murine macrophages express TLR3 and the engagement of this receptor with poly (I:C) results *in vitro* and *in vivo* in the induction of NOS2,

IL-12p40, TNF-α, and IL-6. The combination of poly (I:C) with CpG-ODN is synergistic increasing the secretion of cytokines leading to the activation of an effective antitumor immune response controlling the tumor growth of B16-F_{10} melanoma. Other studies have shown that the maturation of DCs can be directly induced by the engagement of TLR3 by poly (I:C). This stimulation promotes a polarization of T-helper cell responses to a Th1 pattern [66], the production of type I IFN that induces the cross priming of DCs [67] and has been used as an adjuvant therapy to promote immune responses against tumor-associated antigens in clinical trials for different types of cancer [68, 69]. The antitumor effect of poly (I:C) could be enhanced by delivering it inside DCs. For example, phagocytosis of poly (I:C)-electroporated human acute myeloid leukemia (AML) cells induces the activation of DCs by increasing the expression of MHC, CD80, and CD86 and production of TNF-α, IL-6, and type I IFN and Th1 polarization of T cells [70]. In contrast, none of these effects are observed in AML cells passively pulsed with poly (I:C). These results suggest that poly (I:C) transfection increases the immunogenicity of AML cells by activating and inducing the maturation of DCs [70]. Another mechanism used to transport poly (I:C) intracellularly in human DCs is the electroporation of these cells with dsRNA analogues. This procedure results in an induction of CD25, CD40, CD80, CD83, CD86, CCR7, and MHC I and II expression and IFN-α and IL-12p70 production [71]. When DCs are simultaneously electroporated with mRNA coding the melanoma antigen Melan-A, they are able to stimulate higher levels of Melan-A-specific CTLs producing IFN-γ with high cytotoxic activity when compared with DCs activated in the presence of inflammatory cytokines [72, 73]. Other studies have shown that peptide vaccination in conjunction with poly (I:C) enhances $CD8^+$ T cell specific responses. Using the OT-1 model, Salem et al. [74] demonstrated that vaccination with OVA peptide and concomitant administration of poly (I:C) resulted in the expansion, activation, and generation of a memory $CD8^+$ T cell responses capable of protecting a tumor challenge against B16-OVA melanoma and EG.7 lymphoma. These studies demonstrate the capacity of poly (I:C) as an adjuvant for peptide-based vaccines designed to enhance antitumor immunity.

The action of poly (I:C) on tumor immune responses can be also mediated by stimulation of NK cells [75]. A recent study showed that NK cells and IFN-γ are implicated in the inhibition of lung and liver metastasis of B6 melanoma cells following poly (I:C) treatment since depletion of NK cells or blockade of INF-γ abrogated the antitumor effect [76, 77]. Additionally, stimulation with poly (I:C) increases the number of $B220^+$ $CD11c^+$ $NK1.1^+$ cells in spleen, lung, and liver. $B220^+$ $CD11c^+$ $NK1.1^+$ cells are a subset of NK cells also called IKDCs, that express TLR3, have the ability to kill tumor cells, present tumor antigens and produce high amounts of IFN-γ in response to tumors in the absence of exogenous cytokines [76–79]. These cells are critical in controlling and suppressing tumor growth [76–79]. The effects of poly (I:C) to induce NK stimulation have also been seen in humans. Human NK cells in the presence of IL-12 or IL-8 and dsRNA induce the expression of CD69 and CD25 and secretion of IFN-γ and TNF-α [80]. These data suggest that during the inflammatory process, NK cells can be activated by TLR3 ligands that subsequently activate other cells of the innate immune system orchestrating the activation and development of an immune response. Taken together, these studies indicate that the activation of NK cells by poly (I:C) is critical for the effective induction of an antitumor response.

The expression of TLR3 has been reported in several human and murine cancer cell lines [81–84]. Several studies have demonstrated that the engagement of TLR3 expressed in human and murine tumor cell lines by poly (I:C) results in the inhibition of proliferation and induction of apoptosis [81–84]. Based on the immunostimulatory properties and the cytostatic and cytotoxic effects on tumor cells, injections of poly (I:C) or therapies with dsRNA analogs represent a very promising adjuvant for cancer antitumor therapy.

TLR5

TLR5 is specific for the ligand flagellin which is a structural protein found in the flagella of motile bacteria. TLR5 is expressed on immune cells such as monocytes and immature DCs as well as on epithelial cells [85, 86]. Therefore, flagellin activates macrophages, monocytes, and DCs as well as pulmonary and intestinal epithelial cells inducing the release of proinflammatory mediators [87, 88]. Purified or recombinant flagellin causes inflammatory responses on treated cells in vitro [89] and when administered systemically in vivo [90]. The incorporation of TLR-ligands as adjuvants in vaccines could result in more potent and efficacious vaccines. In this context, our group demonstrated that the use of a flagellin fusion protein (flagellin-EGFP) was able to induce the maturation of APCs as measured by the increased surface expression of MHC class II molecules and CD80 [91]. Furthermore, these APCs were able to internalize the flagellin fusion protein and then effectively process and present the antigens since anti-EGFP-specific CD8 T cells effectively killed flagellin fusion pulsed APCs. More importantly, it was shown that this flagellin fusion protein when injected into mice was able to generate a cytotoxic CD8 T cell response which was specific alone to the EGFP [91]. Other studies have shown that immunization of mice with the recombinant-flagellin fused to several proteins resulted in potent antigen-specific T and B cell responses that were equal to or better than responses induced by the same proteins emulsified in Complete Freund's adjuvant. These responses included rapid and consistent antibody responses as well as the development of protective $CD8^+$ T cell responses upon challenge with virulent Listeria monocytogenes [92]. Phase I flagellin from Salmonella called FliC is a monomeric subunit polypeptide and a TLR5 agonist. FliC has been studied extensively, and the regions and residues of FliC important for TLR5 interaction are defined [93, 94]. FliC activates proinflammatory cytokine production and polymorphonuclear granulocyte recruitment in lung [95] and intestinal epithelia [96]. FliC can induce Th1 type inflammatory responses characteristic of TLR activation since it activates mouse macrophages to produce inflammatory mediators human monocytes to produce TNF-α [97]. FliC also induces human monocyte-derived DCs to mature and upregulate costimulatory molecules [98] and to produce IFN-γ, IL-6, TNF-α, and IL-12p-70 [99]. Applequist et al. [100] demonstrated that DNA encoding a TLR5 agonist when injected into mice induces both humoral and cell mediated responses. Mice were vaccinated intradermally with DNA encoding the TLR5 agonist FliC developed localized inflammation at the site of injection with dense infiltrates of neutrophilic granulocytes. Furthermore, when vectors expressing FliC were administered in combination with vectors expressing antigen of interest (in this case OVA), adaptive immune responses were found to increase dramatically with increases in the titers of antigen-specific IgG and IgA antibodies. Antigen-specific IFN-γ producing CD8 T cells were detected by ELISPOT assays from spleen samples of mice that had received a combination of the vectors expressing FliC and antigen. Mice injected with the FliC expressing vectors developed memory responses and were protected when rechallenged with lethal influenza A virus. These aforementioned various vaccination studies illustrate the strong adjuvant activity of flagellin.

Although flagellin could promote tumor immunity, other studies have shown that flagellin could also promote tumor growth. The antitumor effects of flagellin were evaluated in mice transplanted with a weakly immunogenic murine mammary tumor or with its variant tumor stably transfected to express the highly antigenic human Her-2 oncoprotein [101]. Peritumoral injections of flagellin 8 to 10 days later significantly inhibited the growth of the antigenic variant tumor only. This inhibition of tumor growth corresponded with a decreased frequency of T regulatory cells and an increased IFN-γ:IL-4 ratio. In contrast to this finding, when flagellin was administered at the time of tumor injection, the growth of the invariant immunogenic tumors accelerated and this corresponded to the increased frequency of T regulatory cells and the decreased IFN-γ:IL-4 ratio [101]. Therefore, flagellin in this study only activated the adaptive immune response and was shown to have contrasting effects on the adaptive immune response, either fostering a Th1 or a Th2 type response depending on the time it was administered following tumor implantation. A large collection of commensal bacteria reside in the human gut and release various microbial products [102]. CD11c^{+} lamina propria cells (LPC) present in the submucosal layer of the intestine express TLR5 and produce proinflammatory cytokines in response to bacterial flagellin [103]. More so it has been proposed that the adaptor molecule myeloid differentiation factor 88 (MYD88) through which TLR5 signaling occurs, can regulate tumorigenesis in the intestine [104]. Recently, another group [105] investigated whether TLR5-dependent signaling would modulate colonic tumor development in a mouse xenograft model of human colon cancer. Nude mice were subcutaneously implanted with human colon cancer cells (DLD-1) in which the expression of MyD88 or TLR5 had been stably knocked down. They found that lack of MyD88 or TLR5 expression dramatically enhanced tumor growth and inhibited tumor necrosis in mouse xenografts of human colon cancer. Tumors from these knock down mice revealed a reduced production of the neutrophil attracting chemokines epithelial cell-derived neutrophil activating peptide-78, macrophage inflammatory protein-α, and IL-8. However, TLR5 activation by peritumoral flagellin treatment increased tumor necrosis resulting in significant tumor regression. Therefore, in this xenograft mouse model of human colon cancer, flagellin treatment mediated both innate immunity and demonstrated antitumor activity suggesting that in colonic cancers TLR5-dependent signaling could be exploited as a potential target for immunotherapeutic purposes.

To date there are no clinical trials using flagellin as a vaccine adjuvant to cancer immunotherapy. TLR5 is expressed highly on gut epithelia and therefore, it will be important to employ smaller potent molecules of flagellin that will evoke a milder immune reaction. It may be necessary to use pharmacologically inactive prodrugs that are converted to the parent drug once absorbed. Of interest is the notion that flagellin has been selected and it is in clinical development as an adjuvant for influenza vaccine by the pharmaceutical company VaxInnate Inc.

TLR7

TLR7 and TLR8 also referred to as intracellular TLRs, are expressed on the membranes of endosomes and are specific for viral single stranded RNA (ssRNA) and nucleosides [106]. Synthetic agonists known as new chemical entities (NCE) have been generated for TLR7 and TLR8 and are molecular mimics of the natural ligand. Imiquimod is a nucleoside derivative of the imidazoquinoline group of compounds and has been studied more extensively. There are many other derivatives from this family of compounds such as resiquimod, gardiquimod, and isatoribine (7-thia-oxoguanosine) that are TLR7 and TLR8 agonists. All of these derivatives are small molecules with structures resembling nucleic acid bases that are present in the natural ligand of TLR7 and TLR8. TLR7 signals through the adaptor molecule MyD88. These signaling cascades increase the expression of many proinflammatory genes [107] and also control the expression of costimulatory molecules (such as the B7 family members, CD80 and CD86 and the adhesion molecules CD54 and CD83) [108]. Since the discovery that interferons have antiviral properties and are antineoplastic proteins, the search for more potent chemically defined IFN inducers has intensified. Polyribonucleotides were known to induce high serum levels of IFN and showed both antiviral and antitumor activity in experimental models [109]. Scientific and clinical interest in TLR7 and TLR8 for cancer biology originated from earlier studies in which imiquimod was shown to be a potent inhibitor of tumor growth in a wide variety of transplantable murine tumors such as MC-26 colon carcinoma, RIF-1 sarcoma, and Lewis Lung carcinoma [110] and also inhibited tumor metastases [111]. Moreover, imiquimod proved to be a potent inducer of IFN as topical application of imiquimod in mouse models resulted in an increase of specific mRNA coding for IFN-α (the principal cytokine for antiviral activity), IFN-β, TNF-α, IL-1α, IL-1β, IL-6, and IL-12 [112]. Using *in vitro* models imiquimod stimulated human peripheral blood mononuclear cells (PBMCs) to produce a wide range of immunomodulatory cytokines including IFN-α, TNF-α, IL-1α, IL-1β, IL-8, IL-10, and IL-12, GM-CSF, G-CSF, macrophage inhibitory protein (MIP-1α), and the IL-1 receptor antagonists [113]. *In vitro* imiquimod has been described to activate DC by inducing DC maturation along with the release of inflammatory cytokines in a MyD88-dependent manner [114]. Moreover, imiquimod caused the migration of skin Langerhan DCs to regional lymph nodes [115]. Ligation of TLR7 on human myeloid and plasmacytoid DC by imiquimod induces DC maturation and the secretion of inflammatory mediators such as IL-12 (by myeloid DC) and IFN-α (by plasmacytoid DCs) [116, 117]. Imiquimod has proven to be effective in the priming of transgenic cytotoxic T-lymphocytes (CTL) in transgenic TCR mice and even wild type mice. In this context, a transcutaneous immunization regimen was employed whereby the skin was used as a route to deliver topically applied imiquimod containing a specified amount of the relevant specific peptide [118]. Imiquimod delivered epicutaneously with target peptide activated resident skin Langerhan cells and generated potent cytolytic activity in the regional draining lymph nodes. TLR7 is of clinical interest because it can be activated pharmacologically by imidazoquinolines and guanosine analogues. In a clinical case study, a 71-year-old patient diagnosed with cutaneous lymphocytic leukemia (CLL) was given a daily topical treatment with 5% imiquimod [119]. After 6 weeks the cutaneous nodular lesions present on the arms and hands of the patient had disappeared. The functional effects of imiquimod were investigated and it was found that the CLL tumor cells themselves had increased expression of the costimulatory molecules CD80, CD86, CD54, and CD83, and may have potentially activated the tumor reactive T cells directly. Furthermore, the same group continued to investigate the effects of the TLR7 agonists imiquimod and loxoribine on enhancing the immunogeneicity of CLL cells [119]. Imiquimod (S28690) and loxoribine both, enhanced the immunogenicity of CLL cells and they exhibited an activated phenotype, similar to that of activated mature DCs, expressing high surface levels of CD80, CD86, CD83, and CD54, including, CD40 and the MHC class I and II antigens. Additionally, in vitro stimulation of CLL cells with imiquimod and loxoribine, resulted in the release of the inflammatory cytokines predominantly, TNF-α, lymphotoxin, IL-6, and IL-10 and the chemokines CXCL8 and CXCL10 with low amounts of IL-1β and IFN-γ in the supernatants. However, treatment with loxoribine rendered CLL tumor cells more sensitive to killing by chemotherapy. Treatment with imiquimod in another study of basal cell carcinoma induced the expression of opioid growth factor receptor protein on tumor cells and infiltrating cells. Expression of the opioid growth factor receptor following treatment with imiquimod was associated with a good prognosis and correlated with a longer recurrence free period in basal cell carcinoma [120].

Mechanisms explaining the antitumor activity of imiquimod are under discussion. The potential of imiquimod to induce tumor regression in murine cutaneous malignancies by inhibiting angiogenic activity through the release of local IL-18 in conjunction with other antiangiogenic cytokines highlighted a very important biological effect which may prove useful for the treatment of early malignant angiogenesis-dependent proliferative tumors [121] In another study, biopsies taken from patients receiving treatment for basal cell carcinoma with topical imiquimod revealed dense DC infiltrates both of the myeloid DC and plasmacytoid DC phenotype. These DC expressed upregulated levels of perforin, granzyme B, and TNF-related apoptosis inducing ligand (TRAIL) and exhibited lytic ability [122]. Hence, activation of TLR7/8 through imiquimod conferred antitumoricidal activity to inflammatory DCs. The first in phase human trial of a small molecule agonist 852A for TLR7 took place in patients with advanced cancers [123]. 852A is a more potent and selective activator of TLR7 than imiquimod and has 40 times more aqueous solubility allowing it to be easily delivered as a systemic agent. This study concluded that 852A compound was administered safely intravenously and that it was biologically active and promising toward stimulating innate immune responses. Future trials are warranted to assess its therapeutic role in patients with cancer. A recent study [124] administered full length recombinant NY-ESO-1 protein, a cancer testis antigen intradermally into sites that had been preconditioned with imiquimod into patients with malignant melanoma. Imiquimod as a topical adjuvant was tolerated well by patients and the vaccine was able to induce measurable NY-ESO-1 specific antibody and CD4 T cell responses. Dermal inflammatory infiltrates rich in APCs and T cells were also observed. Previously to this, it was shown in humans that topical imiquimod treatment could enhance the immunogenicity of a melanoma peptide vaccine when given with systemic FLT3 ligand [125].

TLR9

In the late 1890s, William Coley, a cancer researcher, injected extracts from *Serratia marcescens* and other bacteria into patients with cancer and was able to get tumor regression, reportedly from the induced inflammatory response [126]. The success of his studies has never been repeated, but in the early 1990s it was determined that bacterial DNA, specifically CpG motifs, caused B cell proliferation in murine models [127, 128]. CpG is unmethylated DNA oligodeoxynucleotides (ODN) composed of CG repeats surrounded by flanking sequences found in bacteria and DNA viruses which acts as the ligand of toll-like receptor 9 (TLR9), a receptor found in the endocytic pathway in APCs and B cells. TLR9 recognizes a consensus sequence as a pattern recognition receptor (PRR), "XCGY" where X and Y are neither cytosine nor guanine on a single stranded CG motif of DNA [129, 130]. There are two main types of CpG, such as A and B. CpG-A, which has a phosphodiester backbone, causes large amounts of IFN-α to be produced by plasmocytoid dendritic cells (pDCs) and activates NK cells, while CpG-B, a synthetic CpG motif, has a more stable phosphorothioate backbone, and is a B cell activator [131, 132]. CpG has been implicated in both mouse and human models to cause a reduction of tumor size in melanoma and other cancer models [133]. It has also been implicated to be a contributing factor in autoimmunity. In mouse models and phase I and II clinical trials, CpG-ODN has shown to be best used as part of a multidrug therapy instead of just a single agent therapy.

CpG-ODN is probably the most studied TLR-ligand for the induction of antitumor responses. The antitumor effect of CpG-ODN had been studied in many syngeneic and transgenic tumor models. Early studies from Wickstrom [134, 135] using a transgenic for c-Myc from an Ig enhancer, which manifested with lymphomas early in their life showed that treatment with CpG-B ODN prevented cancer in 75% of the mice when treatment was begun shortly after weaning. Other models of cancer were examined including syngeneic B16 melanoma in C57BL/6 mice in which CpG-A ODN was administered 3 days prior to B16 challenge with lethal cell numbers and 60% of the mice were protected from tumor growth. However, rechallenge with the tumor did not provide specific protection to the mice [136]. In neuroblastoma models, daily injections of CpG-B ODN caused tumor regression in 50% of the mice [137]. C1498 mouse acute myelogenous leukemia (AML) model described the differences that a particular CpG motif, A or B, have on protection from lethal tumor doses. CpG-B ODN (synthetic CpG) vs. CpG-A ODN (natural form) was used as a preventative measure. CpG-B ODN allowed the mice to survive lethal doses of AML, whereas CpG-A ODN did not allow for mouse survival [138]. This suggests the necessity of using different CpG motifs in different tumor models.

Tolerant mouse models that mimic the natural human condition are in general more difficult to treat. Our group had been using the BALB-neuT mice which are tolerant to neu antigens. After testing the effect of different TLR-ligands (LPS, imiquimod, poly (I:C), flagellin, and CpG-ODN) our results indicate that only intratumoral injections of CpG-ODN into established tumor induced the complete rejection of the tumor in 30% of the BALB-neuT mice [139, 140]. The antitumor effect was significantly enhanced when intratumoral injection of CpG-ODN was combined with depletion of T regulatory cells (Tregs) in which 100% of the animals rejected the tumor. The major drawback of intratumoral injections of CpG-ODN is that not all tumors are physically accessible. In order to target CpG-ODN to the tumor anywhere in the body, we produced a hybrid-molecule between an antibody directed against the neu molecule and CpG-ODN (antineu-CpG). Our results demonstrated that the antineu-CpG retained its dual capacity of: (1) binding to Her-2/neu$^+$ tumor cells; and (2) activating DCs [139]. Treatment with antineu-CpG plus Treg depletion induced tumor rejection in 100% of BALB-neuT mice [139]. The use of the antineu-CpG-ODN will have clinical benefits such as reducing the possible side effects of injecting high doses of CpG-ODN. Our data also indicate that the lower levels of CpG-ODN contained in the hybrid molecule are sufficient to induce an immune response. These results indicate that antineu-CpG-ODN or other similar hybrid molecules provide a new strategy to specifically target CpG-ODN at the tumor site to induce an antitumor response with minimal toxicity.

Due to the success of mouse trials using CpG-ODN as a monotherapy, clinical trials began in humans. Trials using TLR9 agonists are being tried in applications of infectious disease, asthma/allergy in monotherapies, as an adjuvant in vaccines, and primarily in cancer patients. However, because of the differential expression of TLR9 in humans vs. mice, humans only exhibit small tumor regression and protection unlike observations made in mice. One drug which was effective in mice and transferred to humans was PF-3512676 (formerly known as CPG7909). Initially, PF-3512676 was tried in combination with a cytotoxic chemotherapy in a trial with lung cancer patients and was advancing to phase III trial when interim analysis came in indicating the drug combination was no more efficacious than current treatments. This clinical trial along with several others in phase II was shut down as a result. Further trials involving

PF-3512676 were in progress in combination therapies with existing therapies in lymphoma, metastatic breast cancer, renal cell cancer, T cell lymphoma, nonsmall cell lung carinoma (NSCLC), and melanoma. One potentially promising agonist is CpG-28 by University of Paris as a stand alone therapy for glioblastomas after radiotherapy that has preliminary data showing tumor regression and meets safety requirements; as a result this drug is currently in Phase II clinical trials [141].

Overall CpG is not suited for monotherapy (with few exceptions) due to the differences in TLR9 expression in mice and humans. One trial found in mice that use of Rituximab, a CD20 depleting agent, in conjunction with PF-3512676 enhanced the antitumor effects of Rituximab in B cell non-Hodgkin's lymphoma. This drug has been shown to be safe in short and extended use in humans in conjunction with Rituximab in relapsed lymphoma [142]. Current clinical trials using TLR9 agonists include ISS 1018 by Dynavax and IMO-2055 by Idera for use in combination therapies with existing cancer treatments. ISS 1018 given with Irinotecan and Cetuximab is in phase I for metastatic colorectal cancer in patients who relapsed. ISS 1018 is also in phase II given in conjunction with Rituxan in patients with non-Hodgkin's follicular B-cell lymphoma. IM0–2055 is in two phase I trials. One is looking at the safety of adding the CpG agonist to current NSCLC drugs Erlotinib and Bevacizumab as a second line of treatment. NSCLC cells develop resistance to Erlotinib after about 8 months or treatment, usually via a mutation in the receptor the drug targets. The other trial for IMO-2055 is in conjunction with current therapies for colorectal cancer Cetuximab and Irinotecan. Although initial results are promising, these trials have yet to progress to phase III studies where the true fate of CpG lies.

While in mice CpG is promising as a single agent drug, in humans, modifications need to be made as CpG does not evoke a strong enough antitumor response to be optimal as a single drug therapeutic for cancer. The use of this motif may prove to be more efficacious in multitreatment strategies. Synthetic forms have been made to enhance the stability of CpG for effective delivery options to metastatic lesions. Many clinical trials are in the first stages for evaluating the effect of these new compounds in conjunction with multitherapeutic strategies targeting a wide range of cancers. The results of these studies will determine the efficacy of these compounds in inducing an antitumor response.

Summary

Targeting TLRs could serve as mediators that are able to activate and regulate immune responses to control tumor progression. However, it is not clear which is the best TLR-ligand to induce the most effective antitumor response. Based on our own experience using different tumor models and comparing the antitumor of different TLR-ligand, the results indicate that CpG-ODN induces the strongest antitumor response in animal tumor models. However, as indicated above, in humans there are different types of CpG-ODN providing distinct responses. Additionally, it is important to consider the type of tumor to be treated since some of these TLR-ligands might promote tumor growth. Furthermore, not all TLR-ligands will serve the same purpose in promoting an immune response to all tumors. Therefore, it is imperative to further assess and compare the antitumor effect of the different TLR-ligands to particular type of tumors to maximize the antitumor effect and avoid undesirable side effects.

References

1. Imler, J., and Hoffmann, J. (2001) Trends Cell Biol 11, 304
2. Heine, H., and Lien, E. (2003) Int Arch Allergy Immunol 130, 180
3. Schijns, V. (2001) Crit Rev Immunol 21, 75
4. Barton, G., and Medzhitov, R. (2002) Curr Opin Immunol 14, 380
5. Huang, Q., Liu, D., Majewski, P., Schulte, L., Korn, J., Young, R., Lander, E., and Hacohen, N. (2001) Science 294, 870
6. Janeway, C., Jr. (1989) Cold Spring Harb Symp Quant Biol 54, 1
7. Means, T., Golenbock, D., and Fenton, M. (2000) Life Sci 68, 241
8. Kaisho, T., and Akira, S. (2002) Biochim Biophy Acta 1589, 1
9. Takeda, K., and Akira, S. (2003) Cell Microbiol 5, 143
10. Aderem, A., and Ulevitch, R. (2000) Nature 406, 782
11. Means, T., Golenbock, D., and Fenton, M. (2000) Cytokine Growth Factor Rev 11, 219
12. Takeuchi, O., and Akira, S. (2002) Curr Top Microbiol Immunol 270, 155
13. Krieg, A. (2002) Annu Rev Immunol 20, 709
14. Gewirtz, A., and Navas, T. (2001) J Immunol 167, 1882
15. Medzhitov, R., Preston-Hurlburt, P., and Janeway, C., Jr. (1997) Nature 388, 394
16. Lu, Y., Yeh, W., and Ohashi, P. (2008) Cytokine Growth Factor Rev 42, 145
17. Goto, S., Sakai, S., Kera, J., Suma, Y., Soma, G., and Takeuchi, S. (1996) Cancer Immunol Immunother 42, 255
18. Baldridge, J., McGowan, P., Evans, J., Cluff, C., Mossman, S., Johnson, D., and Persing, D. (2004) Expert Opin Biol Ther 4, 1129
19. Johnson, D. (2008) Curr Top Med Chem 8, 64
20. Lee, C., Wu, C., and Shiau, A. (2008) Clin Cancer Res 14, 1905
21. Akazawa, T., Masuda, H., and Saeki, Y. (2004) Cancer Res 64, 757
22. Lamm, D., Thor, D., Harris, S., Reyna, J., Stogdill, V., and Radwin, H. (1980) J Urol 124, 38
23. Perabo, F., and Muller, S. (2004) Urology 64, 409
24. Witjes, J., and Hendricksen, K. (2008) Eur Urol 53, 45
25. Kaasinen, E., Rintala, E., Pere, A., Kallio, J., Puolakka, V., Liukkonen, T., and Tuhkanen, K. (2000) J Urol 164, 47
26. Murata, M. (2008) Cancer Sci 99, 1435
27. Okamoto, M., Oshikawa, T., and Tano, T. (2003) J Natl Cancer Inst 95, 316
28. Oshikawa, T., Okamoto, M., and Tano, T. (2006) J Immunother 29, 143
29. Okamoto, M., Furuichi, S., and Nishioka, Y. (2004) Cancer Res 64, 5461
30. Tano, T., Okamoto, M., Oshikawa, T., Ahmed, S., Sasai, A., and Sato, M. (2005) Gan To Kagaku Ryoho 32, 1562
31. Apetoh, L., Ghiringhelli, F., and Tesniere, A. (2007) Nat Med 13, 1050
32. Apetoh, L., Tesniere, A., Ghiringhelli, F., Kroemer, G., and Zitvogel, L. (2008) Cancer Res 68, 4026
33. Shiratsuchi, A., Watanabe, I., Takeuchi, O., Akira, S., and Nakanishi, Y. (2004) J Immunol 172, 2039
34. Chang, C., Tsai, Y., He, L., Wu, T., and Hung, C. (2007) Cancer Res 67, 10047

35. Fukata, M., and Abreu, M. (2008) Oncogene 27, 234
36. Cochi, K., Ichikura, T., and Kinoshita, M. (2008) Clin Cancer Res 14, 2909
37. Fukata, M., Chen, A., and Vamadevan, A. (2007) Gastroenterology 133, 1869
38. Sun, Q., Liu, Q., Zheng, Y., and Cao, X. (2008) Mol Immunol 45, 2929
39. He, W., Liu, Q., Wang, L., Chen, W., Li, N., and Cao, X. (2007) Mol Immunol 44, 2850
40. Huang, B., Zhao, J., and Li, H. (2005) Cancer Res 65, 5009
41. Kundu, S., Lee, C., and Billips, B. (2008) Prostate 68, 223
42. Pei, Z., Lin, D., Song, X., Li, H., and Yao, H. (2008) Cell Immunol 254, 20
43. Kelly, M., Alvero, A., and Chen, R. (2006) Cancer Res 66, 3859
44. Hold, G., Rabkin, C., and Chow, W. (2007) Gastroenterology 132, 905
45. Achyut, B., Ghoshal, U., Moorchung, N., and Mittal, B. (2007) Hum Immunol 68, 901
46. Zheng, S., Augustsson-Balter, K., and Chang, B. (2004) Cancer Res 64, 2918
47. El-Omar, E., Ng, M., and Hold, G. (2008) Oncogene 27, 244
48. Matsumoto, M., and Seya, T. (2008) Adv Drug Deliv Rev 60, 805
49. Kumar, A., Yang, Y., Flati, V., Der, S., Kadereit, S., Deb, A., Haque, J., Reis, L., Weissmann, C., and Williams, B. (1997) EMBO J 16, 406
50. Khabar, K., Dhalla, M., Siddiqui, Y., Zhou, A., Al Ahdal, M., Der, S., Silverman, R., and Williams, B. (2000) J Interferon Cytokine Res 20, 653
51. Zhou, A., Paranjape, J., Brown, T., Nie, H., Naik, S., Dong, B., Chang, A., Trapp, B., Fairchild, R., Comenares, C., and Silverman, R. (1997) EMBO J 16, 6355
52. Yoneyama, M., Kikuchi, M., Natsukawa, T., Shinobu, N., Imaizumi, T., Miyagishi, M., Taira, K., Akira, S., and Fujita, T. (2004) Nat Immunol 5, 730
53. Yoneyama, M., Kikuchi, M., Matsumoto, K., Imaizumi, T., Miyagishi, M., Taira, K., Foy, E., Loo, Y., Gale, M. J., Akira, S., Yonehara, S., Kato, A., and Fujita, T. (2005) J Immunol 175, 2851
54. Alexopoulou, L., Holt, A., Medzhitov, R., and Flavell, R. (2001) Nature 413, 732
55. Kabelitz, D. (2007) Curr Opin Immunol 19, 39
56. Jiang, Q., Wei, H., and Tian, Z. (2008) J Immunother 31, 555
57. Heinz, S., Haehnel, V., Karaghiosoff, M., Schwarzfischer, L., Muller, M., Krause, S., and Rehli, M. (2003) J Biol Chem 278, 21502
58. Applequist, S., Wallin, R., and Ljunggren, H. (2002) Int Immunol 14, 1065
59. Levy, H., Law, L., and Rabson, A. (1969) Proc Natl Acad Sci USA 62, 357
60. Bart, R., Kopf, A., and Silagi, S. (1971) J Invest Dermatol 56, 33
61. Turner, W., Chan, S., and Chirigos, M. (1970) Proc Soc Exp Biol Med 133, 334
62. Fisher, J., Cooperband, S., and Mannick, J. (1972) Cancer Res 32, 889
63. Droller, M., and Gomolka, D. (1982) Cancer Res 42, 5038
64. Chapekar, M., and Glazer, R. (1986) Cancer Res 46, 1698
65. Whitmore, M., DeVeer, M., Edling, A., Oates, R., Simons, B., Lindner, D., and Williams, B. (2004) Cancer Res 64, 5850
66. Cella, M., Salio, M., Sakakibara, Y., Langen, H., Julkunen, I., and Lanzavecchia, A. (1999) J Exp Med 189, 821
67. Le Bon, A., Etchart, N., Rossmann, C., Ashton, M., Hou, S., Gewert, D., Borrow, P., and Tough, D. (2003) Nat Immunol 4, 1009
68. Khan, A., Heys, S., and Eremin, O. (1995) Eur J Surg Oncol 21, 224
69. Seya, T., Akazawa, T., Uehori, J., Matsumoto, M., Azuma, I., and Toyoshima, K. (2003) Anticancer Res 23, 4369
70. Smits, E., Ponsaerts, P., Van de Velde, A., Van Driessche, A., Cools, N., Lnejou, M., Nijs, G., Van Bockstaele, D., Berneman, Z., and Van Tendeloo, V. (2007) Leukemia 21, 1691
71. McBride, S., Hoebe, K., Georgel, P., and Janssen, E. (2006) J Immunol 177, 6122
72. Fujimura, T., Nakagawa, S., Ohtani, T., Ito, Y., and Aiba, S. (2006) Eur J Immunol 36, 3371
73. Michiels, A., Breckpot, K., Corthals, J., Tuyaerts, S., Bonehill, A., Heirman, C., Thielmans, K., and Aerts, J. (2006) Gene Ther 13, 1027
74. Salem, M., Kadima, A., Cole, D., and Gillanders, W. (2005) J Immunother 28, 220

75. Akazawa, T., Ebihara, T., Okuno, M., Okuda, Y., Shingai, M., Tsujimura, K., Takahashi, T., Ikawa, M., Okabe, M., Inoue, N., Okamoto-Tanaka, M., Ishizaki, H., Miyoshi, J., Matsumoto, M., and Seya, T. (2007) Proc Natl Acad Sci USA 104, 252
76. Bonmort, M., Ullrich, E., Mignot, G., Jacobs, B., Chaput, N., and Zitvogel, L. (2007) Biochimie 89, 872
77. Chan, C., Crafton, E., Fan, H., Flook, J., Yoshimura, K., Sharica, M., Brockstedt, D., Dubensky, T., Stins, M., Lanier, L., Pardoll, D., and Housseau, F. (2006) Nat Med 12, 207
78. Taieb, J., Chaput, N., Menard, C., Apetoh, L., Ullrich, E., Bonmort, M., Pequignot, M., Casares, N., Terme, M., Flament, C., Opolon, P., Lecluse, Y., Metivier, D., Tomasello, E., Vivier, E., Ghiringhelli, F., Martin, F., Klatzmann, D., Poynard, T., Tursz, T., Raposo, G., Yagita, H., Ryffel, B., Kroemer, G., and Zitvogel, L. (2006) Nat Med 12, 214
79. Vremec, D., O'Keeffe, M., Hochrein, H., Fuchsberger, M., Caminschi, I., Lahoud, M., and Shortman, K. (2007) Blood 109, 1165
80. Sivori, S., Falco, M., Della, C., Carlomagno, S., Vitale, M., Moretta, L., and Moretta, A. (2004) Proc Natl Acad Sci USA 101, 10116
81. Jiang, Q., Wei, H., and Tian, Z. (2008) BMC Cancer 8, 12
82. Salaun, B., Lebecque, S., Matikainen, S., Rimoldi, D., and Romero, P. (2007) Clin Cancer Res 13, 4565
83. Salaun, B., Coste, I., Rissoan, M., Lebecque, S., and Renno, T. (2006) J Immunol 176, 4894
84. Huang, B., Zhao, J., Li, H., He, K., Chen, Y., Chen, S., Mayer, L., Unkeless, J., and Xiong, H. (2005) Cancer Res 65, 5009
85. Sebastiani, G., Leveque, G., Lariviere, L., Laroche, L., Skamene, E., Gros, P., and Malo, D. (2000) Genomics 64, 230
86. Zarember, K., and Godowski, P. (2002) J Immunol 168, 554
87. Eaves-Pyles, T., Wong, H., Odoms, K., and Pyles, R. (2001) J Immunol 167, 7009
88. Dwyer, J., and Mackay, I. (1972) Int Arch Allergy Appl Immunol 43, 434
89. Jeon, S., and Arnon, R. (2002) Viral Immunol 15, 165
90. Wyant, T., Tanner, M., and Sztein, M. (1999) Infect Immun 67, 1338
91. Cuadros, C., Lopez-Hernandez, F., Dominguez, A., McClelland, M., and Lustgarten, J. (2004) Infect Immun 72, 2810
92. Huleatt, J., Jacobs, A., Tang, J., Desai, P., Kopp, E., Huang, Y., Song, L., Nakaar, V., and Powell, T. (2007) Vaccine 25, 763
93. Mizel, S., West, A., and Hantgan, R. (2003) J Biol Chem 278, 23624
94. Smith, K., Andersen-Nissen, E., Hayashi, F., Strobe, K., Bergman, M., Barrett, S., Cookson, B., and Aderem, A. (2003) Nat Immunol 4, 1247
95. Liaudet, L., Szabo, C., Engenov, O., Murthy, K., Pacher, P., Virag, L., Mabley, J., Marton, A., Soriano, F., Kirov, M., Bjertnaes, L., and Salzman, A. (2003) Shock 19, 131
96. Gewirtz, A., Navas, T., Lyons, S., Godowski, P., and Madara, J. (2001) J Immunol 167, 1882
97. McDermott, P., Ciacci-Woolwine, F., Snipes, J., and Mizel, S. (2000) Infect Immun 68, 5525
98. Means, T., Hayashi, F., Smith, K., Aderem, A., and Luster, A. (2003) J Immunol 170, 5165
99. Agrawal, S., Agrawal, A., Doughty, B., Gerwitz, A., Blenis, J., Van Dyke, T., and Pulendran, B. (2003) J Immunol 171, 4984
100. Applequist, S., Rollman, E., Wareing, M., Liden, M., Rozell, B., Hinkula, J., and Liunggren, H. (2005) J Immunol 175, 3882
101. Sfondrini, L., Rossini, A., Besusso, D., Merlo, A., Taliabue, E., Menard, S., and Balsari, A. (2006) J Immunol 176, 6624
102. Hooper, L., Wong, M., Thelin, A., Hansson, L., Falk, P., and Gordon, J. (2001) Science 291, 881
103. Uematsu, S., Jang, M., Chevrier, N., Guo, Z., Kumagai, Y., Yamamoto, M., Kato, H., Sougawa, N., Matsui, H., Kuwata, H., Hemmi, H., Coban, C., Kawai, T., Ishii, K., Takeuchi, O., Miyasaka, M., Takeda, K., and Akira, S. (2006) Nat Immunol 7, 868
104. Rakoff-Nahoum, S., and Medzhitov, R. (2007) Science 317, 124
105. Rhee, S., Im, E., and Pothoulakis, C. (2008) Gastroenterology 135, 518
106. Agrawal, S., and Kandimalla, E. (2007) Biochem Soc Trans 35, 1461

107. Akira, S., and Takeda, K. (2004) Nat Rev Immunol 4, 499
108. Spaner, D., and Miller, R. (2005) Leuk Lymphoma 46, 935
109. Field, A., Tytell, A., Lampson, G., and Hilleman, M. (1967) Proc Natl Acad Sci USA 58, 1004
110. Sidky, Y., Borden, E., Weeks, C., Reiter, M., Hatcher, J., and Bryan, G. (1992) Cancer Res 52, 3528
111. Nakaike, S., Yamagishi, T., Samata, K., Nishida, K., Inazuki, K., Ichihara, T., Migita, Y., Otomo, S., Aihara, H., and Tsukagoshi, S. (1989) Cancer Chemother Pharmacol 23, 135
112. Slade, H., Owens, M., Tomai, M., and Miller, R. (1998) Expert Opin Investig Drugs 7, 437
113. Testerman, T., Gerster, J., Imbertson, L., Reiter, M., Miller, R., Gibson, S., Wagner, T., and Tomai, M. (1995) J Leukoc Biol 58, 365
114. Hemmi, H., Kaisho, T., Takeuchi, O., Sato, S., Sanjo, H., Hoshino, K., Horiuchi, T., Tomizawa, H., Takeda, K., and Akira, S. (2002) Nat Immunol 3, 196
115. Suzuki, H., Wang, B., Shivji, G., Toto, P., Amerio, P., Tomai, M., Miller, R., and Sauder, D. (2000) J Invest Dermatol 114, 135
116. Ito, T., Amakawa, R., Kaisho, T., Hemmi, H., Tajima, K., Uehira, K., Ozaki, Y., Tomizawa, H., Akira, S., and Fukuhara, S. (2002) J Exp Med 195, 1507
117. Gibson, S., Lindh, J., Riter, T., Gleason, R., Rogers, L., Fuller, A., Oesterich, J., Gorden, K., Qiu, X., McKane, S., Noelle, R., Miller, R., Kedl, R., Fitzgerald-Bocarsly, P., Tomai, M., and Vasilakos, J. (2002) Cell Immunol 218, 74
118. Rechsteiner, G., and Warger, T. (2005) J Immunol 174, 2476
119. Spaner, D., Shi, Y., White, D., Mena, J., Hammond, C., Tomic, J., He, L., Tomai, M., Miller, R., Booth, J., and Radvanyi, L. (2006) Leukemia 20, 286
120. Urosevic, M., Oberholzer, P., Maier, T., Hafner, J., Laine, E., Slade, H., Benninghoff, B., Burg, G., and Dummer, R. (2004) Clin Cancer Res 10, 4959
121. Majewski, S., Marczak, M., Mlynarczyk, B., Benninghoff, B., and Jablonska, S. (2005) Int J Dermatol 44, 14
122. Stary, G., Bangert, C., Tauber, M., Strohal, R., Kopp, T., and Stingle, G. (2007) J Exp Med 204, 1441
123. Dudek, A., Yunis, C., Harrison, L., Kumar, S., Hawkinson, R., Cooley, S., Vasilakos, J., Gorski, K., and Miller, J. (2007) Clin Cancer Res 13, 7119
124. Adams, S., O'Neill, D., Nonaka, D., Hardin, E., Chiriboga, L., Siu, K., Cruz, C., Angiulli, A., Angiulli, F., Ritter, E., Holman, R., Shapiro, R., Berman, R., Berner, N., Shao, Y., Manches, O., Pan, L., Venhaus, R., Hoffman, E., Jungbluth, A., Gnjatic, S., Old, L., Pavlick, A., and Bhardwaj, N. (2008) J Immunol 181, 776
125. Shackleton, M., Davis, I., Hopkins, W., Jackson, H., Dimopoulos, N., Tai, T., Chen, Q., Jefford, M., Masterman, K., Caron, D., Chen, W., Maraskovsky, E., and Cebon, J. (2004) Cancer Immun 4, 9
126. Wiemann, B., and Starnes, C. (1994) Pharmacol Ther 64, 529
127. Krieg, A. M. (2002) Annu Rev Immunol 20, 709
128. Messina, J., Gilkeson, G., and Pisetsky, D. (1991) J Immunol 147, 1759
129. Bauer, S., Pigisch, S., Hangel, D., Kaufmann, A., and Hamm, S. (2008) Immunobiology 213, 315
130. Ballas, Z., Rasmussen, W., and Krieg, A. (1996) J Immunol 157, 1840
131. Klinman, D. (2004) Rev Immunol 4, 249
132. Iwasaki, A., and Medzhitov, R. (2004) Nature Immunol 5, 987
133. Kunikata, N., Sano, K., Honda, M., Ishii, K., Matsunaga, J., Okuyama, R., Takahashi, K., Watanabe, H., Tamura, G., Tagami, H., and Terui, T. (2004) J Invest Dermatol 123, 395
134. Wickstrom, E. (1997) Antisense Nucleic Acid Drug Dev 7, 225
135. Smith, J., and Wickstrom, E. (1998) J Natl Cancer Inst 90, 1146
136. Ballas, Z., Krieg, A., Warren, T., Rasmussen, W., Davis, H., Waldschmidt, M., and Weiner, G. (2001) J Immunol 167, 4878
137. Carpentier, A., Chen, L., Maltoni, F., and Delattre, J. (1999) Cancer Res 59, 5429
138. Blazar, B., Krieg, A., and Taylor, P. (2001) Blood 98, 1217

139. Sharma, S., Dominguez, A., Manrique, S., Cavallo, F., Sakaguchi, S., and Lustgarten, J. (2008) Cancer Res 68, 7530
140. Sharma, S., Dominguez, A., Hoelzinger, D., and Lustgarten, J. (2008) Cancer Immunol Immunother 57, 549
141. Carpentier, A., Laigle-Donadey, F., Zohar, S., Capelle, L., Behin, A., Tibi, A., Martin-Duverneuil, N., Sanson, M., Lacomblez, L., Tailibert, S., Puybasset, L., Van Effenterre, R., Delattre, J., and Carpentier, A. (2006) Neuro Oncol 8, 60
142. Leonard, J., Link, B., Emmanouilides, C., Gregory, S., Weisdorf, D., Audrey, J., Hainsworth, J., Sparano, J., Tsai, D., Horning, S., Krieg, A., and Weiner, G. (2007) Clin Cancer Res 13, 6168

Manipulating TNF Receptors to Enhance Tumor Immunity for the Treatment of Cancer

Carl E. Ruby and Andrew D. Weinberg

Abstract Members of the TNF receptor superfamily, CD27, CD134, CD137, and GITR, play a major role in the optimal activation of CD4 and CD8 T cells. Signals mediated by these receptors help to define the duration and scope of T cell responses by enhancing the function and survival of recently differentiated effector T cells. In addition to effects on differentiating T cells, recent data also suggest that CD134, CD137, and GITR influence regulatory T cell generation and suppressive activity. The potent immune-modulatory effects of these receptors translate into effective antitumor immunity and successful tumor regression in a number of different preclinical tumor models. On the basis of the effective antitumor responses generated in preclinical models, a number of TNF receptor-based clinical immunotherapeutic interventions have been developed for the treatment of cancer. This chapter will focus on the emergence of clinical approaches for effective tumor immunotherapy by describing the effects of CD27, CD134, CD137, and GITR on T cell-mediated immune responses and preclinical tumor studies.

Introduction

The origins of cancer immunotherapy, the design of immunological approaches for the treatment of cancer, are ultimately tied to a family of receptors known as tumor necrosis factor receptors (TNFRs). Over one hundred years ago, administration of bacterial-derived factors was described to shrink human cancers, an observation that eventually lead to the discovery of a protein that mediated these responses named tumor necrosis factor alpha (TNFα) [1–3]. Once TNFα was isolated and purified, DNA and amino acid homology studies eventually revealed the TNF and TNFR superfamilies [4]. Although the clinical use of systemic TNFα as an anticancer agent has been overtly toxic and not very effective, targeting proteins of the TNFR superfamily expressed on T cells to modulate immune responses offer an alternate

A.D. Weinberg (✉)
Earle A. Chiles Research Institute, Portland Providence Medical Center, Portland, OR 97213
e-mail: andrew.weinberg@providence.org

J. Lustgarten et al. (eds.), *Targeted Cancer Immune Therapy*,
DOI 10.1007/978-1-4419-0170-5_18, © Springer Science+Business Media, LLC 2009

and potentially effective approach for the treatment of cancer. Indeed, stimulation of several TNFR proteins including, CD27, CD134, CD137, and glucocorticoid-induced TNFR-related protein (GITR), has demonstrated the ability to significantly modify T cell responses and to generate productive antitumor immune responses in animal models. Thus, this chapter will focus on the features, function, and ability of these four TNFR proteins to induce effective T cell-mediated antitumor responses and discuss current clinical approaches for cancer immune therapies.

Structural and Signaling Features

The 29 currently identified TNFR proteins, including CD27, CD134, CD137, and GITR, are type I transmembrane monomers, characterized by several extracellular cystine-rich domains (CRDs) and an intracellular signaling domain. Originally, the assembly of the TNFR was thought to be directed by the appropriate TNF trimeric ligand that would recruit the necessary TNFR monomers; however, recent findings suggest that TNFR oligomers are present prior to the ligand binding [5]. In this model, the distal CRDs of at least two TNFR monomers interact to form the preligand assembly domain (PLAD) that significantly increases the affinity of ligand binding and subsequent trimerization of the TNFR. The presence of PLAD on T cells may represent a sensitized state that speeds the formation and strength of signaling through binding TNF-family members during the activation of antigen-specific T cells.

Engagement of CD27, CD134, CD137, and GITR by their cognate TNF protein ligands mediates a signaling cascade involving a number of intracellular kinases, signaling proteins, and transcription factors. Upon cognate ligand binding, the intracellular portion of TNFR proteins mediates signaling via specialized domains that recruit cytoplasmic adaptor proteins, TNF receptor-associated factors (TRAFs). To date six different TRAF molecules have been identified in mammals (TRAF1–6) [6]. While multiple TRAFs can interact with an individual TNFR, TRAFs 1, 2, 3, and 5 commonly interact with the four TNFRs discussed here. Once recruited the TRAFs facilitate activation of the JNK and p38/MAPK kinases, and the transcription factor NF-κB [7, 8]. Activation of these signaling pathways induces transcription of a number of genes involved in T cell growth, division, and survival. It is the activation of these signaling pathways via the TRAF proteins that is a major distinguishing feature of these four costimulatory TNFR proteins, and more importantly is a means for optimal activation of T cells.

T cell activation is generally regarded to occur in two steps: antigen recognition and costimulation. At the heart of the first step, antigen recognition is the presentation of peptide antigen in the context of major histocompatibility complexes (MHC) to a complimentary T cell receptor (TCR) specific for that antigen. The TCR affinity for cognate antigen and the duration of corresponding signaling contribute to the overall strength of the activation signal delivered to the T cell. Successful antigen recognition initiates the proliferation of the T cells, which in the absence of a second costimulatory signal is dramatically altered, resulting in limited T cell division, reduced function, and increased susceptibility to deletion. Costimulation of antigen-primed T cells is predominately delivered by the cell-surface protein, CD28, a member of the immunoglobulin superfamily, as well as proteins from the TNFR superfamily, in particular CD27, CD134, CD137, and GITR. The costimulatory signals provided by these four TNFRs help dictate the optimal strength and duration of a T cell response, ultimately making them attractive targets to enhance immune responses in cancer patients.

Expression

The expression of CD27, CD134, CD137, and GITR is primarily restricted to cells of the immune system and in particular T cells. Their expression, however, is not exclusive to T cells, as other immune cells such as natural killer (NK) cells also express detectable levels of CD27 and CD137 [9, 10]. In addition, B cells can express CD27, dendritic cells (DCs) and eosinophils can express CD137, and CD134 has been observed on neutrophils [11–15]. Yet it is the expression of these TNFRs on T cells that appears to have the greatest impact on an immune response.

The pattern and kinetics of CD27, CD134, CD137, and GITR expression on T cells, both in mice and humans, are important for their function as signaling receptors to direct T cell activation and influence immune responses. The general pattern of T cell expression of these TNFRs can be determined by timing and the state of T cell activation/differentiation as seen in Fig. 1. For instance, naïve T cells express CD27 and GITR, but not CD134 or CD137. Following TCR-activation, expression of CD27 and GITR increases and CD134 and CD137 become detectable with further up-regulation occurring over the course of T cell activation/differentiation. These generalized stages of expression were elucidated from in vitro studies and while helpful, they may not fully account for differences in expression due to the variability

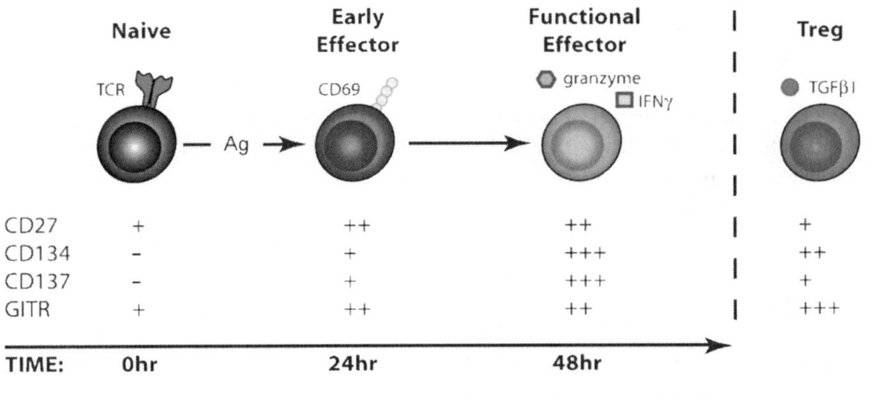

Fig. 1 Generalized expression pattern of CD27, CD134, CD137, and GITR on T cells. Circulating naive T cells express CD27 and GITR at relatively low levels. Upon antigen-activation of naive T cells and differentiation of these cells into effector T cells coincides with the expression of CD134 and CD137 as well as an up-regulation of CD27 and GITR. Optimal levels of these four TNF receptors generally occur 24–48 h after initial antigen-priming. Regulatory T cells (Treg) express all four of these TNF receptors, but GITR is often considered to be particularly high on this T cell subset

of antigen-mediated T cell activation under normal in vivo conditions. Despite the potential variability, CD27, CD134, CD137, and GITR up-regulation occur roughly within 48 h of TCR-binding and can be sustained for several days [7, 8]. During this time the TNFR molecules are available on antigen-primed T cells for stimulation by endogenous ligands or agonistic agents delivered exogenously.

Typical endogenous TNFR signaling requires both the expression of surface bound TNFR protein, and the presence of a cognate ligand at the same time. The cognate ligands for CD27, CD134, CD137, and GITR, are CD70, CD252, CD137L, and GITRL, respectively. Mature or activated antigen-presenting cells (DCs, macrophages, monocytes, and B cells) express levels of CD70, CD252, CD137L, and GITRL sufficient to activate T cells [12, 16–20]. Although expression of these ligands on APCs produces an effective combination of antigen-presentation and costimulation, several of these ligands (CD70, CD252, and GITRL) are also expressed by activated T cells, which may result in T cell–T cell interactions, that prolong TNFR signaling [16, 17, 21]. Finally, expression of TNFR ligands varies and is dependent, in part, on cytokines and pathogen-associated molecules found in a given microenvironment. Thus, in the absence of strong APC maturation signals, antigen presentation may occur with weak expression of TNFR ligands and thereby provide weak costimulation to antigen-specific T cells despite optimal TNFR expression.

Antitumor Responses

Engagement of CD27, CD134, CD137, and GITR on T cells significantly affects the scope, strength, and duration of an immune response and represents a potential means for enhancing antitumor responses. In fact, stimulation of these individual TNFR molecules has been shown in numerous preclinical animal models to enhance T cell activation and generate beneficial tumor immune responses. Such experiments highlight at least two significant T cell-specific mechanisms by which signaling through CD27, CD134, CD137, and GITR successfully mediates antitumor immunity; (1) the enhancement of tumor-specific effector T cell responses and (2) neutralization of the effects of regulatory T cells (Tregs).

By definition, effector T cells are T cells that have been activated by antigen and CD28 to proliferate and differentiate (with the help of cytokines) into cells that produce cytotoxic mediators and/or cytokines that further expand an immune response. CD8 effectors, also known as cytotoxic T lymphocytes (CTLs), produce cytotoxic molecules, granzymes and perforins, which promote the destruction of cells expressing foreign or modified antigens in the form of MHC class I. In addition, effector CD8 and CD4 T cells secrete the cytokines IL-2, TNFα, and IFNγ that mediate effects locally and distally by activating T cells and other cells of the immune system, such as macrophages and B cells. The responding cells, both immune and nonimmune, often work in concert with these cytokine secreting effector cells and cytotoxic effectors to mount an integrated response to a pathogen or tumor. In the case of tumor immunity, both CD4 and CD8 effector T cells are critical for effective antitumor responses, as the presence of effector T cells in large numbers within the tumor represents a positive clinical prognosis [22, 23].

Regulatory T cells (Tregs) are a class of CD4 T cells that regulate normal immune homeostasis, by suppressing aberrant or excessive immune responses. This role is vital in controlling immune responses to self-antigens and maintaining self-tolerance; however, the same effects may have a deleterious effect on tumor immunity. Tregs have been well described and several different subtypes have been identified based on location of origin and mode of immune suppression [24–26]. Generally, the two forms that predominate are natural and induced Tregs, both identified by their expression of the transcription factor Forkhead-Box Protein 3 (FoxP3). Natural Tregs originate from the thymus and are thought to serve as a line of defense against autoimmunity. In contrast, induced Tregs originate at sites of excessive antigen stimulation and/or suppressive cytokines, such as TGFβ1 and IL-10, to keep the immune response in check. Both types of Tregs are influential in modulating tumor immune responses during priming and effector phases, and can be ultimately hijacked by tumors to evade immune-mediated destruction.

Enthusiasm for targeting CD27, CD134, CD137, and GITR as therapeutic interventions has grown out of intriguing results from a number of successful preclinical animal studies. The impact of these preclinical studies has revealed that manipulation of these TNFRs represents a potential strategy to enhance an ongoing antitumor immune response, by either augmenting the effector response and/or neutralizing the effects of Tregs (summarized in Fig. 2). The following sections will describe the effects that signals mediated by CD27, CD134, CD137, and GITR have on T cell function and survey the results of antitumor immune responses mediated by these TNFRs in various models.

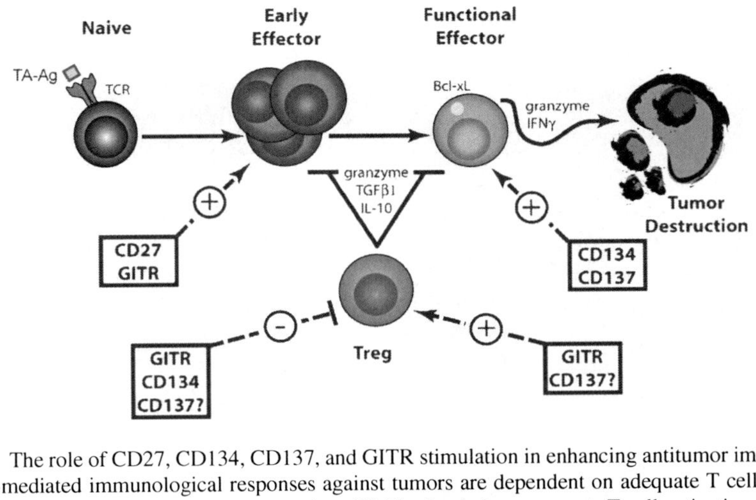

Fig. 2 The role of CD27, CD134, CD137, and GITR stimulation in enhancing antitumor immunity. T cell-mediated immunological responses against tumors are dependent on adequate T cell activation and regulatory T cell (Treg) suppression. CD27-stimulation augments T cell activation early in an antitumor immune response, increasing T cell accumulation. GITR like CD27 mediates costimulatory signals early in an antitumor response, but also can abrogate or boost Treg immunosuppression depending on the immunological model. Acting later in T cell differentiation, CD134 enhances effector T cell survival (Bcl-xL) and function (granzyme and IFNγ) against tumors and abrogates T cell suppression mediated by Tregs. CD137 costimulation also enhances effector T cell survival and function in antitumor immune responses, but its effect on Treg function is not fully understood. Overall, stimulation of each of these TNF receptors can mediate effective tumor destruction

CD27

Costimulatory signals delivered by CD27 mainly impact the survival of recently generated effector T cells, as well as those found at the site of infection. These effects of CD27 ligation, during the initial stages of T cell activation, are a direct consequence of its expression on naïve and TCR-stimulated T cells. Unlike CD134 and CD137 whose expression occurs after antigen stimulation, low levels of CD27 can be found at the time of TCR activation. This arrangement suggests that CD27 provides critical costimulatory signals to T cells coincident with antigen-priming early in T cell activation, as demonstrated when T cells lacking CD27 divided normally after priming, but then failed to expand at later time points [27]. It is likely that CD27 stimulation at these early time points protects developing effector T cells from deletion. Indeed, recent in vitro evidence suggests CD27 stimulation of TCR-primed CD8 T cells sustains levels of IL-7R, which is a classic mediator of T cell homeostasis and survival [28]. Furthermore, genetically modified animals have supplied additional evidence supporting CD27-induced survival of effector T cells. CD27-deficient mice experience decreased numbers of antigen-specific T cells after pathogenic challenge and conversely, mice with constitutively expressed CD70 exhibit an increase in effector T cell numbers following priming [27, 29]. Interestingly, CD70 expression is also up-regulated on activated T cells, thereby resulting in secondary or alternative CD27 signaling mediated by T cell–T cell interactions at sites where effector T cells accumulate. Taken together, CD27 stimulation presumably affects the survival of effector cells shortly after antigen-priming and serves to maintain the effector population both during the early stages of T cell activation, and during the accumulation of effectors at the site of a developing immune response. Complementing the ability of CD27 to enhance effector T cell survival, CD27 has also been shown to enhance effector T cell function by increasing IFNγ production (on a per cell basis) [30]. Collectively, these CD27-mediated biological responses may be a promising target for tumor immunotherapy.

Several approaches that stimulate CD27 directly or boost the level of CD70 have led to tumor regression in a number of animal models. For example, administration of an agonist CD27 antibody 4–7 days after tumor challenge achieved significant tumor-free survival in two different models of lymphoma (BCL_1 and A31) [31]. These results complement two additional studies that used enforced expression of CD70 to induce significant antitumor immunity. In the first study, transgenic CD70 animals completely rejected a transplantable thymoma (EL4) that nontransgenic animals failed to reject [30]. In this study, enforced CD70 expression led to an increase in tumor-associated antigen-specific CD8 T cells infiltrating the tumors. In a second study, a mouse fibroblast cell line that produced a secretable soluble form of biologically active CD70 was coinjected with an unrelated mammary adenocarcinoma (TS/A). This coinjection resulted in significant tumor-free survival that was ascribed to the soluble CD70, as fibroblasts transfected with an irrelevant control gene failed to induce effective tumor immunity in mammary adenocarcinoma-bearing animals [32].

Despite the success of these preclinical therapies based on CD27-stimulation, potential caveats to this intervention have come to light. In at least two instances, tumors (renal cell carcinoma and glioma) were able to escape immune surveillance by expressing CD70 [33, 34]. Escape of the tumors was attributed to CD70-mediated apoptosis of circulating T cells, which is not fully understood. These findings suggest that in a tumor setting CD27 activation may have a deleterious effect on the maintenance and survival of tumor-specific and other responding T cells. In a related study, mice with enforced expression of CD70 experienced rapid conversion of naïve T cells into effector and memory cells that resulted in depletion of naïve T cells in the lymphoid organs [35]. In both of these cases, exhaustion of the T cell pool by persistent/excessive CD27 stimulation may contribute to loss of circulating T cells, thereby resulting in tumor immune escape. Thus, careful control of timing and extent of CD27 stimulation will be the key to the success of this therapy.

GITR

Originally identified on T cells treated with a potent immunosuppressant, GITR has garnered increased attention for its effects on both nonregulatory T cell and Tregs. GITR is expressed on naïve T cells at low levels that then increases following TCR activation; peak levels are achieved within 24 h of initial TCR stimulation. Engagement of the up-regulated GITR on the surface of early CD4 and CD8 effector T cells has been shown to provide costimulation in the form of increased cytokine production, cytotoxicity, and survival [36–38]. Although the expression of GITR on naïve and effector expression mediated significant costimulatory effects on differentiating effector T cells, it was eclipsed by findings demonstrating that Tregs constitutively expressed high levels of GITR.

GITR expression on Tregs indicated that it may play a role in the function of these influential cells. Subsequent studies did in fact show stimulation of GITR on Tregs abrogated their suppressive effect on TCR-activated CD4 T cell responses in vitro, and GITR stimulation in vivo induced or exacerbated autoimmune diseases in several animal models [39–41]. These data formed the foundation to our early understanding of the relationship between GITR and Tregs suppression. However, due to the ability of activated nonregulatory CD4 T cells to also up-regulate GITR expression, it is also possible that engagement of GITR on this population of cells, and not on Tregs, may account for the decrease in suppression in GITR-stimulated cultures. Development of GITR-deficient mice, which have functional Tregs, allowed for detailed investigations into the specific contribution of GITR to responding nonregulatory T cells and Tregs. In two elegant studies, naïve nonregulatory T cells from GITR-intact mice were mixed with GITR-deficient Tregs and stimulated with an agonist GITR antibody. Proliferation of the responding T cells was at or near control levels (no Tregs added) following TCR activation, thereby implicating the responding T cells as the primary target of GITR stimulation [17, 37]. Thus when taken together, these results and earlier ones suggest that GITR engagement can not only reverse the suppressive activity of Tregs, but also provide signals to responding nonregulatory CD4 T cells to make them resistant to Treg suppression. An additional challenge to our understanding of the role of GITR on Treg activity came after it was shown that engagement of GITR on Tregs increased their IL-10 production and proliferation, a stark contrast to GITR abrogating Treg suppression [36, 39]. Therefore, what emerges from the data regarding the effects of GITR on Tregs and normal nonregulatory T cell activation is a delicate balance between augmentation and suppression of T cell responses that relies on GITR modulating the suppressive function of Tregs, and GITR inducing resistance of responding T cells to Treg suppression [42].

In spite of the complexity surrounding the ability of GITR to influence an immune response through responding nonregulatory T cells and suppressive Tregs, a number of studies have shown that GITR stimulation increases antitumor immunity. In these studies an agonist GITR antibody (DTA-1) was delivered systemically at various times before and after tumor challenge in the presence of vaccine or as a monotherapy. When GITR treatment was included in a vaccine regimen using tumor-associated antigens, the responding tumor-associated antigen-specific T cells were increased in number and function. The subsequent rejection of a poorly immunogenic melanoma (B16) was attributed to these GITR-enhanced vaccine-specific T cell responses [43]. In addition to GITR enhancing tumor vaccine approaches, significant tumor-free survival was also conferred in animal models using GITR treatment as a stand-alone therapy against a sarcoma (MethA) and a colon carcinoma (CT26) [44, 45]. In these studies, the agonist GITR antibody showed great efficacy mediating up to 90% survival. A closer inspection of the GITR-treated animals revealed a significant increase in the production of IFNγ by both CD4 and CD8 T cells, as well as an increase in the number of these T cells in the tumor draining lymph nodes and infiltrating the tumors. Furthermore, the Treg frequency after GITR treatment in these animals was diminished. Assessment of the relative contribution of GITR enhancing nonregulatory T cells compared with GITR abrogating Treg activity appeared to favor costimulation of the nonregulatory T cells. It was shown that depletion of Tregs prior to tumor challenge elicited significant tumor-free survival, suggesting early inhibition of Treg activity can release tumor-specific immunity from suppression; yet when agonist GITR antibody was administered prior to tumor challenge tumor-free survival was relatively unchanged compared with untreated controls [44]. Collectively, the preclinical data suggest that administration of agonist GITR antibody provides effective costimulation to tumor-reactive T cells and may dampen the effects of Tregs, together generating a platform for the development of effective tumor immunity with or without a vaccine.

CD134 (OX40)

CD134, also known as OX40, is a potent T cell costimulatory molecule, whose notable effect on T cell activation occurs after antigen-priming and includes enhanced effector T cell survival and function. The costimulatory signals mediated by CD134 are regulated by its transient expression, which is largely restricted to activated CD4 and CD8 T cells. T cell expression of CD134 peaks 24–48 h after TCR engagement and declines to undetectable levels after 120 h [46–48]. Other signals and conditions exert additional control over the expression of OX40 on antigen-activated T cells. These factors include CD28 signaling [49] and localized concentration of antigen. The latter aspect appeared to dictate expression of CD134 on CD8 T cells, as CD134 expression appears to occur only on CD8 T cells in the lymph nodes draining the site of antigen-challenge, where antigen is expected to be at the highest concentration [50, 51].

The engagement of CD134 on CD4 and CD8 T cells has potent effects on the stimulation and survival of effector T cells [52]. This is evident in transgenic mice with enforced CD252, the cognate ligand of CD134 that displayed a dramatic increase in T cell survival and memory T cell generation following immunization [53]. In agreement with the findings from CD252 transgenic mice, CD134-deficient T cells were more susceptible to T cell apoptosis compared with their CD134-intact counterparts [54]. Examination of the underlying mechanism of CD134-mediated improved T cell survival appeared to involve increased NF-κB activity (via direct activation of IκB kinase), and maintenance of intracellular levels of the antiapoptotic proteins Bcl-2 and Bcl-xL [49, 55]. Although CD134 stimulation has been strongly associated with increased T cell survival, there is growing evidence that CD134-mediated costimulation can also greatly enhance both CD4 and CD8 effector T cell function. CD4 T cells stimulated with antigen and agonist anti-CD134 in vivo, recovered from the draining lymph nodes after priming, and restimulated with antigen directly ex vivo produced tenfold greater levels of IFNγ and IL-2 (on a per cell basis) compared with control animals [56, 57]. Additionally, CD8 effector T cell function, measured as increased TNFα, IFNγ, and granzyme B production, was also enhanced following CD134 stimulation [51, 58]. These results suggest that CD134-mediated costimulation of differentiated effector CD4 and CD8 T cells after antigen-priming drives the accumulation of these cells and enhances their function.

In addition to its considerable influence on effector T cells, CD134 affects Tregs. Initial studies from CD134-deficient animals described diminished numbers of natural Tregs in the thymus, hinting that CD134 may have a role in the generation and homeostasis of natural Treg [59]. Additional phenotypic analyses of Tregs established that OX40 was highly expressed on natural, inducible, and Tr1 Tregs, leading to an examination of the function of CD134 within these populations [59–62]. Recently, several studies demonstrated that CD134 stimulation blocked the generation of at least two types of Tregs in culture, inducible and Tr1, a regulatory T cell noted for its prodigious IL-10 production [60–62]. Using combinations of CD134-deficient Tregs or responding nonregulatory T cells, it was found that stimulation of CD134 effectively abrogated the suppression of Tregs in vitro [59, 60, 63]. Additionally, in vivo stimulation of CD134 on Tregs transferred into T cell-deficient Rag-2 mice precipitated the rapid rejection of a skin allograft and exacerbated an experimental model of autoimmunity, verifying the in vitro data that established CD134-mediated abrogation of the suppressive effects of Tregs [59, 60]. Thus, the developing relationship between CD134 and Treg based on these results shows that

CD134 controls checkpoints that direct the generation of Tregs and abrogates Treg suppression of T cell-mediated immune responses.

Beyond its ability to enhance T cell activation and inhibit Treg suppression, a number of preclinical tumor models have shown CD134 stimulation led to suppression of tumor growth and regression of established tumors. CD134 is a convenient target for therapeutic intervention, as it is readily expressed on immune cells found infiltrating a number of tumors [64–66]. The availability of CD134 on potentially tumor-specific T cells has been exploited using either an agonist antibody or a CD252:Ig-fusion protein. Animals challenged with sarcomas (MCA205, MCA303), colon carcinoma (CT26), breast cancer (EMT6), and melanoma (B16), and then treated with CD134-directed therapy, experienced significant improvements in tumor-free survival [64, 66, 67]. The antitumor responses, in these studies, were dose dependent, tumor-specific, and require both CD4 and CD8 T cells, as depletion of either of these populations abrogated tumor-free survival [64]. In a second approach, intratumoral injection of an adenovirus that forced tumor expression of CD252 also promoted tumor regression [68]. Assessment of CD134-stimulated T cell activity in both these models revealed an increase in the secretion of IFNγ and/or IL-2 in both CD4 and CD8 T cells [69–71]. In contrast, analysis of the contribution of CD134-stimulated CD8 T cell in antitumor immunity using CD134-deficient tumor-antigen-specific CD8 T cells demonstrated no significant difference in cytokine production between CD134-deficient and -intact CD8 T cells, though survival of responding CD8 T cells was greater when CD134 was intact [72]. These results suggest the promotion of CD8 T cell survival by CD134 was more important than the enhancement of effector function. Although the relative contribution of increased T cell function and accumulation may be model specific and not yet fully understood, overall CD134-mediated effects on CD4 and CD8 T cells are critical for tumor immunity. The previous studies describe CD134 stimulation as a stand alone therapy, but combining CD134 stimulation with vaccines or cytokine treatments (IL-12) may be another potential means of tumor immunotherapy currently being explored [73, 74].

The significant role of CD134 in Treg generation and function has led to investigations into the contribution of CD134-mediated effects on Tregs in the rejection of established tumors. It has been observed that Tregs residing in tumors express CD134, thereby, representing a potential target for CD134-modulation. Indeed, agonist CD134 antibody treatment of two sarcomas (MCA205 and MCA303) decreased Tregs found infiltrating the tumor without altering Treg levels outside the tumor [75, 76]. To determine if the decline in Tregs seen in the tumors of CD134-stimulated animals could be attributed to an ability of CD134 to block their generation, as previously reported, antigen-specific (ovalbumin) nonregulatory CD4 T cells were transferred into tumor bearing animals at the same time ovalbumin was injected directly into the tumor [76]. Shortly after systemic agonist administration, the number of Tregs was enumerated from the antigen-injected tumors; the number of Tregs in CD134-stimulated animals was significantly less than in controls, suggesting CD134 blocked the generation of Tregs in a tumor setting. In addition to reducing the number of Tregs in the tumor, the remaining Tregs isolated from the tumors of these CD134-stimulated animals exhibited a diminished suppressive capacity [76]. Since CD134 stimulation may effectively dampen Treg suppression and enhance preexistent tumor immunity, it represents an effective immunotherapy.

CD137 (4-1BB)

The costimulatory function of the TNFR CD137 is often compared with that of CD134, yet upon closer inspection CD137 deviates in a number of significant ways. Both are transiently expressed on CD4 and CD8 T cells about 24 h after antigen-priming, but CD137 expression occurs more rapidly and at greater levels on antigen-primed CD8 T cells [77–79]. The kinetics of CD137 up-regulation most likely does not affect early events, such as proliferation, but instead may provide late-acting signals that affect effector T cell function and survival [8]. This could explain why agonist CD137 antibodies failed to boost the division rate of antigen-specific CD8 T cells, but increased the overall number of antigen-specific T cells several days after antigen immunization [18].

While the expression pattern of CD137 is similar to CD134, investigations indicate that CD137 primarily affects CD8 T cells with limited costimulatory effects on CD4 T cells. Early investigations, using agonist-CD137 stimulation or enforced expression of CD137L, demonstrated increased function and survival of both CD4 and CD8 effector T cells. CD137, like CD134, appeared to up-regulate CD4 T cell production of IFNγ and IL-2, CD8 T cell production of IFNγ and granzyme, and survival was enhanced in both T cell populations [80–84]. Activation of NF-κB and maintenance of antiapoptotic factors (e.g., Bcl-xL) underlie T cell survival following engagement of both CD137 and CD134. However, results from mice deficient for CD137 signaling contrasted the earlier results regarding the effects of CD137 on CD4 T cells. In these deficient animals, only CD8 T cell function and survival was affected by the loss of CD137 signaling [80, 83, 85]. These opposing results and additional studies suggest that the preponderance of the CD137-mediated activities appears to be more pronounced in CD8 T cells rather than CD4 T cells [86, 87].

Discovery of CD137 expression by Tregs led to a description of a functional role for CD137 on Treg maintenance and suppression of immunity. Stimulation of CD137 appeared to promote the proliferation of Tregs both in vivo and in vitro, although proliferation was dependent on the form of CD137 stimulation, as CD137L fusion-proteins induced proliferation, but not an agonist CD137 antibody [88–90]. Further examination of the CD137L fusion-protein-expanded population of Tregs revealed that they decreased proliferation of antigen-activated nonregulatory T cells in culture. In vivo these same Tregs prevented the rejection of an allograft, thereby retaining their suppressive nature [88, 89]. Interestingly, stimulation of Treg-CD137 (via agonist antibody) during priming abrogated the suppression of CD137-deficient nonregulatory T cell proliferation by CD137-intact Tregs following TCR-activation [90]. In agreement with data showing CD137-mediated abrogation of Treg activity, agonist CD137-stimulation of Tregs and not nonregulatory T cells exacerbated graft-versus-host disease (GVHD) when transferred into MHC-disparate recipients [90]. The results from these studies suggest that CD137-stimulation not only induces the proliferation of Tregs, but also abrogates Treg suppression during T cell activation. Additional studies are needed to establish more definitive conclusions.

Attempts to target CD137 in tumor-bearing animals to positively affect the generation of antitumor immunity have resulted in tumor regression and improved tumor-free survival. Most studies used agonistic CD137 antibodies to induce tumor immunity [91–93]; however, other successful approaches such as enforced tumor expression of CD137L also mediated the rejection of tumors [94, 95]. The list of tumors that have been shown to regress following agonist CD137 antibody treatment alone continues to grow and includes sarcomas (Ag104A, MCA205), glioma (GL261), lymphoma (EL4), and renal cell carcinoma (RENCA) [91, 92, 96]. In general, CD137-mediated rejection of these tumors appeared to require primarily CD8 T cells and IFNγ. The role of CD4 T cells in CD137-mediated tumor rejection seems to depend on the tumor model, as depletion of CD4 T cells in at least one model failed to affect tumor rejection, but in other tumor models, CD4 T cells were needed for tumor eradication [91, 93, 96]. Interestingly, depletion of CD4 T cells resulted in decreased tumor-specific memory responses in surviving CD137-treated animals, suggesting CD4 T cells are, at least, needed to form memory CD8 T cell responses [96]. On the contrary, IFNγ is required for effective tumor immunity following agonist CD137 treatment [96]. In conjunction with IFNγ, an increase in tumor-specific cytotoxic activity of effector CD8 T cells and an increase in CD8 T cells infiltrating the tumor, also correlated with CD137-enhancement of tumor immunity [97]. Finally, investigations into mechanisms underlying CD137-mediated tumor responses have revealed that signaling via CD137 breaks T cell tolerance to tumor antigens may also confer enhanced survival of tumor-infiltrating T cells by up-regulating the antiapoptotic proteins Bcl-2 and Bcl-xL [92, 98]. In conclusion, the effect of CD137 on tumor immunity is recognized by many to be the most promising potential therapeutic of all the TNFR reviewed here, due in part to its pronounced enhancement of CD8 T cell responses.

Clinical Application

The effective antitumor immunity mediated by CD27, CD134, CD137, and GITR previously highlighted has moved these molecules from preclinical study to the forefront of potential immunotherapeutic agents with a strong likelihood for success in cancer patients. Targeted stimulation of CD134, CD137, and GITR has been recognized to have great potential for broad usage in multiple types of therapeutic regimens especially with the intent to boost T cell stimulation [99]. In addition, successful preclinical studies suggest that these TNFRs have the capacity to be used against a number of different tumor types as stand-alone therapies. Indeed, several clinical approaches based on CD134 and CD137 stimulation are underway, at various clinical levels, in cancer patients; they represent the leading edge of TNFR-based cancer therapy that may in the future include CD27 and GITR.

Current clinical studies involving the stimulation of CD134 and CD137 have involved the therapeutic use of specific agonist monoclonal antibodies. The CD134-specific antibody approved for clinical use is a murine antibody specific for human CD134 that was developed following a study in nonhuman primates [100]. In this study and also in toxicology studies, an anti-CD134 drug increased the number of lymphocytes in the lymph nodes and spleens in primate subjects without overt toxicity, suggesting anti-CD134 could initiate measurable and tolerable immunological changes [100]; ADW (personal communication). The anti-CD134 studies in primates provided the foundation for the design of the current Phase I clinical trial. Advanced stage cancer patients with metastatic or locally advanced tumors have been given the anti-CD134 drug at various doses to assess the toleration of the drug, pharmacokinetics, immunological responses, and tumor regression. The pending results from this clinical study should provide guidance in follow-up Phase II studies and in combination with replacing the immunogenic murine antibody with a humanized antibody, may further optimize any beneficial effects of CD134-stimulation in cancer patients.

CD137-specific monoclonal antibodies for the treatment of cancer are further along in clinical trial than anti-CD134. At this time, there are four trials underway (www.clinicaltrials.gov) designed to assess the fully human monoclonal anti-CD137 drug (BMS-663513) in combination with other established therapies or as a stand-alone. In the stand alone trials, multiple doses of anti-CD137 have been administered to advanced stage cancer patients with various metastatic or locally advanced solid tumors and assessed for toxicity, measurable immune responses, immunological potential, and determination of 6-month progression free survival. Early data suggest that the drug is tolerated with low toxicity, and although clinical data regarding objective clinical responses have yet to be reported and are still accruing, interest in the CD137 drug is high [99, 101]. These promising studies are encouraging and most likely will provide a basis for additional studies and trials.

Looking beyond the current use of agonist antibodies to stimulate CD134 and CD137, other agents are currently being developed to be better tolerated and provide alternate options to induce the optimal activation of these two TNFRs. A humanized CD134 agonist that contains two CD252 trimer domains, required for interaction with CD134, more effectively stimulated T cells in vitro compared with soluble anti-CD134 antibodies [102]. The generation of this promising fusion protein was accomplished by linking the extracellular domain of the human CD252 with conserved domains of the human IgG1 protein, which by design formed hexamers that contained the two CD252 trimer domains. It is hypothesized that this molecule could better mimic the natural in vivo ligation of CD134, imparting a more potent signal than agonist antibodies. In addition to this CD134 specific fusion protein, fusion proteins have also been created to stimulate CD137. Engineered monomers containing the extracellular portion of the human CD137L molecule were designed to form a trimeric structure that interacts with human CD137 [103].

This agonist, like the CD134 multimeric agonist, was highly efficient at costimulating T cells in vitro, and may also be effective at generating antitumor immunity. The ability and ease in which these fusion proteins can be manipulated, may allow for the creation of highly specific features that could be added to these molecules to further target them to tumors. In fact, a mouse CD137L fusion protein was linked to an antibody domain that is specific for proteins found in necrotic tumors and then used to treat a colon carcinoma (CT26) [104]. The antibody-guided CD137 fusion protein increased the infiltration of T cells into the tumor and boosted tumor-free survival compared with a control CD137 fusion protein with a tumor-nonspecific antibody domain. Unfortunately, the antibody-guided CD137 molecule was not as effective as an agonist CD137 antibody and requires continued research and development. Although the TNF fusion protein platform described is in the early stages of development, its inherent ability to be easily manipulated may allow it to emerge as a powerful cancer immunotherapy.

Another approach to stimulate these four TNFRs with the potential to be a superior alternative to the current agonist antibodies is the generation of TNFR-specific aptamers. Aptamers are short DNA or RNA oligonucleotides that assume a specific three-dimensional structure in vivo to bind targets with high affinity and induce a biological response [105]. Aptamers also have the advantage of being highly stable, lack immunogenicity, and may penetrate tissue/tumors better than antibodies. These feature have endeared them to clinical applications and at least one aptamer (AS1411) had entered into clinical trials for the treatment of cancer [105]. Application of aptamer technology to develop TNFR agonists for the treatment of cancer has lead to a functioning bivalent CD137 aptamer. A screen of over 10^{14} RNA sequences identified a CD137-specific aptamer with high binding affinity and the ability to activate T cells in culture better than an agonist CD137 antibody [106]. Linking monomeric CD137 aptamers to form a bivalent molecule was found to bind to CD137 with higher avidity than the base monomeric molecule and induced even greater T cell activation. Subsequent systemic administration of the dimeric CD137 aptamer was observed to mediate significant tumor-free survival in animal models, comparable to the effect of an agonist CD137 antibody. Thus, agonistic TNFR aptamers can be readily synthesized, are cost effective, and are nonimmunogenic, thus representing an attractive alternative to agonist antibodies.

Development of clinical approaches utilizing the molecules CD27 and GITR, at this time, is in the early stages and yet to enter into clinical trials. GITR interventions, similar to CD134 and CD137 drugs, are in part envisioned to be a stand alone therapy with application across multiple tumor types. Recommendation by leading cancer researchers for the production of GITR agonists has given rise to the development of a number of potential agonist molecules [99]. Entry of these agonists into clinical trails appears to be a foregone conclusion, but the form these agonists take, monoclonal antibody or fusion proteins, remains unknown. Unfortunately, the role of CD27 stimulation in the treatment of human cancers is less developed and it is uncertain if this approach will be explored.

Summary

The promise of effective cancer immunotherapy spans over a century and as our understanding of this multifaceted disease and its interface with cells of the immune system has become better understood, this promise seem tantalizing within reach. It is widely accepted that the immune system eradicates developing tumors and keeps the growth of existing tumors in check (equilibrium). However, tumors often escape immune-surveillance. To restore immunological control over tumors, targeting the tumor-associated antigen-specific T cells that mediate tumor destruction is recognized as a viable approach. Expanding the numbers and function of tumor-specific T cells relates to the antitumor immune properties elicited by the TNFRs CD27, CD134, CD137, and GITR. Indeed, stimulation of these TNFRs in preclinical models increases the number of tumor antigen-specific T cells, and increases the activity of these T cells via enhanced effector function and memory cell development. Moreover, a second beneficial effect of systemic stimulation of CD134 and GITR is dampening of the suppressive effects of Tregs, found in high numbers within a tumor. Currently, several clinical trials are underway assessing the efficacy of agonist antibody CD134 and CD137 interventions as cancer therapies. Finally on the horizon, a number of other technologically different approaches are also being developed to activate these two TNFRs, as well as CD27 and GITR that may revolutionize our approach to TNFR stimulation.

References

1. Coley, W. B. (1891) Ann Surg 14, 199
2. O'Malley, W. E., Achinstein, B., and Shear, M. J. (1962) J Natl Cancer Inst 29, 1169
3. Carswell, E. A., Old, L. J., Kassel, R. L., Green, S., Fiore, N., and Williamson, B. (1975) Proc Natl Acad Sci USA 72, 3666
4. Aggarwal, B. B., Moffat, B., and Harkins, R. N. (1984) J Biol Chem 259, 686
5. Chan, F. K. (2007) Cytokine 37, 101
6. Dempsey, P. J., Meise, K. S., and Coffey, R. J. (2003) Exp Cell Res 285, 159
7. Watts, T. H. (2005) Annu Rev Immunol 23, 23
8. Croft, M. (2003) Nat Rev Immunol 3, 609
9. Sugita, K., Hirose, T., Rothstein, D. M., Donahue, C., Schlossman, S. F., and Morimoto, C. (1992) J Immunol 149, 3208
10. Wilcox, R. A., Tamada, K., Strome, S. E., and Chen, L. (2002) J Immunol 169, 4230
11. Maurer, D., Holter, W., Majdic, O., Fischer, G. F., and Knapp, W. (1990) Eur J Immunol 20, 2679
12. Futagawa, T., Akiba, H., Kodama, T., Takeda, K., Hosoda, Y., Yagita, H., and Okumura, K. (2002) Int Immunol 14, 275
13. Wilcox, R. A., Chapoval, A. I., Gorski, K. S., Otsuji, M., Shin, T., Flies, D. B., Tamada, K., Mittler, R. S., Tsuchiya, H., Pardoll, D. M., and Chen, L. (2002) J Immunol 168, 4262
14. Heinisch, I. V., Bizer, C., Volgger, W., and Simon, H. U. (2001) J Allergy Clin Immunol 108, 21
15. Baumann, R., Yousefi, S., Simon, D., Russmann, S., Mueller, C., and Simon, H. U. (2004) Eur J Immunol 34, 2268

16. Tesselaar, K., Xiao, Y., Arens, R., van Schijndel, G. M., Schuurhuis, D. H., Mebius, R. E., Borst, J., and van Lier, R. A. (2003) J Immunol 170, 33
17. Stephens, G. L., McHugh, R. S., Whitters, M. J., Young, D. A., Luxenberg, D., Carreno, B. M., Collins, M., and Shevach, E. M. (20040 J Immunol 173, 5008
18. Diehl, L., van Mierlo, G. J., den Boer, A. T., van der Voort, E., Fransen, M., van Bostelen, L., Krimpenfort, P., Melief, C. J., Mittler, R., Toes, R. E., and Offringa, R. (2002) J Immunol 168, 3755
19. Murata, K., Ishii, N., Takano, H., Miura, S., Ndhlovu, L. C., Nose, M., Noda, T., and Sugamura, K. (2000) J Exp Med 191, 365
20. Oshima, H., Nakano, H., Nohara, C., Kobata, T., Nakajima, A., Jenkins, N. A., Gilbert, D. J., Copeland, N. G., Muto, T., Yagita, H., and Okumura, K. (1998) Int Immunol 10, 517
21. Mendel, I., and Shevach, E. M. (2006) Immunology 117, 196
22. Pages, F., Berger, A., Camus, M., Sanchez-Cabo, F., Costes, A., Molidor, R., Mlecnik, B., Kirilovsky, A., Nilsson, M., Damotte, D., Meatchi, T., Bruneval, P., Cugnenc, P. H., Trajanoski, Z., Fridman, W. H., and Galon, J. (2005) N Engl J Med 353, 2654
23. Zhang, L., Conejo-Garcia, J. R., Katsaros, D., Gimotty, P. A., Massobrio, M., Regnani, G., Makrigiannakis, A., Gray, H., Schlienger, K., Liebman, M. N., Rubin, S. C., and Coukos, G. (2003) N Engl J Med 348, 203
24. Vignali, D. A., Collison, L. W., and Workman, C. J. (2008) Nat Rev Immunol 8, 523
25. Allan, S. E., Broady, R., Gregori, S., Himmel, M. E., Locke, N., Roncarolo, M. G., Bacchetta, R., and Levings, M. K. (2008) Immunol Rev 223, 391
26. Sakaguchi, S., Yamaguchi, T., Nomura, T., and Ono, M. (2008) Cell 133, 775
27. Hendriks, J., Gravestein, L. A., Tesselaar, K., van Lier, R. A., Schumacher, T. N., and Borst, J. (2000) Nat Immunol 1, 433
28. Carr, J. M., Carrasco, M. J., Thaventhiran, J. E., Bambrough, P. J., Kraman, M., Edwards, A. D., Al-Shamkhani, A., and Fearon, D. T. (2006) Proc Natl Acad Sci USA 103, 19454
29. Couderc, B., Zitvogel, L., Douin-Echinard, V., Djennane, L., Tahara, H., Favre, G., Lotze, M. T., and Robbins, P. D. (1998) Cancer Gene Ther 5, 163
30. Arens, R., Schepers, K., Nolte, M. A., van Oosterwijk, M. F., van Lier, R. A., Schumacher, T. N., and van Oers, M. H. (2004) J Exp Med 199, 1595
31. French, R. R., Taraban, V. Y., Crowther, G. R., Rowley, T. F., Gray, J. C., Johnson, P. W., Tutt, A. L., Al-Shamkhani, A., and Glennie, M. J. (2007) Blood 109, 4810
32. Cormary, C., Gonzalez, R., Faye, J. C., Favre, G., and Tilkin-Mariame, A. F. (2004) Cancer Gene Ther 11, 497
33. Diegmann, J., Junker, K., Loncarevic, I. F., Michel, S., Schimmel, B., and von Eggeling, F. (2006) Neoplasia 8, 933
34. Wischhusen, J., Jung, G., Radovanovic, I., Beier, C., Steinbach, J. P., Rimner, A., Huang, H., Schulz, J. B., Ohgaki, H., Aguzzi, A., Rammensee, H. G., and Weller, M. (2002) Cancer Res 62, 2592
35. Tesselaar, K., Arens, R., van Schijndel, G. M., Baars, P. A., van der Valk, M. A., Borst, J., van Oers, M. H., and van Lier, R. A. (2003) Nat Immunol 4, 49
36. Kanamaru, F., Youngnak, P., Hashiguchi, M., Nishioka, T., Takahashi, T., Sakaguchi, S., Ishikawa, I., and Azuma, M. (2004) J Immunol 172, 7306
37. Ronchetti, S., Zollo, O., Bruscoli, S., Agostini, M., Bianchini, R., Nocentini, G., Ayroldi, E., and Riccardi, C. (2004) Eur J Immunol 34, 613
38. Igarashi, H., Cao, Y., Iwai, H., Piao, J., Kamimura, Y., Hashiguchi, M., Amagasa, T., and Azuma, M. (2008) Biochem Biophys Res Commun 369, 1134
39. Uraushihara, K., Kanai, T., Ko, K., Totsuka, T., Makita, S., Iiyama, R., Nakamura, T., and Watanabe, M. (2003) J Immunol 171, 708
40. McHugh, R. S., Whitters, M. J., Piccirillo, C. A., Young, D. A., Shevach, E. M., Collins, M., and Byrne, M. C. (2002) Immunity 16, 311
41. Shimizu, J., Yamazaki, S., Takahashi, T., Ishida, Y., and Sakaguchi, S. (2002) Nat Immunol 3, 135
42. Shevach, E. M., and Stephens, G. L. (2006) Nat Rev Immunol 6, 613
43. Cohen, A. D., Diab, A., Perales, M. A., Wolchok, J. D., Rizzuto, G., Merghoub, T., Huggins, D., Liu, C., Turk, M. J., Restifo, N. P., Sakaguchi, S., and Houghton, A. N. (2006) Cancer Res 66, 4904

44. Ko, K., Yamazaki, S., Nakamura, K., Nishioka, T., Hirota, K., Yamaguchi, T., Shimizu, J., Nomura, T., Chiba, T., and Sakaguchi, S. (2005) J Exp Med 202, 885
45. Zhou, P., L'Italien, L., Hodges, D., and Schebye, X. M. (2007) J Immunol 179, 7365
46. Fujita, T., Ukyo, N., Hori, T., and Uchiyama, T. (2006) Immunol Lett 106, 27
47. Gramaglia, I., Weinberg, A. D., Lemon, M., and Croft, M. (1998) J Immunol 161, 6510
48. Weinberg, A. D., and Montler, R. (2005) Curr Drug Targets Inflamm Allergy 4, 195
49. Rogers, P. R., Song, J., Gramaglia, I., Killeen, N., and Croft, M. (2001) Immunity 15, 445
50. Ruby, C. E., Redmond, W. L., Haley, D., and Weinberg, A. D. (2007) Eur J Immunol 37, 157
51. Lee, S. W., Park, Y., Song, A., Cheroutre, H., Kwon, B. S., and Croft, M. (2006) J Immunol 177, 4464
52. Prell, R. A., Evans, D. E., Thalhofer, C., Shi, T., Funatake, C., and Weinberg, A. D. (2003) J Immunol 171, 5997
53. Murata, K., Nose, M., Ndhlovu, L. C., Sato, T., Sugamura, K., and Ishii, N. (2002) J Immunol 169, 4628
54. Gramaglia, I., Jember, A., Pippig, S. D., Weinberg, A. D., Killeen, N., and Croft, M. (2000) J Immunol 165, 3043
55. Song, J., So, T., and Croft, M. (2008) J Immunol 180, 7240
56. Weinberg, A. D., Vella, A. T., and Croft, M. (1998) Semin Immunol 10, 471
57. Kaleeba, J. A., Offner, H., Vandenbark, A. A., Lublinski, A., and Weinberg, A. D. (1998) Int Immunol 10, 453
58. Redmond, W. L., Gough, M. J., Charbonneau, B., Ratliff, T. L., and Weinberg, A. D. (2007) J Immunol 179, 7244
59. Takada, Y., and Aggarwal, B. B. (2004) J Immunol 173, 1066
60. Vu, M. D., Xiao, X., Gao, W., Degauque, N., Chen, M., Kroemer, A., Killeen, N., Ishii, N., and Chang Li, X. (2007) Blood 110, 2501
61. So, T., and Croft, M. (2007) J Immunol 179, 1427
62. Ito, T., Wang, Y. H., Duramad, O., Hanabuchi, S., Perng, O. A., Gilliet, M., Qin, F. X., and Liu, Y. J. (2006) Proc Natl Acad Sci USA 103, 13138
63. Valzasina, B., Guiducci, C., Dislich, H., Killeen, N., Weinberg, A. D., and Colombo, M. P. (2005) Blood 105, 2845
64. Weinberg, A. D., Rivera, M. M., Prell, R., Morris, A., Ramstad, T., Vetto, J. T., Urba, W. J., Alvord, G., Bunce, C., and Shields, J. (2000) J Immunol 164, 2160
65. Kjaergaard, J., Tanaka, J., Kim, J. A., Rothchild, K., Weinberg, A., and Shu, S. (2000) Cancer Res 60, 5514
66. Morris, A., Vetto, J. T., Ramstad, T., Funatake, C. J., Choolun, E., Entwisle, C., and Weinberg, A. D. (2001) Breast Cancer Res Treat 67, 71
67. Ali, S. A., Ahmad, M., Lynam, J., McLean, C. S., Entwisle, C., Loudon, P., Choolun, E., McArdle, S. E., Li, G., Mian, S., and Rees, R. C. (2004) Vaccine 22, 3585
68. Andarini, S., Kikuchi, T., Nukiwa, M., Pradono, P., Suzuki, T., Ohkouchi, S., Inoue, A., Maemondo, M., Ishii, N., Saijo, Y., Sugamura, K., and Nukiwa, T. (2004) Cancer Res 64, 3281
69. Gri, G., Gallo, E., Di Carlo, E., Musiani, P., and Colombo, M. P. (2003) J Immunol 170, 99
70. Biagi, E., Dotti, G., Yvon, E., Lee, E., Pule, M., Vigouroux, S., Gottschalk, S., Popat, U., Rousseau, R., and Brenner, M. (2005) Blood 105, 2436
71. Dannull, J., Nair, S., Su, Z., Boczkowski, D., DeBeck, C., Yang, B., Gilboa, E., and Vieweg, J. (2005) Blood 105, 3206
72. Song, A., Tang, X., Harms, K. M., and Croft, M. (2005) J Immunol 175, 3534
73. Murata, S., Ladle, B. H., Kim, P. S., Lutz, E. R., Wolpoe, M. E., Ivie, S. E., Smith, H. M., Armstrong, T. D., Emens, L. A., Jaffee, E. M., and Reilly, R. T. (20060 J Immunol 176, 974
74. Ruby, C. E., Montler, R., Zheng, R., Shu, S., and Weinberg, A. D. (2008) J Immunol 180, 2140
75. Gough, M. J., Ruby, C. E., Redmond, W. L., Dhungel, B., Brown, A., and Weinberg, A. D. (2008) Cancer Res 68, 5206
76. Piconese, S., Valzasina, B., and Colombo, M. P. (20080 J Exp Med 205, 825
77. Takahashi, C., Mittler, R. S., and Vella, A. T. (1999) J Immunol 162, 5037

78. Wen, T., Bukczynski, J., and Watts, T. H. (2002) J Immunol 168, 4897
79. Taraban, V. Y., Rowley, T. F., O'Brien, L., Chan, H. T., Haswell, L. E., Green, M. H., Tutt, A. L., Glennie, M. J., and Al-Shamkhani, A. (20020 Eur J Immunol 32, 3617
80. Dawicki, W., and Watts, T. H. (2004) Eur J Immunol 34, 743
81. Cannons, J. L., Lau, P., Ghumman, B., DeBenedette, M. A., Yagita, H., Okumura, K., and Watts, T. H. (2001) J Immunol 167, 1313
82. DeBenedette, M. A., Wen, T., Bachmann, M. F., Ohashi, P. S., Barber, B. H., Stocking, K. L., Peschon, J. J., and Watts; T. H. (1999) J Immunol 163, 4833
83. Tan, J. T., Whitmire, J. K., Ahmed, R., Pearson, T. C., and Larsen, C. P. (1999) J Immunol 163, 4859
84. Tan, J. T., Whitmire, J. K., Murali-Krishna, K., Ahmed, R., Altman, J. D., Mittler, R. S., Sette, A., Pearson, T. C., and Larsen, C. P. (2000) J Immunol 164, 2320
85. Kwon, B. S., Hurtado, J. C., Lee, Z. H., Kwack, K. B., Seo, S. K., Choi, B. K., Koller, B. H., Wolisi, G., Broxmeyer, H. E., and Vinay, D. S. (2002) J Immunol 168, 5483
86. Shuford, W. W., Klussman, K., Tritchler, D. D., Loo, D. T., Chalupny, J., Siadak, A. W., Brown, T. J., Emswiler, J., Raecho, H., Larsen, C. P., Pearson, T. C., Ledbetter, J. A., Aruffo, A., and Mittler, R. S. (1997) J Exp Med 186, 47
87. Sun, Y., Chen, H. M., Subudhi, S. K., Chen, J., Koka, R., Chen, L., and Fu, Y. X. (2002) Nat Med 8, 1405
88. Zheng, G., Wang, B., and Chen, A. (2004) J Immunol 173, 2428
89. Elpek, K. G., Yolcu, E. S., Franke, D. D., Lacelle, C., Schabowsky, R. H., and Shirwan, H. (2007) J Immunol 179, 7295
90. Choi, B. K., Bae, J. S., Choi, E. M., Kang, W. J., Sakaguchi, S., Vinay, D. S., and Kwon, B. S. (2004) J Leukoc Biol 75, 785
91. Melero, I., Shuford, W. W., Newby, S. A., Aruffo, A., Ledbetter, J. A., Hellstrom, K. E., Mittler, R. S., and Chen, L. (1997) Nat Med 3, 682
92. Wilcox, R. A., Flies, D. B., Zhu, G., Johnson, A. J., Tamada, K., Chapoval, A. I., Strome, S. E., Pease, L. R., and Chen, L. (20020 J Clin Invest 109, 651
93. Strome, S. E., Martin, B., Flies, D., Tamada, K., Chapoval, A. I., Sargent, D. J., Shu, S., and Chen, L. (20000 J Immunother 23, 430
94. Mogi, S., Sakurai, J., Kohsaka, T., Enomoto, S., Yagita, H., Okumura, K., and Azuma, M. (2000) Immunology 101, 541
95. Ye, Z., Hellstrom, I., Hayden-Ledbetter, M., Dahlin, A., Ledbetter, J. A., and Hellstrom, K. E. (2002) Nat Med 8, 343
96. Miller, R. E., Jones, J., Le, T., Whitmore, J., Boiani, N., Gliniak, B., and Lynch, D. H. (2002) J Immunol 169, 1792
97. Ju, S. A., Lee, S. C., Kwon, T. H., Heo, S. K., Park, S. M., Paek, H. N., Suh, J. H., Cho, H. R., Kwon, B., Kwon, B. S., and Kim, B. S. (2005) Immunol Cell Biol 83, 344
98. Kroon, H. M., Li, Q., Teitz-Tennenbaum, S., Whitfield, J. R., Noone, A. M., and Chang, A. E. (2007) J Immunother 30, 406
99. Cheever, M. A. (2007) http://web.ncifcrf.gov/research/brb/workshops.asp
100. Weinberg, A. D., Thalhofer, C., Morris, N., Walker, J. M., Seiss, D., Wong, S., Axthelm, M. K., Picker, L. J., and Urba, W. J. (2006) J Immunother 29, 575
101. Lynch, D. H. (2008) Immunol Rev 222, 277
102. Morris, N. P., Peters, C., Montler, R., Hu, H. M., Curti, B. D., Urba, W. J., and Weinberg, A. D. (2007) Mol Immunol 44, 3112
103. Rabu, C., Quemener, A., Jacques, Y., Echasserieau, K., Vusio, P., and Lang, F. (2005) J Biol Chem 280, 41472
104. Zhang, N., Sadun, R. E., Arias, R. S., Flanagan, M. L., Sachsman, S. M., Nien, Y. C., Khawli, L. A., Hu, P., and Epstein, A. L. (2007) Clin Cancer Res 13, 2758
105. Ireson, C. R., and Kelland, L. R. (2006) Mol Cancer Ther 5, 2957
106. McNamara, J. O., Kolonias, D., Pastor, F., Mittler, R. S., Chen, L., Giangrande, P. H., Sullenger, B., and Gilboa, E. (2008) J Clin Invest 118, 376

Index

U

V